THE WASHINGTON MANUAL® OF CARDIO-ONCOLOGY

A Practical Guide for Improved Cancer Survivorship

THE WASHINGTON MANUAL® OF CARDIO-ONCOLOGY
A Practical Guide for Improved Cancer Survivorship

Editor

Daniel J. Lenihan, MD, FACC, FESC, FIC-OS
President, International Cardio-Oncology Society
Tampa, Florida

Associate Editors

Joshua D. Mitchell, MD, MSCI, FACC, FIC-OS
Assistant Professor of Medicine
Director, Cardio-Oncology Fellowship
Cardio-Oncology Center of Excellence
Cardiovascular Division, Department of Medicine
Washington University School of Medicine
St. Louis, Missouri

Kathleen W. Zhang, MD, FACC, FIC-OS
Assistant Professor of Medicine
Associate Program Director, Cardiology Fellowship
Cardio-Oncology Center of Excellence
Washington University School of Medicine
St. Louis, Missouri

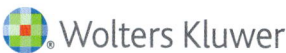

Philadelphia • Baltimore • New York • London
Buenos Aires • Hong Kong • Sydney • Tokyo

Acquisitions Editor: Keith Donnellan, James P. Sherman
Senior Development Editor: Ashley Fischer
Editorial Coordinator: Venugopal Loganathan
Marketing Manager: Kirsten Watrud
Senior Production Project Manager: Alicia Jackson
Manager, Graphic Arts & Design: Stephen Druding
Senior Manufacturing Coordinator: Beth Welsh
Prepress Vendor: S4Carlisle Publishing Services

Copyright © 2023 Department of Medicine, Washington University School of Medicine, Published by Wolters Kluwer.

All rights reserved. This book is protected by copyright. No part of this book may be reproduced or transmitted in any form or by any means, including as photocopies or scanned-in or other electronic copies, or utilized by any information storage and retrieval system without written permission from the copyright owner, except for brief quotations embodied in critical articles and reviews. Materials appearing in this book prepared by individuals as part of their official duties as U.S. government employees are not covered by the above-mentioned copyright. To request permission, please contact Wolters Kluwer at Two Commerce Square, 2001 Market Street, Philadelphia, PA 19103, via email at permissions@lww.com, or via our website at shop.lww.com (products and services).

9 8 7 6 5 4 3 2 1

Printed in Mexico

Library of Congress Cataloging-in-Publication Data

ISBN-13: 978-1-975180-44-7

ISBN-10: 1-975180-44-5

Cataloging-in-Publication data available on request from the Publisher.

This work is provided "as is," and the publisher disclaims any and all warranties, express or implied, including any warranties as to accuracy, comprehensiveness, or currency of the content of this work.

This work is no substitute for individual patient assessment based upon healthcare professionals' examination of each patient and consideration of, among other things, age, weight, gender, current or prior medical conditions, medication history, laboratory data and other factors unique to the patient. The publisher does not provide medical advice or guidance and this work is merely a reference tool. Healthcare professionals, and not the publisher, are solely responsible for the use of this work including all medical judgments and for any resulting diagnosis and treatments.

Given continuous, rapid advances in medical science and health information, independent professional verification of medical diagnoses, indications, appropriate pharmaceutical selections and dosages, and treatment options should be made and healthcare professionals should consult a variety of sources. When prescribing medication, healthcare professionals are advised to consult the product information sheet (the manufacturer's package insert) accompanying each drug to verify, among other things, conditions of use, warnings and side effects and identify any changes in dosage schedule or contraindications, particularly if the medication to be administered is new, infrequently used or has a narrow therapeutic range. To the maximum extent permitted under applicable law, no responsibility is assumed by the publisher for any injury and/or damage to persons or property, as a matter of products liability, negligence law or otherwise, or from any reference to or use by any person of this work.

shop.lww.com

Dedication

We dedicate this initial *The Washington Manual® of Cardio-Oncology* to all our patients who trusted us with their lives as we helped them through their cancer war. It is these patients who we serve and strive to provide optimal cardioprotection during their arduous cancer journey. We are also deeply indebted to our faculty colleagues in many medical disciplines at Washington University in St. Louis who provide outstanding patient care and have shared their extensive expertise in this text. We have been graced with many superior fellows who have trained with us in Cardio-Oncology, mostly from Washington University, who have contributed to the book and also stimulated us to learn, teach, and research on a continuous basis. Additionally, we are extremely thankful for the love and support of our spouses and families through all aspects of our careers in medicine. Lastly, we are honored to produce this Manual largely at the encouragement of Doug Mann, MD, who has been our leader, friend, mentor, and confidante over the past 20 years. We want to thank Doug from the bottom of our hearts and will always cherish his presence in our lives.

Daniel J. Lenihan, MD, FACC, FESC, FIC-OS
Kathleen W. Zhang, MD, FACC, FIC-OS
Joshua D. Mitchell, MD, MSCI, FACC, FIC-OS

Contributors

Jose A. Alvarez-Cardona, MD
Assistant Professor of Medicine
Cardiovascular Division, Department of Medicine
Section of Advanced Heart Failure and Cardiac Transplantation
Section of Cardio-Oncology
Washington University School of Medicine
St. Louis, Missouri

Ankit Bhatia, MD, FACC
Advanced Heart Failure Cardiologist
Section of Advanced Heart Failure and Transplant Cardiology
The Christ Hospital Heart and Vascular Physicians
The Christ Hospital Health Network
Cincinnati, Ohio

Courtney M. Campbell, MD, PhD
Cardio-Oncology and Cardiac Amyloidosis Fellow
Instructor of Medicine
Cardiovascular Division, Department of Medicine
Washington University School of Medicine
Cardio-Oncology Center of Excellence
St. Louis, Missouri

Rahul A. Chhana, MD
Fellow, Cardiovascular Medicine
Department of Medicine
Washington University School of Medicine
St. Louis, Missouri

Fahrettin Covut, MD
Clinical Fellow
Divisions of Hematology and Medical Oncology,
Department of Medicine
Washington University,
St Louis, Missouri

Phillip S. Cuculich, MD
Associate Professor
Internal Medicine (Cardiology) and Radiation Oncology
Washington University School of Medicine
St. Louis, Missouri

Christopher Fine, MD
Instructor of Medicine
Division of Cardiology
Department of Medicine
National Jewish Health | SCL Health
Denver, Colorado

Scott R. Goldsmith, MD
Clinical Fellow
Division of Oncology
Washington University School of Medicine
St. Louis, Missouri

Jesus Jimenez, MD
Instructor in Medicine
Cardiovascular Division, Department of Internal Medicine
Washington University School of Medicine
St. Louis, Missouri

Benjamin J. Kopecky, MD, PhD
Instructor of Medicine
Division of Oncology, Department of Medicine
Section of Advanced Heart Failure and Cardiac Transplant
Washington University
St. Louis, Missouri

Michael Kramer, MD, PhD
Fellow
Department of Hematology/Oncology
Washington University in St. Louis
St. Louis, Missouri

Ronald J. Krone, MD, FACC, FSCAI
Professor of Medicine
Cardiovascular Division, Department of Medicine
Washington University School of Medicine
St. Louis, Missouri

Douglas A. Kyrouac, MD
Cardiology Fellow
Department of Cardiology
UT Southwestern Medical Center
Dallas, Texas

Gregory M. Lanza, MD, PhD
Professor of Medicine and Bioengineering
Department of Medicine
Washington University School of Medicine
St. Louis, Missouri

Daniel J. Lenihan, MD, FACC, FESC, FIC-OS
President, International Cardio-Oncology Society
Tampa, Florida

Brandon W. Lennep, MD
Assistant Professor of Medicine
Division of Cardiology & Cardiovascular Disease, Department of Internal Medicine
University of Mississippi Medical Center
Jackson, Mississippi

Ann Mahoney, BSN, RN
Amyloidosis, Cardiology-Oncology Clinical Coordinator
Department of Cardiology
Washington University School Of Medicine
St. Louis, Missouri

Manuel Rivera Maza, MD
Fellow in Cardiovascular Disease
Cardiovascular Division, John T. Milliken Department of Medicine
Washington University
St. Louis, Missouri

Krasimira M. Mikhova, MD
Fellow, Clinical Cardiac Electrophysiology
Division of Oncology, Department of Medicine
Barnes-Jewish Hospital/Washington University School of Medicine
St. Louis, Missouri

Joshua D. Mitchell, MD, MSCI, FACC, FIC-OS
Assistant Professor of Medicine
Director, Cardio-Oncology Fellowship
Cardio-Oncology Center of Excellence
Cardiovascular Division, Department of Medicine
Washington University School of Medicine
St. Louis, Missouri

J. Westley Ohman, MD, FACS
Assistant Professor of Vascular Surgery
Associate Program Director for Vascular Training
Washington University School of Medicine
St. Louis, Missouri

Marissa Olson, PharmD
Clinical Pharmacy Specialist Bone Marrow Transplant/Hematologic Malignancies
Department of Pharmacy
Barnes-Jewish Hospital
St. Louis, Missouri

Arick Park, MD, PhD
Fellow, Advanced Heart Failure and Transplant
Department of Cardiovascular Medicine
Washington University in St. Louis
St. Louis, Missouri

Iskra Pusic, MD, MSCI
Associate Professor
Division of Oncology, Department of Medicine
Washington University School of Medicine
St. Louis, Missouri

Nishath Quader, MD
Associate Professor of Medicine
Department of Medicine, Division of Cardiology
Washington University School of Medicine
St. Louis, Missouri

Tarun Ramayya, MD
Physician
Department of Cardiology
Washington University School of Medicine
St. Louis, Missouri

Molly Rater, MSN
Cardio-Oncology Nurse Practitioner
Department of Cardiology
Washington University School of Medicine
St. Louis, Missouri

Mario Rodriguez Rivera, MD
Fellow, Cardiovascular Medicine
Department of Medicine
Barnes-Jewish Hospital, Washington University School of Medicine
St. Louis, Missouri

Kristen Sanfilippo, MD, MPHS
Assistant Professor
Division of Hematology, Department of Medicine
Washington University School of Medicine
Staff Physician
Department of Medicine, Hematology/Oncology
John Cochran St. Louis VA Medical Center
St. Louis, Missouri

Walter B. Schiffer, MD
Resident
Department of Internal Medicine
Washington University School of Medicine
St. Louis, Missouri

Karen Sneed, RN, BSN
Cardio-Oncology Clinical Nurse Coordinator
Department of Cardiology
Washington University School of Medicine
St. Louis, Missouri

Debra Spoljaric, MSN
Nurse Practitioner
Department of Surgery
Washington University
St. Louis, Missouri

Keith E. Stockerl-Goldstein, MD
Professor of Medicine
Division of Oncology/Section of BMT & Leukemia
Washington University School of Medicine/Barnes-Jewish Hospital/Siteman Cancer Center
St. Louis, Missouri

Tushar Tarun, MD
Assistant Professor
Division of Cardiovascular Medicine
Department of Internal Medicine
University of Arkansas for Medical Sciences
Little Rock, Arkansas

Prashanth D. Thakker, MD
Assistant Professor of Medicine
Cardiovascular Division, Department of Medicine
Washington University School of Medicine
St. Louis, Missouri

Justin M. Vader, MD, MPHS
Associate Professor of Medicine
Heart Failure/Transplant Section, Cardiovascular Division
Washington University School of Medicine
St. Louis, Missouri

Srilakshmi Vallabhaneni, MD, FACC
Assistant Professor of Medicine
Division of Cardiology, Department of Internal Medicine
University of Texas Southwestern Medical Center
Dallas, Texas

Holly Wiesehan, MSN, AGACNP
Nurse Practitioner
Department of Hematology
Washington University School of Medicine
St. Louis, Missouri

Jonathan D. Wolfe, MD
Fellow in Cardiovascular Disease
Division of Cardiology, Department of Medicine
Washington University School of Medicine/Barnes Jewish Hospital
St. Louis, Missouri

Jeannette Wong-Siegel, MD, MPH
Pediatric Cardiology Fellow
Department of Pediatrics
St. Louis Children's Hospital
St. Louis, Missouri

Pamela K. Woodard, MD
Hugh Monroe Wilson Professor of Radiology
Professor of Biomedical Engineering; Head Cardiac MRI/CT
Mallinckrodt Institute of Radiology,
Washington University School of Medicine,
St. Louis, Missouri

Kathleen W. Zhang, MD, FACC, FIC-OS
Assistant Professor of Medicine
Associate Program Director, Cardiology Fellowship
Cardio-Oncology Center of Excellence
Washington University School of Medicine
St. Louis, Missouri

Preface

THE WASHINGTON MANUAL® OF CARDIO-ONCOLOGY: A PRACTICAL GUIDE FOR IMPROVED CANCER SURVIVORSHIP

It is with great honor and reverence that we, in collaboration with our expert colleagues, present this concise yet comprehensive manual summarizing the current world of Cardio-Oncology! We fondly remember the *Washington Manual® for Internal Medicine* as the "go-to" handbook for new interns, used to become proficient in Internal Medicine in short order and also to get through rounds without excessive embarrassment (*I won't tell you which edition I was using ... DJL*). Over the years, there has been seemingly unanimous respect for these practical guides in the practice of Internal Medicine. Now, in the year 2021, we hope to utilize the Washington Manual® series to bring the complex and ever-evolving field of Cardio-Oncology to the white coat pockets of physicians for generations to come.

The concept of Cardio-Oncology has only been a clinical entity for about 20 years and, at the outset, was mostly limited to the diagnosis and management of anthracycline-related cardiotoxicity. Since that time, the emergence of novel cancer therapies and improved cancer outcomes has greatly extended the life span for patients with cancer. In response, the field of Cardio-Oncology has expanded to account for adverse cardiovascular effects of a vast array of cancer therapies that may occur over an extended period of time. In many cases, cancer has become a chronic disease not unlike diabetes or hypertension, with therapy-related cardiovascular toxicities that require long-term surveillance.

For this *Washington Manual of Cardio-Oncology*, we assembled an outstanding team of contributors who provide exceptional clinical cardiovascular care for cancer patients. Many of these colleagues have cared for our own patients, and we can attest to the energy, thoughtfulness, and intellect that each one of these individuals brings to Cardio-Oncology care. Within this Manual, our colleagues have concisely summarized their respective areas within Cardio-Oncology with attention to practical and actionable teaching points that can be utilized in everyday practice. We believe that this Manual will be the most invaluable resource for the day-to-day practice of Cardio-Oncology available to date.

One major challenge in writing and editing this book has now become very evident. We cannot cover every detail that may enter into the decision-making paradigm for each complex patient challenge. Instead, we organized the book in a manner that would be easily accessible, authoritative, and concise. We start out the book with a general approach to a patient with cancer who may be at risk for cardiovascular complications. We then transition into several chapters of specific cancer therapeutics and their relation to cardiovascular disease including cardiac dysfunction, valvular heart disease, vascular disease, ischemic heart disease, pericardial disease, thrombosis and embolism, cardiac masses, hypertension, arrhythmias, and management of intravascular devices and then finish this section with autonomic dysfunction. The next several chapters focus on common and effective tools to detect cardiovascular toxicity with echocardiography, cardiac biomarkers, as well as cardiac magnetic resonance imaging. We then focus on comprehensive care of cancer survivorship, hematopoietic cell transplantation, the importance of pharmacy expertise, and the concept of permissive cardiotoxicity and close this section with the need for a multidisciplinary approach utilizing advanced practice provider expertise. The last section of the book focuses on amyloidosis, an area that frequently falls within the Cardio-Oncologist's purview because of the overlap between light chain amyloidosis (a hematologic malignancy) and cardiac amyloidosis (an underdiagnosed cause of heart failure). We conclude the book with a contemporary discussion of the considerations of advanced heart failure therapy in a patient with active cancer or previously treated for cancer.

We hope you will enjoy this first edition of the *Washington Manual® of Cardio-Oncology*. Given the rapidly evolving nature of Cardio-Oncology, we hope to have an updated second edition available to you in the near future!

Daniel J. Lenihan, MD (Senior Editor)
Joshua D. Mitchell, MD (Associate Editor)
Kathleen W. Zhang, MD (Associate Editor)

Foreword

It is a pleasure to be able to write the foreword for the first edition of the *Washington Manual® of Cardio-Oncology*, which I am certain will be a great resource for all practitioners interested in the newly emerging discipline of Cardio-Oncology.

The manual is organized logically and begins with a general approach to evaluating Cardio-Oncology patients. Following this incisive overview, there are a series of chapters that highlight the role of biomarkers to detect cardiotoxicity, as well as the development of cardiac dysfunction, valvular heart disease, vascular disease, pericardial disease, thromboembolic disorders, hypertension, autonomic dysfunction, advanced heart failure and arrhythmias that may occur following treatment with chemotherapeutic regimens. There are separate chapters that cover the diagnosis and management of cardiac masses, management of intravascular devices, pre-operative assessment of Cardio-Oncology patients, and an important chapter on how to avoid drug-drug interactions in Cardio-Oncology patient. Three chapters are dedicated to the role of cardiac imaging in managing patients during and after therapy, including the use of echocardiography, magnetic resonance imaging and nuclear cardiology. The use of multidisciplinary teams and advanced practice providers is also discussed. Given the recent advances in the diagnosis and management of amyloidosis, the manual has 3 separate chapters that cover the general approach to the patient and treatment strategies for AL and ATTR amyloidosis. Certainly, there are a number of excellent, comprehensive articles and book chapters that cover similar topics in Cardio-Oncology; however, the *Washington Manual® of Cardio-Oncology* is the only resource that puts all of the information one needs to know at their fingertips, and in their pocket!

Dr. Daniel J. Lenihan, who is the lead editor for the book, and Drs. Zhang and Mitchell have done a masterful job of organizing and editing the first edition of the *Washington Manual® of Cardio-Oncology*. I am quite certain that the book will prove to be a useful and reliable source of concise information for trainees and cardiovascular health care providers alike who care for patients afflicted with cardiovascular complications that arise from treatment of their cancers. I am proud to endorse this book, which I believe will prove to be an outstanding addition to the family of Washington Manuals in cardiology subspecialty consultation and echocardiography.

Douglas L. Mann, MD

Contents

Dedication v
Contributors vii
Preface xi
Foreword xiii

1 A Practical Approach to the Evaluation of a Cardio-Oncology Patient 1
Daniel J. Lenihan, Joshua D. Mitchell, and Jose A. Alvarez-Cardona

2 Cardiac Dysfunction: Traditional Chemotherapy, Human Epidermal Growth Factor Receptor 2–Based Therapy, and Radiation 26
Srilakshmi Vallabhaneni, Ronald J. Krone, and Kathleen W. Zhang

3 Cardiac Dysfunction: Small-Molecule Kinase Inhibitors, Immune-Based Therapies, and Proteasome Inhibitors 48
Jesus Jimenez and Jose A. Alvarez-Cardona

4 Valvular Heart Disease 64
Manuel Rivera Maza, Kathleen W. Zhang, and Nishath Quader

5 Vascular Disease in Cardio-Oncology 76
Prashanth D. Thakker and Ronald J. Krone

6 Evaluation for Ischemic Heart Disease in Cardio-Oncology 89
Arick Park and Joshua D. Mitchell

7 Pericardial Diseases in Malignancy 103
Rahul A. Chhana and Joshua D. Mitchell

8 Cancer-Associated Thrombosis and Embolism 114
Fahrettin Covut, Daniel J. Lenihan, and Kristen Sanfilippo

9 Cardiac Masses   125
Jonathan D. Wolfe and Daniel J. Lenihan

10 Hypertension   140
Tarun Ramayya and Kathleen W. Zhang

11 Arrhythmias   150
Krasimira M. Mikhova and Phillip S. Cuculich

12 Intravascular Devices and Thrombotic Complications   167
Douglas A. Kyrouac, J. Westley Ohman, and Joshua D. Mitchell

13 Autonomic Dysfunction   179
Walter B. Schiffer and Daniel J. Lenihan

14 Echo Techniques for Cardiac Safety During and After Cancer Treatment   192
Christopher Fine and Joshua D. Mitchell

15 Biomarkers as a Tool For Cardiac Safety   208
Courtney M. Campbell and Daniel J. Lenihan

16 MRI Techniques to Monitor Cardiac Safety During and After Cancer Treatment   223
Srilakshmi Vallabhaneni, Pamela K. Woodard, Gregory M. Lanza, and Daniel J. Lenihan

17 Cancer Survivorship: Adverse Outcomes and Other Long-term Cardiovascular Considerations   238
Jeannette Wong-Siegel, Debra Spoljaric, and Daniel J. Lenihan

18 Hematopoietic Cell Transplantation   249
Tushar Tarun, Michael Kramer, and Iskra Pusic

19 Drug-Drug Interactions and the importance of a PharmD   257
Marissa Olson

20 Permissive Cardiotoxicity   268
Brandon W. Lennep and Joshua D. Mitchell

21 Multidisciplinary Approach to Cardio-Oncology and the Use of Advanced Practice Provider   280
Molly Rater, Holly Wiesehan, Ann Mahoney, and Karen Sneed

22 Cardiac Amyloidosis: General Diagnostic Approach   287
Walter B. Schiffer and Kathleen W. Zhang

23 Light Chain Amyloidosis: Latest Treatment Strategies   299
Scott R. Goldsmith and Keith E. Stockerl-Goldstein

24 Cardiac Amyloidosis: Latest Treatment Strategies for Transthyretin Amyloidosis   310
Mario Rodriguez Rivera and Justin M. Vader

25 Cancer Survivors and Advanced Heart Failure Therapies   321
Benjamin J. Kopecky, Ankit Bhatia, and Jose A. Alvarez-Cardona

Index   *333*

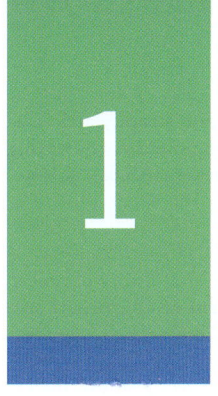

A Practical Approach to the Evaluation of a Cardio-Oncology Patient

Daniel J. Lenihan, Joshua D. Mitchell, and Jose A. Alvarez-Cardona

There has been an explosion of interest regarding many aspects of cancer care in the past two decades internationally. This trend is in large part because of the increased survival from an initial cancer diagnosis, such that cancer has become a chronic disease to be managed over many years in contrast to the long-held belief that a cancer diagnosis is a death sentence in the near term for an individual patient. The other major consideration is that cancer therapeutics have developed rapidly and have had remarkable successes in previously treatment-resistant cancers. The initial three pillars of cancer treatment such as **chemotherapy, surgery, and radiation** have now been expanded to five and include **targeted therapy and immunotherapy**. As a result of this enhanced complexity and success, Cardio-Oncology (CO) has become an essential supportive discipline for patients undergoing contemporary cancer therapy.

This chapter seeks to highlight **a systematic approach to maximize the cardiac status of any patient with cancer being treated with potentially cardiotoxic cancer therapeutics to minimize any cardiovascular (CV) limitation for optimal cancer therapy**.

GENERAL PRINCIPLES

- **Cancer therapy, including radiation, chemotherapy, targeted agents, and immunotherapy, can have substantial effects on the vasculature**, as well as any **cardiac structure** including the myocardium, valvular, electrical system, and pericardium.
- Patients seen **within the realm of CO are often complex with significant comorbidities that can directly affect their CV care**. Thrombocytopenia, commonly as a result of chemotherapy or the underlying disease, often influences CV treatment decisions.
- A **collaborative multidisciplinary team, including cardiologists and hematologists/oncologists, is essential for best overall patient management**. The team should work together to select the best cancer therapy for a given patient's overall survival, limiting and mitigating CV toxicity if possible, and minimizing treatment interruptions.
- **Cardiac risk factors (CRFs) should be assessed and treated in all patients**.
- Screening programs help identify patients at highest risk and those with early CV toxicity. Early treatment of left ventricular (LV) dysfunction has been shown to limit major CV adverse events.

- Patients at **highest risk for cardiotoxicity may benefit from prophylactic cardioprotective medications that can include β-blockers, angiotensin-converting enzyme inhibitors (ACE-Is) and angiotensin receptor blockers (ARBs), aldosterone antagonists, aspirin, anticoagulants, and statins**.

Definition

- CO broadly addresses the CV care of a patient with cancer or a history of cancer, and includes the **prevention of, screening for, and treatment of CV toxicity secondary to the short- or long-term effects of their cancer therapy** (see Chapter 17 on Cancer Survivorship).
- The **importance of having CO specialists has grown as a direct result of the explosion of new cancer therapies with varying mechanisms of action and adverse effects** on the CV system.
- **CV toxicity refers to damage to the heart and/or vasculature**. For patients undergoing cancer treatment, or for those with a history of exposure, clinicians should have a high index of suspicion that the cancer therapy could be a contributing factor.
- CV toxicity can be clinically apparent immediately, years, or even decades after anticancer therapy.

Classification

- **CV toxicity can be classified using the Common Terminology Criteria for Adverse Events (CTCAE) version 5 developed by the National Cancer Institute for codification of adverse events during oncology trials** (https://ctep.cancer.gov/protocolDevelopment/adverse_effects.htm). In the classification scheme, adverse events are graded from 1 (mild) to 5 (death).
- Because of discrepancies in definitions and reporting with CTCAE, events are often underreported in oncology trials.[1] Patients encountered in clinical practice, as opposed to research trials, also have a higher incidence of CV comorbidities, placing them at higher risk for CV events. Post-marketing analysis, therefore, often reveals higher incidence/prevalence of adverse CV events than anticipated during the oncology trials. Some adverse effects, such as myocarditis associated with checkpoint inhibitors, may go unrecognized until after the drug is used clinically outside of a trial.
- Although anticancer therapies can have wide-ranging CV toxic effects, most classification schemes have focused initially on LV dysfunction or heart failure (HF). **Various cutoffs for evaluating cardiac dysfunction have been defined in addition to the CTCAE criteria** (Table 1-1), which can complicate comparative reporting of events.

Epidemiology

- As of January 2016, there were 15.5 million cancer survivors, a number expected to grow by 31% to 20.3 million by 2026.[2]
- CV events are second only to malignancy in their impact on morbidity and mortality among cancer survivors in general.[3]
- In older patients diagnosed with breast cancer, CV death has been found to be even more prevalent than death because of the cancer itself.[4]
- **The cumulative incidence of HF continues to steadily increase yearly following anthracycline and trastuzumab therapy, measuring 20.1% at 5 years.**[5]
- The incidence and prevalence of CV disease are generally higher in patients being treated outside of clinical trials.

TABLE 1-1 Cardiotoxicity Classification Criteria for HF and LV Dysfunction

	Severity		
	Mild	**Moderate**	**Severe**
Cardiac Review and Evaluation Committee, Definition of Chemotherapy-Induced Cardiotoxicity[64]	Any one of the following: (1) reduction of LVEF, either global or specific in the interventricular septum (2) symptoms of congestive HF (3) signs associated with HF, such as S3 gallop, tachycardia, or both (4) reduction in LVEF from baseline to ≥5% to <55% in the presence of signs or symptoms of HF, or a reduction in LVEF ≥10% to <55% without signs or symptoms of HF		
NYHA Classification	**Class I** No symptoms	**Class II** Mild symptoms and slight limitation during ordinary activity	**Class III** Marked limitation because of symptoms, even with less than ordinary activity / **Class IV** Symptoms at rest
ACCF/AHA Stages of HF[65]	**Stage A** At high risk for HF but without structural disease or symptoms of HF	**Stage B** Structural heart disease but without signs or symptoms of HF	**Stage C** Structural heart disease with prior or current symptoms of HF / **Stage D** Refractory HF requiring specialized interventions
CTCAE v5.0 Ejection Fraction Decreased[a]		**Grade 2** Resting EF 50%–40%; 10%–19% drop from baseline	**Grade 3** Resting EF 39%–20%; ≥20% drop from baseline / **Grade 4** Resting EF <20%

(continued)

TABLE 1-1 Cardiotoxicity Classification Criteria for HF and LV Dysfunction (*continued*)

	Severity		
	Mild	**Moderate**	**Severe**
CTCAE v5.0 LV Systolic Dysfunction[a]		**Grade 3** Symptomatic because of drop in EF responsive to intervention	**Grade 4** Refractory or poorly controlled HF because of drop in EF; intervention such as ventricular assist device, intravenous vasopressor support, or heart transplant indicated
CTCAE v5 Heart Failure[a]	**Grade 1** Asymptomatic with laboratory (eg, BNP) or cardiac imaging abnormalities	**Grade 2** Symptoms with moderate activity or exertion	**Grade 3** Symptoms at rest or with minimal activity or exertion; hospitalization; new onset of symptoms

Severe column, Grade 4 (Heart Failure row): Life-threatening consequences; urgent intervention indicated (eg, continuous intravenous therapy or mechanical hemodynamic support)

	Severity		
	Mild	**Moderate**	**Severe**
U.S. FDA Package Insert Guidelines to Hold Cancer Therapy because of LV Dysfunction		**Trastuzumab**[66] ≥16% absolute decrease in LVEF or ≥10% drop to below institutional limits of normal	**Pertuzumab**[67] ≥10% drop in LVEF to <50% for early breast cancer, ≥10% drop in LVEF to 40%-45% for metastatic breast cancer, or drop to <40%
2014 Echo Guidelines for Subclinical LV Dysfunction[56]		**Subclinical LV dysfunction** >15% relative drop in GLS from baseline	**CRTCD** Drop in LVEF of >10 percentage points to a level <53%. Should be confirmed by repeat testing
2016 ESC Position Statement[68]	**Mild (Asymptomatic)** LVEF <50% or LVEF reduction >10% from baseline, should be repeated within 3-4 weeks		**Moderate (Symptomatic from HF)** LVEF <50%
2017 ASCO Guideline[7]	Cardiotoxicity not specifically defined		
		All Cancer Therapy	
2020 ESMO Guideline[69]	**Mild (Asymptomatic)** LVEF >15% from baseline if LVEF >50%		**Moderate** Symptomatic HF regardless of LVEF
		Anthracycline or Trastuzumab Related	
			Moderate LVEF ≥10% from baseline, or any drop of LVEF to <50% but ≥40% **Severe** LVEF <40%

(continued)

TABLE 1-1 Cardiotoxicity Classification Criteria for HF and LV Dysfunction (*continued*)

	Severity			
	Mild	**Moderate**	**Severe**	
2021 ICOS Universal Definition Asymptomatic CTRCD (with or without additional biomarkers)	**Mild** New LVEF reduction to ≥50% AND new fall in GLS by >15% ± new rise in cardiac biomarkers[b]	**Moderate** New LVEF reduction to >10% and to 40%-49% New LVEF reduction by <10% and to 40%-49% AND new fall in GLS by >15% ± new rise in cardiac biomarkers[b]	**Severe** New LVEF reduction to <40%	
2021 ICOS Universal Definition Symptomatic CTRCD (with LVEF and supportive diagnostic biomarkers)	**Mild** Mild HF symptoms, no intensification of therapy required	**Moderate** Need for outpatient intensification of diuretic and HF therapy	**Severe** HF hospitalization	**Very Severe** Requiring inotropic support, mechanical circulatory support, or consideration for transplantation

ACCF, American College of Cardiology Foundation; ASCO, American Society of Clinical Oncology; AHA, American Heart Association; BNP, brain natriuretic peptide; CTCAE, Common Terminology Criteria for Adverse Events; CTRCD, cancer-therapy–related cardiac dysfunction; EF, ejection fraction; ESC, European Society of Cardiology; ESMO, European Society for Medical Oncology; GLS, global longitudinal strain; HF, heart failure; ICOS, International Cardio-Oncology Society; LVEF, left ventricular ejection fraction; NYHA, New York Heart Association; U.S. FDA, United States Food and Drug Administration.

[a]Oncology trial investigators can choose to classify a given event under "ejection fraction decreased," "LV systolic dysfunction," or "Heart Failure" with associated grades if they decide the adverse effect is related to the intervention. This contributes to difficulty in comparing results of trials and effects of cancer therapies. Grade 1 to Grade 4 (mild to severe). Death = Grade 5. No Grade 5 for "ejection fraction decreased." Ref: Common Terminology Criteria for Adverse Events (CTCAE) v5.0. Accessed May 24, 2021. https://ctep.cancer.gov/protocoldevelopment/electronic_applications/ctc.htm.

[b]Cardiac troponin I/T >99th percentile, BNP ≥35 pg/mL, NT-proBNP ≥125 pg/mL.

Etiology
- CV disease is highly prevalent in patients being treated with cancer because of common risk factors (age, tobacco use, etc.) as well as on- and off target effects of anticancer therapies.
- Documented **CV adverse events include, but are not limited to, arrhythmias and QTc prolongation, fulminant myocarditis, severe systolic LV dysfunction, constrictive pericarditis, hypertension (HTN) and subsequent LV dysfunction, arterial (ATE) and venous thromboembolism (VTE), and even sudden cardiac death**, just to name a few.

Risk Factors
- CV toxicity from anthracyclines and radiation is directly related to the total dose or exposure. Mediastinal radiation ≥30 Gy (with the heart in the treatment field), doxorubicin ≥ 250 mg/m^2 (or epirubicin ≥600 mg/m^2), and the combination of anthracyclines or radiation at any dose have been identified as particularly significant risk factors for LV dysfunction and HF.[6]
- In addition to the increased relative risk for the development of cardiac dysfunction related to specific anticancer therapies, **traditional CRFs increase the likelihood of CV toxicity from any anticancer treatment**.
- Risk factors for the development of HF include older age, traditional CRFs, baseline LV dysfunction or prior HF, history of atherosclerotic CV disease, valvular heart disease, frailty, and poor cardiorespiratory fitness.
- **Presence of HTN is a specifically multiplicative risk in the presence of other risks**. For example, HTN leads to a relative increased risk of coronary artery disease (CAD) requiring treatment 24-fold over radiation alone, and it leads to a relative risk of HF 44-fold over anthracycline alone in childhood survivors of cancer.[7]
- For childhood survivors of cancer within 5 years of their cancer diagnosis, a CV risk calculator can be found at https://ccss.stjude.org/tools-and-documents/calculators-and-other-tools/ccss-cardiovascular-risk-calculator.html (accessed May 26, 2021).[8,9]
- A risk score for incident HF within 3 years of receiving trastuzumab for breast cancer has also been developed and includes adjuvant chemotherapy, age, and presence of CAD, atrial fibrillation/flutter, diabetes mellitus, HTN, and renal failure.[10]
- These risk scores may not apply to all patients with cancer undergoing all different varieties of cancer treatment (Fig. 1-1).

History
- All patients should receive a comprehensive screening for traditional CV risk factors (HTN, smoking, diabetes mellitus, dyslipidemia, physical activity, diet, obesity) and receive guideline-directed treatment as indicated.
- **The CO history should be tailored to the specific CV concern but should always include**:
  - **Underlying cancer prognosis**
  - **Previous treatments received**
  - **Ongoing and planned therapy**
- Information on past/present treatment regimen should include cumulative dose of anthracycline and mediastinal radiation.
- All patients should be screened for history of:
  - Cardiomyopathy, HF, or LV dysfunction

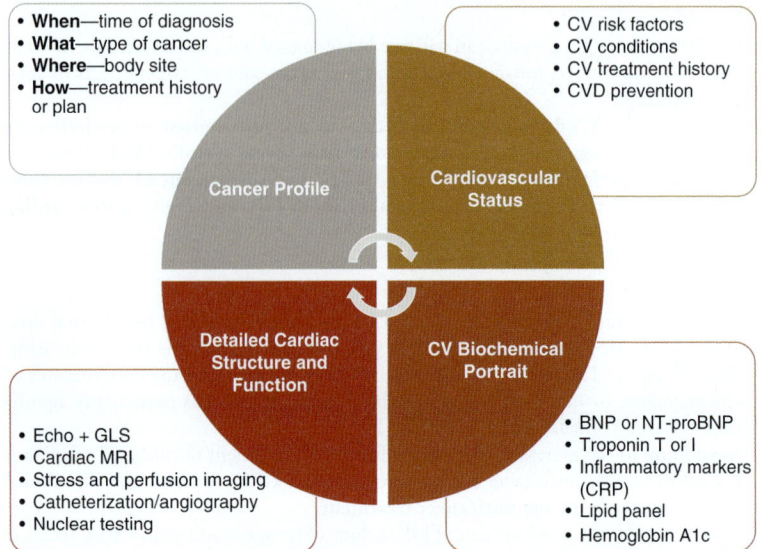

Figure 1-1. General approach to cardio-oncology (CO) patient. One suggested approach to carefully addressed important cardiovascular (CV) issues prior to initiating cancer therapy and identifying any cardiac risk factors (CRFs) or specific CV toxicity risk factors related to an underlying cancer or the treatment chosen. BNP, B-type natriuretic peptide; CRP, C-reactive protein; CVD, cardiovascular disease; GLS, global longitudinal strain; MRI, magnetic resonance imaging; NT-proBNP, N-terminal pro–brain natriuretic peptide

- CAD
- Arrhythmia or QT prolongation including symptoms of presyncope/syncope
- ATE or VTE

PATHOPHYSIOLOGY AND SPECIFIC TOXICITIES

- Although extensive, Table 1-2 should not be considered an all-inclusive list of CV toxicities. CV adverse effects may only be noted during post-marketing surveillance and the actual risk may be higher in patients outside of clinical trials.
- Clinicians treating patients with cancer should always maintain an index of suspicion that the underlying therapy can contribute to an adverse CV event.

Alkylating Agents
- **Examples**: cyclophosphamide, ifosfamide, cisplatin, melphalan
- **Mechanism of action**: Adds methyl, alkyl, or other side groups to DNA leading to DNA fragments, cross-linking, and/or nucleotide mispairing, ultimately leading to cell death
- **Main CV adverse effects**:
  - Hemorrhagic myopericarditis
  - Symptomatic cardiomyopathy

TABLE 1-2 Anticancer Therapies with CV Complications

	Cancer use	Common types of CV toxicity
Anthracyclines • Doxorubicin, epirubicin	Breast, sarcoma, lung, bladder, gastric, prostate, leukemia, lymphoma, others	HF, LVD, arrhythmias
Alkylating agents • Cyclophosphamide, cisplatin, melphalan	Breast, lymphoma, multiple myeloma, sarcoma, stem cell transplant, lung bladder, esophageal	HF, LVD, arrhythmias, myopericarditis
Antimetabolite agents • Fluorouracil, capecitabine	Breast, colon, gastric, pancreatic, head and neck	Coronary vasospasm, ischemia, arrhythmias
Antimicrotubule agents • Docetaxel, paclitaxel	Breast, lung, prostate, gastric, head and neck, ovarian, cervical, gastric, esophageal	HF, LVD, arrhythmias (bradyarrhythmia)
HER2-targeted therapies • Trastuzumab, pertuzumab	Breast, gastric, esophageal	HF, LVD
Small-molecule TKIs • Dabrafenib, dasatinib, imatinib, pazopanib, ponatinib, sorafenib, sunitinib, ibrutinib, axitinib	Melanoma, renal cell, thyroid, sarcoma, gastrointestinal stromal cell tumor, neuroendocrine tumor, lymphoma, colorectal, leukemia, pancreatic	Hypertension, QT prolongation, arterial thromboembolism and VTE, ischemia/atherosclerosis, edema, arrhythmias, pleural effusion
Immune checkpoint inhibitors • Nivolumab, ipilimumab, pembrolizumab	Melanoma, lung, kidney, bladder, head and neck, lymphoma	Myocarditis, arrhythmia, LVD, sudden cardiac death, vasculitis, pericarditis

(*continued*)

TABLE 1-2 Anticancer Therapies with CV Complications (continued)

	Cancer use	Common types of CV toxicity
Proteasome inhibitors • Bortezomib, carfilzomib	Multiple myeloma	HF, LVD, VTE, hypertension, acute coronary syndrome, pulmonary hypertension (carfilzomib)
Selective estrogen receptor modulators • Tamoxifen	Breast	VTE, QT prolongation
Aromatase inhibitors • Anastrozole, letrozole, exemestane	Breast	VTE, hyperlipidemia, hypertension
Luteinizing hormone releasing hormone agonists • Goserelin, leuprolide	Breast, endometrial, prostate	Ischemia, VTE, stroke, HF, LVD, QT prolongation
Antiandrogens • Bicalutamide	Prostate	Hypertension
Chimeric antigen receptor (CAR) T-cell therapy • Tisagenlecleucel	B-cell acute lymphoblastic leukemia, large B-cell lymphoma	Cytokine release syndrome, tachycardia, arrhythmia, hypotension, hypertension, HF, capillary leak syndrome
Bleomycin	Squamous cell carcinoma, melanoma, sarcoma, testicular, lymphoma	Ischemia, pericarditis, stroke, pulmonary toxicity
Tretinoin	Leukemia	HF, LVD
Arsenic trioxide	Leukemia	QT prolongation

HER2, human epidermal growth factor receptor 2; HF, heart failure; LVD; TKI, tyrosine kinase inhibitors; VTE, venous thromboembolism.

- VTE and ATE
- **HTN, hyperlipidemia, and Raynaud phenomenon with cisplatin in patients with testicular cancer**[11]

Androgen Deprivation Therapy, Antiandrogens, Androgen Receptor Blockers

- **Examples**:
  - Gonadotropin-releasing hormone (GnRH) agonists: goserelin, histrelin, leuprolide, triptorelin
  - GnRH antagonists: degarelix
  - Antiandrogens: bicalutamide, enzalutamide, flutamide, nilutamide
- **Mechanism of action**: Modulates the gonadotropin-testosterone axis to reduce testosterone levels to castration levels. Can result in overproduction of other adrenal hormones such as aldosterone
- **Main CV adverse effects: metabolic syndrome, CAD, myocardial infarction (MI) including acute coronary syndrome (ACS), HTN**
  - The exact CV impact of androgen deprivation therapy remains controversial. Androgen deprivation therapy consistently results in an unfavorable metabolic profile although there have been conflicting studies as to the degree to which it increases CV events above that of baseline risk factors.[12]
- Because of the mechanism of action, an aldosterone antagonist would be uniquely suited to treat associated HTN, although this has not been directly studied.

Anthracyclines

- **Examples**: daunorubicin, doxorubicin, epirubicin, idarubicin, mitoxantrone
- **Mechanism of action**: Inhibits topoisomerase II, inducing DNA strand breaks and ultimately resulting in apoptosis
- **Main adverse CV effects**:
  - **LV dysfunction—7% at dose of 150 mg/m^2 of doxorubicin**[13]
  - **HF—26% at dose of 550 mg/m^2 of doxorubicin**[13]
- Inhibition of topoisomerase IIb in cardiac tissue has been implicated in causing LV dysfunction.
- Anthracyclines also lead to generation of free radicals and reactive oxygen species with resultant oxidative damage.
- Toxicity is dose-dependent with $\geq$250 mg/m^2 of doxorubicin equivalent ($\geq$600 mg/m^2 of epirubicin) found to be a threshold for increased risk for toxicity (conversion rates and thresholds for toxicity are specific to the anthracycline used).
- As a general rule of thumb, patients receive 50 mg/m^2 of doxorubicin per cycle of chemotherapy in breast cancer and lymphoma.
- **Dexrazoxane is Food and Drug Administration (FDA) approved to prevent cardiotoxicity from anthracyclines**. Evidence suggests that dexrazoxane may achieve its cardioprotective benefit from its antioxidant properties and interfering with the effect of anthracyclines on topoisomerase IIb in the heart.[14]
- Carvedilol may achieve part of its cardioprotective benefit because of its antioxidant properties, a characteristic not shared by metoprolol.

Checkpoint Inhibitors (Programmed Death 1/Programmed Cell Death Ligand 1 and Cytotoxic T-lymphocyte-Associated Antigen 4 Inhibitors)

- **Examples**: ipilimumab, nivolumab, pembrolizumab
- **Mechanism of action**: Programmed Death 1 (PD-1)/Programmed Cell Death Ligand 1 (PDL-1) and Cytotoxic T-lymphocyte-Associated Antigen 4 (CTLA-4) serve

as checkpoints on the immune system. Some cancers are able to activate these receptors to turn the immune system off. By inhibiting these checkpoints, the immune system is activated and attacks the cancer.
- **Main adverse CV effects**:
  - **Myocarditis is rare (1%) but can be fatal.**[15-17]
  - **HF can occur with or without signs of myocarditis (case studies, no systematic reports).**
  - Serious arrhythmia[18,19]
- Because of the activated immune system, immune-mediated side effects can occur throughout the body, including the heart.
- **Expert opinion currently favors early administration of high-dose corticosteroids for treatment.**[20] **Higher intensity immunosuppression therapy has been attempted with limited success.**

Chimeric Antigen Receptor T-Cell Therapy

- **Examples**: axicabtagene ciloleucel, tisagenlecleucel
- **Mechanism of action**: T cells are genetically engineered to produce chimeric antigen receptors that target tumor cells.
- **Main adverse CV effects**:
  - Tachycardia
  - Arrhythmia (axicabtagene ciloleucel)
  - Cardiac arrest: 4%; cardiac failure: 6% to 7%
- **Up to 94% of patients will have symptoms of the cytokine release syndrome (CRS), which can be fatal in ~4%.**[21]

Fluoropyrimidine

- **Examples**: 5-fluorouracil (5-FU), capecitabine
- **Mechanism of action**: Inhibits the synthesis of thymidine, a nucleoside (pyrimidine) required for the construction of DNA
- **Main CV adverse effects**:
  - Coronary vasospasm, MI, ACS[22]

Human Epidermal Growth Factor Receptor 2 Targeted Therapies

- **Examples**: trastuzumab, pertuzumab, lapatinib
- **Mechanism of action**: Recombinant humanized monoclonal antibodies against human epidermal growth factor receptor 2 (HER2, aka ErbB2). HER2 promotes cell proliferation through growth signaling pathways.
- **Main adverse CV effect** (trastuzumab, pertuzumab):
  - **LV dysfunction (reduction in LV ejection fraction [EF] >10%)**
    - **Trial data**: 9.4% at 65 months; 18.6% in combination with anthracycline[23]
  - HF
    - Trial data: 2.0% in combo with anthracyclines[23]; retrospective cohort alone 12% at 5 years; 20% at 5 years with trastuzumab + anthracycline[6]
- **HER2 is also present in cardiac tissue and likely is important in the stress response as well as cardiac repair mechanisms in the heart.**[24]
- Lapatinib is a tyrosine kinase inhibitor (TKI) that affects the HER2 signaling pathway. It is uncommonly associated with LV dysfunction or HF. Pertuzumab has similar CV risk to trastuzumab and may not have significant additive risk when used in conjunction with trastuzumab.

Immunomodulatory Agents
- **Examples**: thalidomide, lenalidomide, pomalidomide
- **Mechanism of action**: The drugs have antiangiogenic and immunomodulatory properties that include T-cell activation and reduced production of proinflammatory cytokines.[25] Drugs in this class are synthetically derived from thalidomide.
- **Main adverse CV effects**[26,27]:
  - **VTE**
  - ATE
    - MI and cerebrovascular events are reported with lenalidomide and dexamethasone
  - Sinus bradycardia with thalidomide (not commonly seen with newer metabolites):
    - 26% including asymptomatic patients, 3% with severe or life-threatening bradycardia (Phase II trial)[28]
- **Consider prophylactic anticoagulation for VTE prevention in patients with multiple myeloma on lenalidomide**.

PI3K/AKT/mTOR Inhibitor
- **Examples**: everolimus, idelalisib, temsirolimus
- **Mechanism of action**: Inhibits the phosphatidylinositol 3-kinase (PI3K)/protein kinase B (AKT)/mammalian target of rapamycin (mTOR) signaling cascade, resulting in reduced cell growth, proliferation, and angiogenesis
- **Main CV adverse effects**: The phosphatidylinositol 3-kinase (PI3K)/protein kinase B (AKT)/mammalian target of rapamycin (mTOR) signaling cascade is important in a number of cellular processes including tissue metabolism and glucose homeostasis. There was over a 50% incidence of hyperglycemia, hypercholesterolemia, and hypertriglyceridemia in clinical trials, though new onset of diabetes mellitus was <1% and hyperglycemia in patients being treated for cancer is common in general.[29]

Proteasome Inhibitors
- **Examples**: bortezomib, carfilzomib, ixazomib
- **Mechanism of action**: The proteasome is responsible for degradation of proteins within the cell. Inhibiting the proteasome subsequently leads to apoptosis.
- **Main adverse CV effects**:
  - HF
    - Few reports with bortezomib
    - 4% in systematic review of clinic trials of carfilzomib[30]
  - HTN
    - **18% in systematic review of carfilzomib**[30]
- **Carfilzomib has been associated with increased incidence of HF and MI compared to bortezomib**.[31]

Tyrosine Kinase Inhibitors
- See also vascular endothelial growth factor (VEGF) signaling pathway (VSP) inhibitors, HER2 antagonists, and mTOR inhibitors.
- **Examples**:
  - MEK (mitogen-activated protein kinase) inhibitors: trametinib, selumetinib
  - BRAF inhibitors: vemurafenib, dabrafenib
  - ABL kinase inhibitors: imatinib, dasatinib, ponatinib, nilotinib
  - BTK (Bruton tyrosine kinase) inhibitor: ibrutinib
  - EGFR (endothelial growth factor receptor) inhibitors: erlotinib, cetuximab, lapatinib
  - ALK (anaplastic lymphoma kinase) inhibitors: ceritinib, crizotinib, alectinib, brigatinib

- **Mechanism of Action**: Inhibit tyrosine kinases directly or by inhibiting the kinase receptor, blocking downstream cell signaling. There are several tyrosine kinase targets to date, and some drugs can affect multiple targets.
- **Main adverse CV effects** (not consistent across class, relatively more toxic drugs listed as examples):
  - **ATE (ponatinib)**
  - **Atrial fibrillation (ibrutinib)**
  - **Atherosclerosis (nilotinib)**
  - **Bleeding (ibrutinib)**
  - **Bradyarrhythmia (trametinib, alectinib, crizotinib)**
  - **Edema (imatinib)**
  - **HTN (ibrutinib, trametinib, nilotinib)**
  - **LV dysfunction (ponatinib, trametinib)**
  - **QT prolongation (dabrafenib, nilotinib, trametinib)**
  - **VTE (ponatinib, erlotinib, trametinib, nilotinib)**

Vascular Endothelial Growth Factor Signaling Pathway Inhibitors

- Includes VEGF receptor inhibitors and antiangiogenic TKIs
- **Examples**: bevacizumab, pazopanib, sunitinib, sorafenib, axitinib, vandetanib, regorafenib, cabozantinib, ziv-aflibercept, ramucirumab, lenvatinib
- **Mechanism of action**: Inhibit angiogenesis through the VEGF pathway. Bevacizumab directly binds the VEGF receptor, whereas drugs such as sunitinib are TKIs that block downstream signaling.
- **Main adverse CV effects**[32,33]: **Side effects are generally a class effect, although HTN and LV dysfunction are lower with some medications such as bevacizumab than with the antiangiogenic multikinase TKIs such as sunitinib. QT prolongation is specific to the medication, with vandetanib reporting the highest incidence of significant QT prolongation, although the incidence is still low (<3%).**
  - HTN
  - LV dysfunction
  - ATE event
  - VTE event
  - QT prolongation

Select Other Medications and Cardiovascular Adverse Effects

- Arsenic trioxide: **QT prolongation** (38%); retrospective analysis[34]
- Decitabine (hypomethylating agent): <5% incidence of cardiac failure, MI, atrial fibrillation, supraventricular tachycardia
- Docetaxel/Paclitaxel (antimicrotubules): **autonomic dysfunction** (incidence not well defined)
- Ribociclib (CDK4/CDK6 inhibitor): **QT prolongation**[35]
- Rituximab (anti-CD20 antibody): hypotension in 10% (infusion reaction), Grade 3 or 4 in 1%
- Tretinoin: arrhythmias, HF[36]
- Vorinostat (histone deacetylase inhibitor): QT prolongation >500 ms[37]

Radiation (Chest/Mediastinal)

- **Mechanism of action**: Damages DNA directly and through free radical production, leading to cell death

- **Main CV adverse effects**:
  - Arrhythmia 16% (9-year median follow-up)
  - **Autonomic dysfunction 30% to 45% (19-year median follow-up)**[38]
  - **CAD 19% to 20% (9- to 20-year median follow-up)**[39,40]
  - **HF 11% to 12% (9- to 20-year median follow-up)**[39,40]
  - **Pericardial disease 5% (9-year median follow-up)**[40]
  - **Pacemaker/implantable cardioverter-defibrillator (ICD) malfunction 3%**[41]
  - **Valvular heart disease 11% to 31% (9- to 20-year median follow-up)**[39,40]
- **Mediastinal radiation ≥30 Gy (with the heart in the treatment field) and the combination of anthracyclines or radiation at any dose has been identified as especially high-risk factors for LV dysfunction.**[7]
- More recent radiation protocols have incorporated a number of different measures to reduce toxicity. It is expected that the cardiac impact will be lower in the future, although the degree of which it will be lower is unknown.

PREVENTION

- Preventive measures should always include assessing for CRFs accompanied by guideline-directed treatment.

ABCDEs of Prevention

- **The ABCDEs have had a couple of modifications for use in screening to prevent CV disease and can be a useful tool generally in patients with cancer.**[42]
  - **A**: Awareness of risks of heart disease, Aspirin
  - **B**: Blood pressure, Biomarkers
  - **C**: Cholesterol, Cigarette/tobacco cessation
  - **D**: Diet and weight management, Dose of chemotherapy or radiation, Diabetes mellitus prevention/treatment
  - **E**: Exercise, Echocardiography

Coronary Vasospasm

- **Secondary prevention of vasospasm** associated with fluoropyrimidines (5-FU, capecitabine) can be achieved with bolus administration as opposed to continuous infusion of 5-FU as well as use **of calcium channel blockers (eg, nifedipine, diltiazem) and nitrates.**[43]
- Any use of diltiazem should be carefully considered because of its interactions with the cytochrome P450 system and associated risk of adverse drug interactions as well as its association with worsening LV function in patients with HF.
- **Given their underlying endothelial dysfunction, all patients should be considered for treatment for CAD including aspirin, statin, and clopidogrel if indicated.**

Left Ventricular Dysfunction

- Patients on VSP inhibitors, specifically, are at high risk for developing HTN, which may lead to subsequent LV dysfunction.
- In high-risk patients for LV dysfunction, doxorubicin cardiotoxicity can be limited through continuous infusion instead of bolus dosing and the use of liposomal formulation.[44]

- **Dexrazoxane is the only agent with specific FDA approval for the prevention of anthracycline cardiotoxicity and is generally considered for patients receiving over 300 mg/m² of doxorubicin or equivalent.** A Cochrane meta-analysis found that it successfully reduced incident HF without affecting progression-free or overall survival.[45]
- Studies have also found potential benefit for the use of some ACE-I, ARB, and β-blockers including carvedilol, enalapril, and candesartan for the prevention of LV dysfunction.[46-48] Metoprolol has not shown benefit.[47]
- Limited direct evidence supports possible use of statins and aldosterone antagonists. It is unknown if the hormonal, antiandrogen, effects of spironolactone have a clinical impact in tumors tied to the hormonal axis (prostate, breast, etc.).
- Patients at the highest risk for LV dysfunction, based on patient characteristics or treatment regimen, are likely to derive the most benefit from protective medications. Patients with elevated troponin showed benefit from enalapril and carvedilol, for instance, in reducing LV dysfunction.[46] Additional studies are still needed for optimal patient selection.

Thrombosis

- **Patients with multiple myeloma on lenalidomide should be considered for thromboembolism prophylaxis with anticoagulation.**[26,27]

Torsades de Pointes

- Several chemotherapy drugs have the potential to prolong the QTc interval, notably arsenic trioxide as well as certain TKIs (dabrafenib, nilotinib, trametinib, vandetanib), the histone deacetylase inhibitor vorinostat, and the CDK4/CDK6 inhibitor ribociclib.
- Ribociclib specifically requires an FDA-mandated electrocardiogram (ECG) on C1D1 (Cycle 1 Day 1), C1D14, and C2D1 per FDA guidelines.[35]
- Patients with cancer are routinely exposed to other QT prolonging medicines such as antiemetics, which could place them at higher risk for arrhythmia.
- ECGs and possibly topical telemetry should be considered for patients initiated on new QT prolonging medications or with clinical status changes such as electrolyte abnormalities. Electrolytes should be monitored and replaced as needed to reduce the risk for arrhythmia.

DIAGNOSIS OF CARDIOVASCULAR ADVERSE EVENTS DURING CANCER THERAPY

Clinical Presentation

- Full discussion of cancer therapeutic–based monitoring strategies can be found in Chapters 2, 3, 14 to 16, 18, and 22.
- Clinical signs and symptoms of CV toxicity can develop immediately or be delayed as far as decades later.
- Cardiologists may be consulted prior to treatment for preoperative assessment, during chemotherapy initiation because of immediate adverse effects, or in survivorship clinic for monitoring or treatment of long-term sequelae.
- During cancer treatment, patients are at high risk for orthostatic hypotension and should be monitored for symptoms of presyncope/syncope.

Physical Examination
- A few noteworthy comments relevant to the differential diagnosis in patients with cancer:
  - Isolated elevated jugular venous pressure (JVP) can occur after administration of intravenous fluids even in a patient without documented LV dysfunction.
  - Graft-versus-host disease (GVHD) (see Chapter 18) and radiation pneumonitis can mimic pulmonary edema on lung auscultation and x-ray, although other signs of HF would be absent.
- Importantly, cardiac tamponade remains a critical clinical diagnosis and physical examination should assess for patient distress, tachycardia, elevated JVP, and pulsus paradoxus.

Diagnostic Criteria
- Diagnostic criteria for CV adverse events are generally consistent with the diagnostic criteria for CV events in patients without cancer. In addition to cancer therapy–related cardiac dysfunction (CTRCD), all common etiologies of CV adverse events should still be considered (eg, ischemic cardiomyopathy).
- **The diagnosis of subclinical LV dysfunction and cardiotoxicity in patients with cancer does also incorporate global longitudinal strain (GLS) (Table 1-1) and/or use of biomarkers. Patients with subclinical LV dysfunction should be considered for cardioprotective medications.**

Screening and Diagnostic Testing
- In addition to the standard evaluation for any patient for HF, ACS, or other CV disease, screening and diagnostic testing specific to patients with cancer are presented below.
- Patients receiving cancer treatment should receive appropriate monitoring during and after treatment. CV disease can become evident years after therapy is completed.
- **Patients on VSP inhibitors should check their blood pressure regularly** (Fig. 1-2).

Laboratories
- Both standard clinical cardiac biomarkers, troponin and NP (B-type natriuretic peptide [BNP], N-terminal pro–brain natriuretic peptide [NT-proBNP]) levels have shown some promise in detecting subclinical cardiotoxicity and predicting future events.[31,49-51] The optimal timing for testing in all cancers and with specific anticancer therapy has not been fully defined.
- Baseline cardiac biomarkers can be helpful prior to initiation of cancer therapy, allowing one to identify patients at highest risk[52-55] (Chapter 15).

Imaging
- Echocardiogram (or potentially MRI) should be considered (Chapters 14 and 16):
  - At baseline for patients scheduled to undergo cancer therapy associated with high risk of HF or LV dysfunction
  - For patients with signs (elevated JVP, edema) or symptoms (orthopnea, paroxysmal nocturnal dyspnea, dyspnea on exertion) of HF
  - Routine surveillance in patients at moderate to high risk of LV dysfunction (high baseline CV risk, regimen with HER-2 antagonist and/or anthracycline, mediastinal radiation)
  - 6 to 12 months after completion of cancer therapy at moderate to high risk of LV dysfunction even in asymptomatic patients

Overview of monitoring strategies for patients treated with cardiotoxic therapy

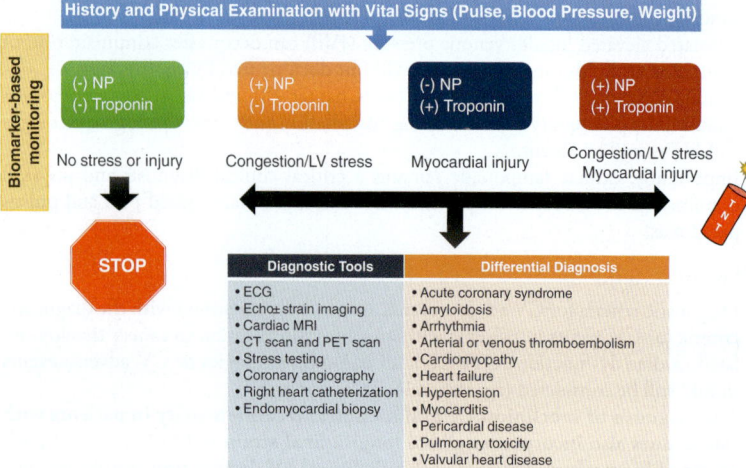

Figure 1-2. Monitoring strategies to detect and treat cardiovascular (CV) adverse events. After carefully considering the baseline cardiac risk factors (CRFs) and the cancer treatment–specific risks, as well as initiating primary and secondary prevention strategies to manage these identified risks, it is important to consider how to monitor for CV adverse events. The most important initial step is to follow vital signs (heart rate [HR], blood pressure [BP], and weights) depending on the cancer treatment that will begin. For therapies known to affect the BP, daily home measurement by the patient is a reasonable expectation. If the cancer therapeutic requires monitoring for the development of heart failure (HF), a combination of biomarker and imaging strategies is employed. If any CV toxicity is identified during treatment, careful CV-based medical management is necessary. CT, computed tomography; ECG, electrocardiography; LV, left ventricular; MRI, magnetic resonance imaging; PET, positron emission tomography.

- Echo is generally the test of choice because of cost and availability, although MRI has some advantages particularly with reproducibility.
- In patients undergoing Echo, the addition of GLS is recommended if feasible.[56]

Electrocardiography
- A baseline ECG should be obtained in all patients to screen for conduction disorders (including QT prolongation) as well as signs of prior MI or other significant cardiac disease.
- ECGs and possibly telemetry should be used to monitor patients initiated on new QT prolonging medications or with clinical status changes such as electrolyte abnormalities.

TREATMENT OF SPECIFIC CARDIAC DISEASES

- Treatment for CV events (HF, ACS) in the cancer population mirrors treatment in the noncancer population, but comorbidities (such as thrombocytopenia, orthostatic hypotension) often limit management options.

- In patients with active cancer, treatment goals should always include **minimizing stoppages or cessation of cancer therapy**.
- In patients with planned or current treatment for cancer and indication for coronary evaluation, the expected treatment course and platelet trend should be considered when making management decisions.
- Radial approach for invasive coronary evaluation can be considered to minimize bleeding in patients with thrombocytopenia.

Medications

- Patients with HF with reduced EF (HFrEF) should receive guideline-directed medical therapy as with all other patients.
- **LV dysfunction** not meeting criteria for HFrEF (EF >40% and less than institutional normal) is treated more aggressively in order to reduce ongoing decline in function and potentially allow for continued cancer treatment if needed.
- **In patients with thrombocytopenia requiring antiplatelets or anticoagulation**, the following practice recommendations[57,58] are based on expert opinion and review of the available literature. Decisions should be individualized based on patient-specific risk factors and goals of care.
  - Aspirin in patients with CAD for platelets >30k
  - Dual antiplatelet therapy in indicated patients post-PCI with platelets >50k
  - In patients with acute VTE, full-dose low-molecular-weight heparin (LMWH) anticoagulation for platelets >50k, 50% dose for platelets 30 to 50k. Hold for platelets <30k.
  - In patients with nonacute VTE, 75% LMWH anticoagulation dose for platelets 50 to 100k, 50% or lower dose for platelets 30 to 50k
- For treatment of **HTN, cardioprotective medications (ACE-I/ARB or carvedilol) should be considered as first line for antihypertensives in all patients undergoing treatment with the potential for LV dysfunction. These patients are considered Stage A HF patients (at risk) per the HF guidelines**.
- Given increased arterial stiffness and resistive load seen during treatment with sunitinib,[59] patients may also benefit from **vasodilator therapy such as dihydropyridine calcium channel blockers as well as combined α and β blockade (eg, carvedilol) for the treatment of HTN** associated with antiangiogenic TKIs.
- **Non-dihydropyridines (diltiazem, verapamil) inhibit the cytochrome P450 system and affect the metabolism of TKIs and other cancer therapies**. They should be avoided or used with caution in patients with cancer after checking all drug-drug interactions (see Chapter 19).
- See also Table 1-2.

Other Nonpharmacologic Therapies (Lifestyle)

Diet

- In addition to diet's role in CV disease, dietary excesses have been linked to the development of cancer.
- Saturated fats may reduce survival from cancer in addition to increasing the risk for CV disease.
- Eating sufficient fruits and vegetables as well as foods high in fiber is linked to a lower risk of certain cancers, whereas certain processed and red meat, as well as high levels of smoked food, have been linked to an increased risk of colorectal and stomach cancer, respectively.

- Patients with cancer can frequently have poor nutrition because of anorexia or adverse effects of cancer treatment on the gastrointestinal mucosa. In these patients, maximizing calories often becomes the priority.
- Certain diets, such as lower fiber, may also be recommended to counteract symptoms of diarrhea or trouble digesting food.

Activity
- Peak exercise capacity, as measured by peak oxygen consumption, is often substantially reduced in patients with cancer, and patients can benefit from interventions improving their exercise capacity.
- In women with nonmetastatic breast cancer, the incidence of CV events is reduced proportionately with increasing amounts of exercise.[60]
- Exercise has also been shown to reduce breast cancer–related death and all-cause mortality.[61]
- Given the wide range in capabilities and comorbidities of individual patients, experts have recommended tailoring the exercise plan to the individual patient and giving specific recommendations (number of times per week, duration) when able.[62]

SPECIAL CONSIDERATIONS/PULLING IT ALL TOGETHER

- Care should be individualized to the patient's goals of care and quality of life. Some patients may simply be focused on relieving or reducing symptoms, whereas others may want more aggressive CV care.
- Delay in recognition of CV adverse events can significantly worsen prognosis and recovery.

REFERRAL

Referral to a CO specialist is preferred in any patient with significant baseline CV risk or with plans for therapy with intermediate to high risk for cardiotoxicity.[63] These CV specialists will have the most experience working with the oncologist in selecting the optimal treatment regimen and mitigating any potential CV adverse events.

PATIENT EDUCATION

- All patients should be educated on their cancer regimen, potential toxicities, and recommended follow-up (Fig. 1-3).
- Emphasizing all important factors in maintaining overall CV health is paramount. The American Heart Association Life's Simple 7 is a useful guide that advocates for a healthy weight, tobacco cessation, a healthy diet, regular physical activity as well as blood pressure, cholesterol, and glucose management. Patients can be directed to their website.
- The American College of Cardiology is also developing a number of patient resources through CardioSmart at https://www.cardiosmart.org/Heart-Conditions/Cardio-Oncology.

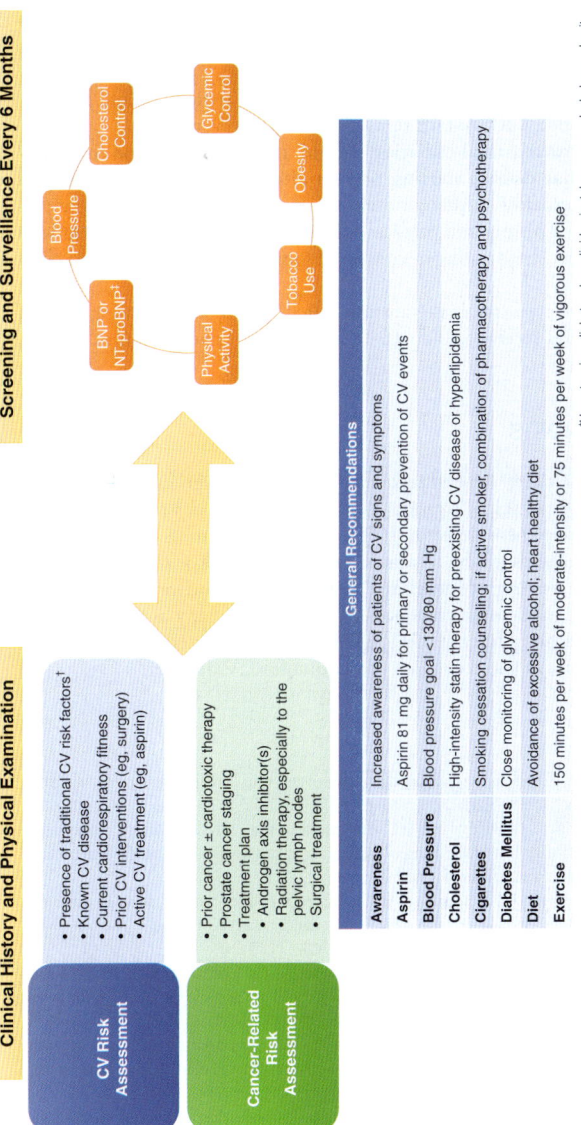

Figure 1-3. The comprehensive approach to a patient with prostate cancer considering cardiovascular (CV) impact of cancer therapy. The holistic approach to a patient is illustrated here in reference to a patient with prostate cancer. Baseline CV assessment should be complete with ascertainment of all cardiac risk factors (CRFs) and then understanding the cancer-based treatment choices and the potential CV impact. A reasonable monitoring strategy is put in place and followed in the future. Maintaining CV health is emphasized at every opportunity. (Derived from Bhatia N, Santos M, Jones LW, et al. Cardiovascular effects of androgen deprivation therapy for the treatment of prostate cancer: ABCDE steps to reduce cardiovascular disease in patients with prostate cancer. *Circulation.* 2016;133:537-541; Hu JR, Duncan MS, Morgans AK, et al. Cardiovascular effects of androgen deprivation therapy in prostate cancer: contemporary meta-analyses. *Arterioscler Thromb Vasc Biol.* 2020;40:e55-e64.)

MONITORING/FOLLOW-UP

- Close follow-up, ideally within 2 weeks, is recommended after discharge from the hospital in patients being treated for cancer. In such patients, delays in care can contribute to increased or more prolonged stoppages of cancer therapy. Such stoppages can have a significant impact on mortality.
- Patients on cancer therapies with known potential for CV toxicity should have ongoing evaluation of their CRF and for signs of CV adverse events.
- **Patients with prior mediastinal radiation should undergo evaluation for CAD/ischemia and valvular disease starting 5 years after completion of therapy at regular intervals thereafter**. Although there are no data to recommend any particular screening test, a history and physical examination should be completed with consideration for other stress testing or computed tomography angiography as clinically appropriate.
- Patients who have received cancer therapy associated with moderate to high risk of LV dysfunction should receive an Echo 6-12 months after completion of therapy, even if asymptomatic.

OUTCOME/PROGNOSIS

- Prognosis varies significantly depending on cancer type and stage, as well as whether the cancer is refractory to initial treatment options. The patient's prognosis should be considered in management decisions by the multidisciplinary team.
- **It is important to note that new treatment options can allow for much longer survival even in the setting of metastatic disease**. Patients with metastatic renal cell cancer can be controlled for years on VSP inhibitor therapy as can metastatic breast cancer patients on hormonal therapy. These patients can continue to benefit from appropriate primary and secondary prevention for CV disease.

REFERENCES

1. Groarke JD, Cheng S, Moslehi J. Cancer-drug discovery and cardiovascular surveillance. *N Engl J Med.* 2013;369:1779-1781.
2. Bluethmann SM, Mariotto AB, Rowland JH. Anticipating the "Silver Tsunami": prevalence trajectories and comorbidity burden among older cancer survivors in the United States. *Cancer Epidemiol Biomarkers Prev.* 2016;25:1029-1036.
3. Armstrong GT, Kawashima T, Leisenring W, et al. Aging and risk of severe, disabling, life-threatening, and fatal events in the childhood cancer survivor study. *J Clin Oncol.* 2014;32:1218-1227.
4. Patnaik JL, Byers T, DiGuiseppi C, Dabelea D, Denberg TD. Cardiovascular disease competes with breast cancer as the leading cause of death for older females diagnosed with breast cancer: a retrospective cohort study. *Breast Cancer Res.* 2011;13:R64.
5. Bowles EJ, Wellman R, Feigelson HS, et al. Risk of heart failure in breast cancer patients after anthracycline and trastuzumab treatment: a retrospective cohort study. *J Natl Cancer Inst.* 2012;104:1293-1305.
6. Armenian SH, Lacchetti C, Barac A, et al. Prevention and monitoring of cardiac dysfunction in survivors of adult cancers: American Society of Clinical Oncology clinical practice guideline. *J Clin Oncol.* 2017;35:893-911.
7. Armstrong GT, Oeffinger KC, Chen Y, et al. Modifiable risk factors and major cardiac events among adult survivors of childhood cancer. *J Clin Oncol.* 2013;31:3673-3680.

8. Chow EJ, Chen Y, Hudson MM, et al. Prediction of ischemic heart disease and stroke in survivors of childhood cancer. *J Clin Oncol.* 2018;36:44-52.
9. Chow EJ, Chen Y, Kremer LC, et al. Individual prediction of heart failure among childhood cancer survivors. *J Clin Oncol.* 2015;33:394-402.
10. Ezaz G, Long JB, Gross CP, Chen J. Risk prediction model for heart failure and cardiomyopathy after adjuvant trastuzumab therapy for breast cancer. *J Am Heart Assoc.* 2014;3:e000472.
11. Kerns SL, Fung C, Monahan PO, et al. Cumulative burden of morbidity among testicular cancer survivors after standard cisplatin-based chemotherapy: a multi-institutional study. *J Clin Oncol.* 2018;36:1505-1512.
12. Bhatia N, Santos M, Jones LW, Beckman JA, Penson DF, Morgans AK, Moslehi J. Cardiovascular effects of androgen deprivation therapy for the treatment of prostate cancer: ABCDE steps to reduce cardiovascular disease in patients with prostate cancer. *Circulation.* 2016;133(5):537-541. doi: 10.1161/CIRCULATIONAHA.115.012519.
13. Swain SM, Whaley FS, Ewer MS. Congestive heart failure in patients treated with doxorubicin: a retrospective analysis of three trials. *Cancer.* 2003;97:2869-2879.
14. Van Tine BA, Hirbe AC, Oppelt P, et al. Interim analysis of the phase ii study: noninferiority study of doxorubicin with upfront dexrazoxane plus olaratumab for advanced or metastatic soft-tissue sarcoma. *Clin Cancer Res.* 2021;27:3854-3860.
15. Johnson DB, Balko JM, Compton ML, et al. Fulminant myocarditis with combination immune checkpoint blockade. *N Engl J Med.* 2016;375:1749-1755.
16. Heinzerling L, Ott PA, Hodi FS, et al. Cardiotoxicity associated with CTLA4 and PD1 blocking immunotherapy. *J Immunother Cancer.* 2016;4:50.
17. Mahmood SS, Fradley MG, Cohen JV, et al. Myocarditis in patients treated with immune checkpoint inhibitors. *J Am Coll Cardiol.* 2018;71:1755-1764.
18. Ball S, Ghosh RK, Wongsaengsak S, et al. Cardiovascular toxicities of immune checkpoint inhibitors: JACC review topic of the week. *J Am Coll Cardiol.* 2019;74:1714-1727.
19. Schiffer WB, Deych E, Lenihan DJ, Zhang KW. Coronary and aortic calcification are associated with cardiovascular events on immune checkpoint inhibitor therapy. *Int J Cardiol.* 2021;322:177-182.
20. Zhang L, Zlotoff DA, Awadalla M, et al. Major adverse cardiovascular events and the timing and dose of corticosteroids in immune checkpoint inhibitor-associated myocarditis. *Circulation.* 2020;141:2031-2034.
21. Alvi RM, Frigault MJ, Fradley MG, et al. Cardiovascular events among adults treated with chimeric antigen receptor T-cells (CAR-T). *J Am Coll Cardiol.* 2019;74:3099-3108.
22. Polk A, Vaage-Nilsen M, Vistisen K, Nielsen DL. Cardiotoxicity in cancer patients treated with 5-fluorouracil or capecitabine: a systematic review of incidence, manifestations and predisposing factors. *Cancer Treat Rev.* 2013;39:974-984.
23. Slamon D, Eiermann W, Robert N, et al. Adjuvant trastuzumab in HER2-positive breast cancer. *N Engl J Med.* 2011;365:1273-1283.
24. Odiete O, Hill MF, Sawyer DB. Neuregulin in cardiovascular development and disease. *Circ Res.* 2012;111:1376-1385.
25. Kotla V, Goel S, Nischal S, et al. Mechanism of action of lenalidomide in hematological malignancies. *J Hematol Oncol.* 2009;2:36.
26. Palumbo A, Rajkumar SV, Dimopoulos MA, et al. Prevention of thalidomide-and lenalidomide-associated thrombosis in myeloma. *Leukemia.* 2008;22:414-423.
27. Musallam KM, Dahdaleh FS, Shamseddine AI, Taher AT. Incidence and prophylaxis of venous thromboembolic events in multiple myeloma patients receiving immunomodulatory therapy. *Thromb Res.* 2009;123:679-686.
28. Rajkumar SV, Gertz MA, Lacy MQ, et al. Thalidomide as initial therapy for early-stage myeloma. *Leukemia.* 2003;17:775-779.
29. Potocki M, Breidthardt T, Mueller A, et al. Copeptin and risk stratification in patients with acute dyspnea. *Crit Care.* 2010;14:R213.
30. Waxman AJ, Clasen S, Hwang W, et al. Carfilzomib-associated cardiovascular adverse events: a systematic review and meta-analysis. *JAMA Oncol.* 2018;4:e174519.

31. Cornell RF, Ky B, Weiss BM, et al. Prospective study of cardiac events during proteasome inhibitor therapy for relapsed multiple myeloma. *J Clin Oncol.* 2019;37:1946-1955.
32. Li W, Croce K, Steensma DP, McDermott DF, Ben-Yehuda O, Moslehi J. Vascular and metabolic implications of novel targeted cancer therapies: focus on kinase inhibitors. *J Am Coll Cardiol.* 2015;66:1160-1178.
33. Narayan V, Wang L, Putt M, et al. Risk of left ventricular systolic dysfunction with sunitinib therapy in patients with metastatic renal cell carcinoma: a prospective cohort study. *J Clin Oncol.* 2016;34:e16104.
34. Barbey JT, Pezzullo JC, Soignet SL. Effect of arsenic trioxide on QT interval in patients with advanced malignancies. *J Clin Oncol.* 2003;21:3609-3615.
35. Ribociclib (Kisqali). Package insert. Novartis Pharmaceuticals Corporation; 2017.
36. Tretinoin. Package insert. Roche Laboratories Inc; 2004.
37. Porta-Sánchez A, Gilbert C, Spears D, et al. Incidence, diagnosis, and management of QT prolongation induced by cancer therapies: a systematic review. *J Am Heart Assoc.* 2017;6(12):e007724.
38. Groarke JD, Tanguturi VK, Hainer J, et al. Abnormal exercise response in long-term survivors of Hodgkin lymphoma treated with thoracic irradiation: evidence of cardiac autonomic dysfunction and impact on outcomes. *J Am Coll Cardiol.* 2015;65:573-583.
39. van Nimwegen FA, Schaapveld M, Janus CP, et al. Cardiovascular disease after Hodgkin lymphoma treatment: 40-year disease risk. *JAMA Intern Med.* 2015;175:1007-1017.
40. Maraldo MV, Giusti F, Vogelius IR, et al. Cardiovascular disease after treatment for Hodgkin's lymphoma: an analysis of nine collaborative EORTC-LYSA trials. *Lancet Haematol.* 2015;2:e492-e502.
41. Zaremba T, Jakobsen AR, Sogaard M, Thogersen AM, Riahi S. Radiotherapy in patients with pacemakers and implantable cardioverter defibrillators: a literature review. *Europace.* 2016;18:479-491.
42. Montazeri K, Unitt C, Foody JM, Harris JR, Partridge AH, Moslehi J. ABCDE steps to prevent heart disease in breast cancer survivors. *Circulation.* 2014;130:e157-e159.
43. Clasen SC, Ky B, O'Quinn R, Giantonio B, Teitelbaum U, Carver JR. Fluoropyrimidine-induced cardiac toxicity: challenging the current paradigm. *J Gastrointest Oncol.* 2017;8:970-979.
44. Smith LA, Cornelius VR, Plummer CJ, et al. Cardiotoxicity of anthracycline agents for the treatment of cancer: systematic review and meta-analysis of randomised controlled trials. *BMC Cancer.* 2010;10:337.
45. van Dalen EC, Caron HN, Dickinson HO, Kremer LC. Cardioprotective interventions for cancer patients receiving anthracyclines. *Cochrane Database Syst Rev.* 2011;2011:CD003917.
46. Cardinale D, Colombo A, Sandri MT, et al. Prevention of high-dose chemotherapy-induced cardiotoxicity in high-risk patients by angiotensin-converting enzyme inhibition. *Circulation.* 2006;114:2474-2481.
47. Gulati G, Heck SL, Ree AH, et al. Prevention of cardiac dysfunction during adjuvant breast cancer therapy (PRADA): a 2 × 2 factorial, randomized, placebo-controlled, double-blind clinical trial of candesartan and metoprolol. *Eur Heart J.* 2016;37:1671-1680.
48. Bosch X, Rovira M, Sitges M, et al. Enalapril and carvedilol for preventing chemotherapy-induced left ventricular systolic dysfunction in patients with malignant hemopathies: the OVERCOME trial (preventiOn of left Ventricular dysfunction with Enalapril and caRvedilol in patients submitted to intensive ChemOtherapy for the treatment of Malignant hEmopathies). *J Am Coll Cardiol.* 2013;61:2355-2362.
49. Cardinale D, Sandri MT, Colombo A, et al. Prognostic value of troponin I in cardiac risk stratification of cancer patients undergoing high-dose chemotherapy. *Circulation.* 2004;109:2749-2754.
50. Ky B, Putt M, Sawaya H, et al. Early increases in multiple biomarkers predict subsequent cardiotoxicity in patients with breast cancer treated with doxorubicin, taxanes, and trastuzumab. *J Am Coll Cardiol.* 2014;63:809-816.
51. Lenihan DJ, Stevens PL, Massey M, et al. The utility of point-of-care biomarkers to detect cardiotoxicity during anthracycline chemotherapy: a feasibility study. *J Cardiac Fail.* 2016;22:433-438.

52. Curigliano G, Cardinale D, Dent S, et al. Cardiotoxicity of anticancer treatments: epidemiology, detection, and management. *CA Cancer J Clin.* 2016;66:309-325.
53. Lipshultz SE, Rifai N, Sallan SE, et al. Predictive value of cardiac troponin T in pediatric patients at risk for myocardial injury. *Circulation.* 1997;96:2641-2648.
54. Cardinale D, Sandri MT, Martinoni A, et al. Myocardial injury revealed by plasma troponin I in breast cancer treated with high-dose chemotherapy. *Ann Oncol.* 2002;13:710-715.
55. Kilickap S, Barista I, Akgul E, et al. cTnT can be a useful marker for early detection of anthracycline cardiotoxicity. *Ann Oncol.* 2005;16:798-804.
56. Plana JC, Galderisi M, Barac A, et al. Expert consensus for multimodality imaging evaluation of adult patients during and after cancer therapy: a report from the American Society of Echocardiography and the European Association of Cardiovascular Imaging. *J Am Soc Echocardiogr.* 2014;27:911-939.
57. Chang HM, Moudgil R, Scarabelli T, Okwuosa TM, Yeh ETH. Cardiovascular complications of cancer therapy: best practices in diagnosis, prevention, and management: part 1. *J Am Coll Cardiol.* 2017;70:2536-2551.
58. Saccullo G, Marietta M, Carpenedo M, et al. Platelet cut-off for anticoagulant therapy in cancer patients with venous thromboembolism and thrombocytopenia: an expert opinion based on RAND/UCLA Appropriateness Method (RAM). *Blood.* 2013;122:581.
59. Narayan V, Keefe S, Haas N, et al. Prospective evaluation of sunitinib-induced cardiotoxicity in patients with metastatic renal cell carcinoma. *Clin Cancer Res.* 2017;23:3601-3609.
60. Jones LW, Habel LA, Weltzien E, et al. Exercise and risk of cardiovascular events in women with nonmetastatic breast cancer. *J Clin Oncol.* 2016;34:2743-2749.
61. Lahart IM, Metsios GS, Nevill AM, Carmichael AR. Physical activity, risk of death and recurrence in breast cancer survivors: a systematic review and meta-analysis of epidemiological studies. *Acta Oncol.* 2015;54:635-654.
62. Gilchrist SC, Barac A, Ades PA, et al. Cardio-oncology rehabilitation to manage cardiovascular outcomes in cancer patients and survivors: a scientific statement from the American Heart Association. *Circulation.* 2019;139:e997-e1012.
63. Adusumalli S, Alvarez-Cardona J, Khatana SM, et al. Clinical practice and research in cardio-oncology: finding the "Rosetta Stone" for establishing program excellence in cardio-oncology. *J Cardiovasc Transl Res.* 2020;13:495-505.
64. Seidman A, Hudis C, Pierri MK, et al. Cardiac dysfunction in the trastuzumab clinical trials experience. *J Clin Oncol.* 2002;20:1215-1221.
65. Hunt SA, Baker DW, Chin MH, et al. ACC/AHA guidelines for the evaluation and management of chronic heart failure in the adult: executive summary. A report of the American College of Cardiology/American Heart Association Task Force on Practice Guidelines (Committee to revise the 1995 Guidelines for the Evaluation and Management of Heart Failure). *J Am Coll Cardiol.* 2001;38:2101-2113.
66. Trastuzumab (Herceptin). Package insert. Genentech, Inc; 2010.
67. Pertuzumab (Perjeta). Package insert. Genentech, Inc; 2012.
68. Zamorano JL, Lancellotti P, Rodriguez Munoz D, et al. 2016 ESC Position Paper on cancer treatments and cardiovascular toxicity developed under the auspices of the ESC Committee for Practice Guidelines: The Task Force for cancer treatments and cardiovascular toxicity of the European Society of Cardiology (ESC). *Eur Heart J.* 2016;37:2768-2801.
69. Curigliano G, Lenihan D, Fradley M, et al. Management of cardiac disease in cancer patients throughout oncological treatment: ESMO consensus recommendations. *Ann Oncol.* 2020;31:171-190.

2 Cardiac Dysfunction: Traditional Chemotherapy, Human Epidermal Growth Factor Receptor 2–Based Therapy, and Radiation

Srilakshmi Vallabhaneni, Ronald J. Krone, and Kathleen W. Zhang

GENERAL PRINCIPLES

- Anthracyclines, cyclophosphamide, human epidermal growth factor receptor 2 (HER-2) inhibitors, and radiation therapy are well-established cancer therapies that have been associated with cardiac dysfunction, specifically heart failure (HF) and cardiomyopathy.
- Cancer therapy–related cardiac dysfunction is a serious adverse event that leads to interruption of cancer treatment and potentially even severe HF or death.
- Optimization of cardiovascular care before, during, and after cancer therapy can mitigate cancer therapy–related cardiac dysfunction, minimizing treatment interruptions and allowing the patient to receive effective cancer treatment.
- Early identification of cancer therapy–related cardiac dysfunction is essential as it allows for early implementation of medical HF therapy.

DEFINITION OF CARDIAC DYSFUNCTION

- Several definitions of cancer therapy–related cardiac dysfunction have been proposed, based predominantly on changes in left ventricular ejection fraction (LVEF) on treatment[1] (Table 2-1).
- A more comprehensive definition including signs and symptoms of HF, cardiac biomarkers (troponin and natriuretic peptides), and LV global longitudinal strain (GLS, a measure of cardiac deformation) may be more relevant in clinical practice.
- **We define cancer therapy–related cardiac dysfunction as a decline in LVEF by >10% to a value <50%, or in the setting of new signs and/or symptoms of HF (ie, exertional dyspnea, orthopnea, lower extremity edema, elevation of the jugular venous pulsation) along with elevated cardiac biomarkers.**

SPECIFIC DRUGS AND THERAPIES

Anthracyclines

- Anthracyclines (doxorubicin, daunorubicin, idarubicin, epirubicin, mitoxantrone) are derived from the *Streptomyces* bacterium and exert anticancer effects by

TABLE 2-1 Definitions of Cancer Therapy–Related Cardiac Dysfunction

National Cancer Institute/CTCAE[1]

Grade 1: asymptomatic elevation in biomarkers or imaging abnormalities
Grade 2: heart failure symptoms with mild exertion
Grade 3: heart failure symptoms with moderate exertion
Grade 4: life-threatening symptoms requiring hemodynamic support
Grade 5: death

U.S. Food and Drug Administration[1]

>20% decrease in LVEF when baseline LVEF is normal, OR
>10% decrease in LVEF to less than lower limit of normal or absolute value of <45%

Cardiac Review and Evaluation Committee[1]

Decrease in LVEF that is global or more severe in the septum AND
Decline in LVEF of at least 5% to <55% with HF signs or symptoms, OR
Decline in LVEF of at least 10% to <55% without HF signs or symptoms

Herceptin Adjuvant (HERA) Trial[1]

≥10% decrease in LVEF to <50%

Breast Cancer International Research Group (BCIRG)[1]

>10% decline in LVEF

American Society of Echocardiography/European Association of CV Imaging[2]

>10% decrease in LVEF to <53%
>15% relative decline in GLS compared to baseline strain

European Society of Cardiology (ESC)[3]

>10% decline in LVEF to <50%
>15% relative decline in GLS compared to baseline strain

European Society of Medical Oncology (ESMO)[10]

>10% decline in LVEF to <50%
>20% absolute decline in LVEF
>12% relative decline/>5% absolute decline in GLS compared to baseline

CTCAE, Common Terminology Criteria for Adverse Events; CV, cardiovascular; GLS, global longitudinal strain; HF, heart failure; LVEF, left ventricular ejection fraction.

intercalating with DNA and inhibiting topoisomerase II from repairing breaks in the DNA strand.
- Anthracyclines are among the most effective anticancer treatments available and remain essential components of therapy for leukemia, lymphoma, breast cancer, and sarcoma.
- Potential mechanisms of anthracycline cardiotoxicity include generation of reactive oxygen species, incorporation of iron into the mitochondrial respiratory pathway leading to damage to the cell membrane, and DNA damage by topoisomerase suppression.[4,5] Other potential targets include cardiac fibroblasts, endothelial cells, and cardiac progenitor cells.

Human Epidermal Growth Factor Receptor 2 Inhibitors

- HER-2 is a cellular protein receptor that is overexpressed in certain solid organ tumors and promotes tumor growth, proliferation, and survival.
- HER-2 inhibitors (trastuzumab, pertuzumab, lapatinib, neratinib) are the mainstay of therapy for HER-2-positive malignancies (primarily breast and gastric cancers).
- Because of the expression of HER-2 on myocardial cells, HER-2 inhibitors disrupt cardiac energy metabolism, mitochondrial function, and cellular homeostasis, resulting in LV dysfunction.

Cyclophosphamide

- Cyclophosphamide is an alkylating agent that induces cellular apoptosis by forming DNA cross-links.
- The precise mechanism of cyclophosphamide-induced cardiotoxicity is not well established. Cyclophosphamide metabolites are thought to cause oxidative stress and endothelial cell damage with extravasation of toxic metabolites and resultant myocardial damage.

Radiation

- Radiation therapy, especially for thoracic malignancies when used alone or in conjunction with other treatments, is associated with cardiovascular complications including coronary artery disease, carotid and subclavian stenosis, valvular heart disease, cardiomyopathy, pericardial disease, and conduction abnormalities.
- Radiation therapy–induced cardiotoxicity is multifactorial and related to inflammatory vascular damage causing accelerated atherosclerosis, myocardial fibrosis, and subsequent systolic and diastolic dysfunction.

EPIDEMIOLOGY/RISK FACTORS FOR CARDIAC DYSFUNCTION

- **Older age, traditional cardiovascular risk factors, preexisting cardiac disease, and previous or concurrent cardiotoxic cancer therapy are general risk factors for cancer therapy–related cardiac dysfunction** (Table 2-2).

Anthracyclines

- **The risk of cardiac dysfunction increases with the cumulative anthracycline dose administered, with incidence of 3% to 5% at 400 mg/m^2 that increases to 18% to 48% at 700 mg/m^2.**[6] Cumulative anthracycline doses that exceed established drug-specific cutoffs (Table 2-3) are associated with increased risk for cardiac dysfunction.
- Breast cancer patients are particularly susceptible to anthracycline-induced cardiac dysfunction because of concurrent or sequential HER-2 inhibitor and/or radiation therapy. Sarcoma patients are also at increased risk because of high cumulative anthracycline doses administered.
- Traditionally, anthracycline-induced cardiotoxicity has been classified into three distinct types based on retrospective studies: acute (occurring after a single dose or course of therapy), early-onset chronic (within 1 year of completion of therapy), late-onset chronic (presenting more than 1 year after completion of therapy).
- Currently, anthracycline-induced cardiotoxicity is considered a continuous phenomenon starting at the time of exposure and continuing for months to years. This

TABLE 2-2	Risk Factors for Cancer Therapy–Related Cardiac Dysfunction

High-dose anthracyclines (doxorubicin >250 mg/m^2, daunorubicin >400-550 mg/m^2, epirubicin >600 mg/m^2, idarubicin >160 mg/m^2, mitoxantrone >200 mg/m^2)

High-dose radiation therapy (≥30 Gy) when the heart is in the treatment field

Lower dose anthracyclines followed by HER-2 therapy

Lower dose anthracycline or HER-2 inhibitor therapy AND
- Lower dose radiation therapy (<30 Gy)
- Age ≥ 65 years
- ≥2 cardiovascular risk factors (smoking, hypertension, diabetes mellitus, dyslipidemia, chronic kidney disease, obesity)

Preexisting cardiac disease (heart failure, history of myocardial infarction, ≥ moderate valvular disease)

Elevated cardiac biomarkers prior to initiation of chemotherapy

Prior mediastinal or chest radiation therapy

Prior anthracycline or HER-2 inhibitor therapy

Gy, gray; HER-2, human epidermal growth factor receptor 2.
Data from Armenian SH, Lacchetti C, Barac A, et al. Prevention and monitoring of cardiac dysfunction in survivors of adult cancers: American Society of Clinical Oncology clinical practice guideline. *J Clin Oncol.* 2017;35(8):893-911.

hypothesis is supported by studies showing early elevation of troponins after anthracycline administration with subsequent reduction in LVEF.[7]

Human Epidermal Growth Factor Receptor 2 Inhibitors
- In clinical trials of trastuzumab monotherapy, incidence of HF ranges from 1% to 4%, whereas incidence of asymptomatic reduction in LVEF ranges from 10% to 15%.[8]
- The risk of cardiomyopathy increases in patients receiving concurrent or prior exposure to anthracyclines, aged ≥50 years, or with obesity.
- **HER-2 inhibitor–related cardiomyopathy is usually reversible after cessation of therapy and initiation of HF therapy.**

Cyclophosphamide
- Cyclophosphamide-induced cardiotoxicity occurs in 7% to 28% of patients receiving a total dose of >150 mg/kg.[9]
- The incidence of cardiomyopathy is higher with high-dose protocols; however, it is not related to cumulative dose. The risk is higher in patients with lymphoma, prior radiation to chest, older age, and prior reduced ejection fraction. The incidence of fatal cardiomyopathy is reported to be 2% to 17% and is dependent on the chemotherapy regimen and patient characteristics.

TABLE 2-3 Incidence of Cardiomyopathy and Other Cardiovascular Toxicities With Most Commonly Used Chemotherapy Agents

Cancer treatment class	Cardiomyopathy incidence	Other types of CV toxicities	Cancer indication
Anthracyclines	7%-65%	Supraventricular tachycardia Ventricular tachycardia Pericarditis	Hodgkin lymphoma, non-Hodgkin lymphoma, leukemia, sarcoma, breast cancer
Doxorubicin			
400 mg/m^2	3%-5%		
550 mg/m^2	7%-26%		
700 mg/m^2	18%-48%		
Daunorubicin (>400 mg/m^2)	9.9%		
Idarubicin (>90 mg/m^2)	5%-18%		
Epirubicin (>900 mg/m^2)	0.9%-11.4%		
Mitoxantrone (>120 mg/m^2)	2.6%		
Liposomal anthracyclines (>900 mg/m^2)	2%		
HER2-targeted therapies			HER-2-positive breast cancer and gastric malignancies
Trastuzumab	3%-28%		
Pertuzumab	3%-8%		
Ado-trastuzumab emtansine	1%-2%		
Fam-trastuzumab deruxtecan	1%		
Lapatinib	2%-5%		
Fluoropyrimidines		Coronary vasospasm	Adenocarcinoma Head and neck, GI (liver, colon, pancreas), breast cancer
5-fluorouracil capecitabine	1.9%-8%		
Alkylating agents			Leukemia, breast cancer, sarcoma
Cyclophosphamide	7%-28%	Myopericarditis	
Thoracic radiation	13% (high dose)	Valvular heart disease Pericardial disease Coronary artery disease	Hodgkin lymphoma, breast cancer, lung cancer

CV, cardiovascular; GI, gastrointestinal; HER2, human epidermal growth factor receptor 2.

- Mild to moderate HF is largely reversible within few weeks to months of discontinuation of cyclophosphamide.

Radiation
- **Radiation-induced cardiotoxicity is observed 5 to 10 years after radiation therapy and the risk persists for at least 25 years after initial treatment.**
- The 25-year cumulative incidence of cardiomyopathy is 7.9% in patients receiving combined mediastinal radiation and anthracycline-based chemotherapy.[10]

CLINICAL PRESENTATION OF CARDIAC DYSFUNCTION

History
- Dyspnea and reduced exercise tolerance are the primary early clinical manifestations of cancer therapy–induced cardiac dysfunction. Other clinical findings may include ventricular or supraventricular arrhythmias. Signs and symptoms of HF are late clinical manifestations.
- HER-2 inhibitor–related cardiac dysfunction is frequently asymptomatic.

Physical Examination
- The cardiac physical examination may be normal in patients with asymptomatic LV dysfunction. Findings of decompensated HF include elevated jugular venous pulsation, lower extremity edema, crackles on lung examination, and S3 gallop.
- Systolic or diastolic murmurs related to valvular heart disease may be heard especially in patients with prior radiation therapy.

Diagnostic Testing
- A 12-lead electrocardiogram is recommended for all patients undergoing evaluation for cancer therapy–related cardiac dysfunction.
- Serum testing for natriuretic peptides (brain natriuretic peptide [BNP] or N-terminal pro B-type natriuretic peptide [NT-proBNP]) and troponin levels can help to detect cardiac injury.
- **Transthoracic echocardiography (TTE) is recommended to screen for functional and structural cardiac abnormalities. Acquisition of two-dimensional (2D) LVEF, three-dimensional (3D) LVEF, and GLS is recommended to maximize confidence in the quantitative assessment of LV function, particularly when abnormal LV function would necessitate interruption in cancer therapy.**
- Cardiac magnetic resonance imaging (CMR) may be pursued to confirm LV function and to rule out alternate causes of cardiomyopathy.
- Coronary artery disease should be excluded as an alternative cause of HF and LV dysfunction. Noninvasive evaluation with cardiac computed tomography angiography or myocardial perfusion imaging with regadenoson is reasonable when the pretest probability for coronary disease is low.

TREATMENT OF CARDIAC DYSFUNCTION

- **Prompt initiation of guideline-directed HF therapy is essential for patients with symptomatic HF and asymptomatic cardiac dysfunction.**
  - β-Blockers (especially carvedilol) and inhibitors of the renin–angiotensin–aldosterone system are preferred as initial therapy.

- Bisoprolol or metoprolol succinate is preferable in the presence of hypotension, and bisoprolol in the presence of bronchospasm. Ivabradine can also be considered for heart rate lowering in the presence of hypotension.
- Angiotensin receptor-neprilysin inhibitors should be used if tolerated by blood pressure.
- Eplerenone is the preferred mineralocorticoid receptor antagonist in patients with estrogen-receptor positive breast cancer because of the theoretical risk of pro-estrogenic effects with spironolactone.
- Loop diuretics should be used to optimize fluid status.
- The risk/benefit profile of continued cardiotoxic cancer therapy should be discussed with the treating oncologist.
- **In general, anthracycline and HER-2 inhibitor therapy should be interrupted in patients who develop symptomatic HF or asymptomatic cardiac dysfunction to allow for optimization of HF therapy.**
  - Reassessment of cardiac function after several weeks of HF therapy is recommended prior to potentially retreating with cardiotoxic cancer therapy.
  - HER-2 inhibitor–related cardiac dysfunction is usually reversible with treatment discontinuation. HER-2 inhibitor therapy can be reintroduced in patients on optimal HF therapy with LVEF >40% and New York Heart Association (NYHA) class I or II symptoms.
  - In patients who require continuation of anthracycline therapy, addition of dexrazoxane should be considered.
- The use of implantable cardioverter defibrillator therapy should be considered in the context of the patient's overall cancer prognosis.
- In cancer survivors with advanced HF because of cancer therapy, referral to a Heart Failure and Transplantation specialist may be appropriate.

OUTCOMES/PROGNOSIS

Anthracyclines
- Historically, anthracycline-induced cardiotoxicity was considered irreversible with poor cardiovascular outcomes compared to other etiologies of cardiomyopathy.[11] However, this is based on older data with limited HF therapies; recent studies suggest that it is reversible with early detection and prompt initiation of HF therapy. Continuation of cardioprotective therapy is essential even after recovery of LV function to prevent recurrence of cardiac dysfunction.[12]
- Patients with anthracycline-induced cardiotoxicity have shown to have reduced peak oxygen consumption (VO_{2max}) on cardiopulmonary exercise testing, which can be used as a predictor for survival and to monitor recovery of function.[13]

Human Epidermal Growth Factor Receptor 2 Inhibitors
- Cardiotoxicity with HER-2 inhibitors is usually reversible. HER-2 inhibitor therapy can generally be restarted after improvement in LV function, with close cardiac monitoring and continuation of HF therapy.

Cyclophosphamide
- Mild to moderate HF with cyclophosphamide is largely reversible; however, cardiogenic shock is associated with high case fatality rate.

Radiation Therapy
- Diastolic dysfunction is generally well tolerated, and systolic dysfunction from radiation therapy alone is uncommon.
- Patients requiring surgical intervention for radiation therapy–associated coronary artery disease, valvular heart disease, or pericardial constriction are at increased surgical risk as compared to patients without history of chest radiation.

PREVENTION OF CARDIAC DYSFUNCTION

- **Pretreatment cardiovascular evaluation is recommended for primary prevention of cancer therapy–related cardiac dysfunction.**
  - Aggressive cardiovascular risk factor modification should be implemented (smoking cessation, blood pressure control, lipid management, weight control, glycemic control, and therapeutic lifestyle modification).
  - A baseline TTE with measurement of 2D LVEF, 3D LVEF, and GLS should be obtained for all patients.
  - If high-dose anthracycline therapy is planned, pretreatment consultation with cardio-oncology is recommended.
- Modification of cancer therapy administration may mitigate the risk of cardiac dysfunction.
  - Radiation strategies to minimize the total heart dose (ie, when possible reduce the volume and dose of incidental cardiac irradiation, standard fractionation, deep inspiration breath hold, prone positioning) should be implemented.
  - Liposomal anthracycline formulations have longer plasma half-life and decreased volume of distribution compared to nonliposomal formulation and reduce the likelihood of cardiotoxicity.[14]
  - If possible, limiting the maximum anthracycline dose or switching to a non-anthracycline-based regimen should be pursued in patients with preexisting cardiac dysfunction or significant cardiovascular risk factors.
- Dexrazoxane is an iron chelator that protects against anthracycline-related cardiac dysfunction, although concerns have been raised regarding possible reduction in cancer treatment efficacy.[15,16]
  - Dexrazoxane is approved by the U.S. Food and Drug Administration for the prevention of cardiotoxicity in patients with breast cancer who have reached a cumulative doxorubicin dose of 300 mg/m^2 (or equivalent) and require additional anthracyclines.
  - In patients with breast cancer, dexrazoxane reduces the risk of clinical HF and cardiac events without significant impact on cancer outcomes.[16] Similarly, dexrazoxane was associated with no cardiac dysfunction and no reduction in progression-free survival in sarcoma patients receiving high-dose doxorubicin.[17]
  - A potential role for dexrazoxane in patients at high risk for anthracycline-related cardiac dysfunction should be discussed with the treating oncologist.
- Other adjunctive therapies may also reduce the risk of cancer therapy–related cardiac dysfunction.
  - Regular exercise minimizes loss of muscle mass and improved cardiorespiratory fitness during cancer therapy and is recommended.[18]
  - There is conflicting evidence regarding the utility of β-blockers, inhibitors of the renin–angiotensin–aldosterone system, and statins for primary prevention of

cardiac dysfunction (Table 2-4).[19-27] Patients with standard clinical indications for these therapies (ie, hypertension, diabetes mellitus, atherosclerotic cardiovascular disease) should be treated.

SURVEILLANCE STRATEGIES FOR CARDIAC DYSFUNCTION

- Patients should be assessed for new-onset HF symptoms (ie, dyspnea, lower extremity edema, orthopnea) at each treatment visit, especially on anthracycline and HER-2 inhibitor therapy. New HF symptoms should be evaluated with cardiac biomarkers (troponin and BNP/NT-proBNP), cardiac imaging (TTE or CMR), and referral to Cardio-Oncology.
- **Regular cardiac surveillance using cardiac biomarkers (troponin and BNP) and/or cardiac imaging (TTE and/or CMR) is recommended during anthracycline and HER-2 inhibitor therapy** (Figs. 2-1 and 2-2). **Mode and frequency of cardiac surveillance is dependent on baseline cardiovascular risk as determined by clinical history, laboratory testing, and echocardiography.**
- A surveillance TTE is recommended by the American Society of Clinical Oncology 12 months after completing anthracycline chemotherapy.[28]
- After radiation therapy, screening TTE and functional noninvasive stress testing are recommended every 5 years after completion of therapy in high-risk patients and 10 years after exposure in others with repeat testing every 5 years thereafter to evaluate myocardial function, valvular function, and coronary ischemia.[29]

Cardiac Biomarkers

- Troponin is highly sensitive and specific for active myocardial injury and has prognostic value for cardiac risk stratification in patients undergoing cardiotoxic cancer therapy.
- Natriuretic peptides (BNP/NT-proBNP) are highly sensitive for the detection of LV dysfunction or diastolic dysfunction and may detect congestion and injury after cardiotoxic chemotherapy prior to detectable changes in LVEF.[28]
- The optimal frequency of cardiac biomarker surveillance is unknown. Our approach is detailed in Figures 2-1 and 2-2.

Transthoracic Echocardiography

- Measurement of 2D LVEF, 3D LVEF, and GLS should be performed as part of echocardiographic surveillance for cancer therapy–related cardiac dysfunction.
- Biplane method of disks (modified Simpson rule) should be used to determine 2D LVEF, and contrast enhancement should be utilized when visualization of the endocardial border is limited.
- 3D LVEF is more reliable and reproducible than 2D LVEF for serial measurements, although 3D imaging requires excellent image quality.[30]
- Strain imaging is more sensitive than LVEF for the detection of subclinical myocardial dysfunction, although measurements vary by software manufacturer.[31] Serial studies should therefore be performed using the same strain software manufacturer.
- **Variable image quality, interobserver variability, and intra-observer reproducibility are important limitations of echocardiography as a surveillance tool for cancer**

TABLE 2-4 Clinical Trials for Primary Prevention of Cancer Therapy–Related Cardiotoxicity

Author (year/study design)	N	Cancer type/cardio-toxic chemotherapy	Cardioprotective intervention	Primary outcome/ follow-up	Results
β-Blockers					
Kalay et al (2006/RCT)[32]	50	Breast cancer/ lymphoma/other Adriamycin or epirubicin	Carvedilol 12.5 mg once daily ($n = 25$) Control ($n = 25$)	LVEF Follow-up: 6 months	**No LVEF ↓** Baseline to follow-up Carvedilol group: 70.5%-60.7% ($P = .3$) Control group: 68.9%-52.3% ($P < .001$)
Nabati et al (2017/RCT)[33]	91	Breast cancer Doxorubicin	Carvedilol (3.125-6.25 mg twice daily) ($n = 46$) Control ($n = 45$)	LVEF Follow-up: 6 months	**No LVEF ↓** • Baseline vs follow-up Carvedilol group: 58.72 ± 4.69% to 57.44 ± 7.52% Control group: 61.13 ± 4.97% to 51.67 ± 6.01% ($P < .001$) • Troponin-I, ng/mL: 0.073-vs-0.146 ($P = .036$)

(continued)

TABLE 2-4 Clinical Trials for Primary Prevention of Cancer Therapy–Related Cardiotoxicity (*continued*)

Author (year/study design)	N	Cancer type/cardiotoxic chemotherapy	Cardioprotective intervention	Primary outcome/follow-up	Results
Avila et al (2018/RCT)[23] (CECCY)	200	Breast cancer Doxorubicin/cyclophosphamide	Carvedilol (target dose 25 mg twice daily) (n = 96) Control (n = 96)	Prevention of ≥10% LVEF reduction at 6 months (secondary outcomes—troponin-I, BNP, diastolic dysfunction) Follow-up: 6 months	**No change in LVEF (≥10%), lower elevation of troponin, ↓ diastolic function** <ul><li>Carvedilol-vs-placebo-14.5%-vs-13.5% (*P* = 1)</li><li>% of patients with troponin-I ≥0.04: 26%-vs-41.6% (*P* = .003)</li><li>% patients with abnormal diastolic function: 28.5%-vs-37.2% (*P* = .039)</li></ul>
ACEI/ARB					
Cardinale et al (2006/RCT)[20]	114	Breast cancer, sarcoma, myeloma, Hodgkin/non-Hodgkin lymphoma, acute myeloid leukemia High-dose chemotherapy	Enalapril 20 mg daily (n = 56) Control (n = 58)	Absolute LVEF decrease >10% to a decline below normal Follow-up: 12 months	**No LVEF ↓** Enalapril-vs-placebo: 0%-43%, *P* < .001

Study	N	Cancer/Chemotherapy	Intervention	Outcome Measure	Results
Boekhout et al (2016/RCT)[27]	210	Breast cancer Anthracyclines/Trastuzumab	Candesartan (32 mg daily) ($n = 103$) Control ($n = 103$)	Decline in LVEF of ≥15% or absolute value <45% Follow-up: 21 months	**No change in LVEF decline of ≥15% or absolute value <45** % patients with primary outcome: Candesartan-vs-placebo-19%-vs-16% ($P = .58$)
Janbabai et al (2017/RCT)[34]	69	Breast cancer, lymphoma, sarcoma, Wilms tumor, lung cancer Anthracyclines	Enalapril (5-10 mg twice daily) ($n = 34$) Control ($n = 35$)	Change in LVEF from baseline Follow-up: 6 months	**No LVEF ↓** LVEF baseline to follow-up ($P < .001$) • Control group: 59.6 ± 5.7 to 46.3 ± 7 ($P < .001$) • Enalapril group: 59.4 ± 7 to 59.9 ± 7.8 ($P = .58$)
ACEI/ARB or β-blockers					
Georgakopoulos (2010/RCT)[21]	147	Lymphoma Anthracyclines	Metoprolol tartrate (target dose 100 mg daily) ($n = 42$) or enalapril (target dose 20 mg daily) ($n = 43$) Control ($n = 40$)	Clinical cardiotoxicity—HF with two or more of the following • Cardiomegaly on CXR • Basilar rales • S3 gallop • PND, orthopnea or DOE Follow-up: 36 months	• **No significant HF** in metoprolol or enalapril compared to control group (overall HF incidence: 6 patients [4.8%]) • **No change in LVEF** compared to baseline

(*continued*)

TABLE 2-4 Clinical Trials for Primary Prevention of Cancer Therapy–Related Cardiotoxicity (continued)

Author (year/study design)	N	Cancer type/cardiotoxic chemotherapy	Cardioprotective intervention	Primary outcome/follow-up	Results
Gulati et al (2016/RCT) (PRADA)[24]	130	Breast cancer Anthracyclines with or without trastuzumab	Metoprolol succinate (100 mg daily) or candesartan (32 mg daily) 30 (combination), 32 (candesartan), 32 (metoprolol), 33 (placebo)	Change in LVEF by CMR Follow-up: 16 months	**No LVEF ↓** • placebo-vs-candesartan-2.6%-vs-0.8%, $P = .026$ No difference in metoprolol vs placebo
Pituskin et al (2017/RCT)[22] MANTICORE	99	Breast cancer Trastuzumab	Bisoprolol ($n = 31$)/perindopril ($n = 33$) control ($n = 30$)	Left ventricular remodeling (LVEDVI on CMR) Follow-up: 12 months	**No LVEF ↓** • bisoprolol +8 ± 9 mL/m^2, perindopril +7 ± 14 mL/m^2, placebo +4 ± 11 mL/m^2 ($P = .36$) • LVEF change from baseline to follow-up: Bisoprolol: 62 ± 4 to 61 ± 4, Perindopril: 62 ± 5 to 59 ± 6, placebo: 61 ± 5 to 56 ± 4 ($P < .001$-compared to baseline and for other groups)

| Guglin et al (2019/RCT)[35] | 464 | Breast cancer Trastuzumab | Carvedilol extended release (10 mg) (n = 156) or lisinopril (10 mg) (n = 156) Control (n = 152) | LVEF decrease of ≥10%, or >5% if LVEF below 50% Follow-up: 24 months | • **No change in rate of cardiotoxicity**: carvedilol 29%-vs-lisinopril 30%-vs-placebo 32%
• In anthracycline group event rate when compared to placebo
• placebo 47%
• carvedilol 31% (P = .008)
• lisinopril 37% (P = .002)
• Fewer interruptions in trastuzumab for those on cardioprotection |

ACEI+β-blockers

| Bosch et al (2013/RCT) (OVERCOME)[19] | 90 | Hematologic Anthracyclines | Enalapril (target dose 10 mg twice daily) + carvedilol (target dose 25 mg twice daily) (n = 45) Control (n = 45) | LVEF Follow-up: 6 months | **No LVEF change between the two groups** No change in LVEF in intervention group Control group: −3.1% change by echocardiography (P = .04)/ −3.4% change by CMR (P = .09) |

(continued)

TABLE 2-4 Clinical Trials for Primary Prevention of Cancer Therapy–Related Cardiotoxicity *(continued)*

Author (year/study design)	N	Cancer type/cardiotoxic chemotherapy	Cardioprotective intervention	Primary outcome/follow-up	Results
Leong et al (2019/prospective uncontrolled) (SCHOLAR)[36]	20	Breast cancer Doxorubicin+ Trastuzumab	Ramipril/candesartan + carvedilol/bisoprolol	LVEF <40% with heart failure symptoms or LVEF <35% Follow-up: 12 months	2 patients (10%), no deaths
Lynce et al (2019/prospective uncontrolled) (SAFE-HEART)[37]	31	Breast cancer Trastuzumab ($n=$ 15), pertuzumab (combination, $n=$ 14) or ado-trastuzumab emtansine ($n=2$)	Ramipril/candesartan + carvedilol	Completion of chemotherapy without asymptomatic drop in LVEF (LVEF drop of >10% points from baseline or <35%) or cardiac events (HF, MI, arrhythmias, cardiac death) Follow-up: 6 months after completion of chemotherapy	27 (90%) completed planned therapy, 2 patients with CE, 1 patient with asymptomatic drop in LVEF

Aldosterone antagonists					
Akpek et al (2015/RCT)[38]	83	Breast cancer Anthracyclines	Spironolactone 25 mg daily ($n = 43$) Control group ($n = 40$)	Change in LVEF compared to baseline Follow-up: 6 months	**No LVEF ↓, no TNI or BNP ↑** LVEF baseline to follow-up: • Spironolactone −67 ± 6.1% to 65.7 ± 7.4% ($P = .094$) • control group 67.7 ± 6.3% to 53.6 ± 6.8% ($P < .001$)
Device therapy					
Singh et al (2019/ prospective uncontrolled) (MADIT-CHIC)[39]	30	Breast cancer/lymphoma/leukemia, sarcoma Anthracyclines	Cardiac resynchronization therapy	Change in LVEF compared to baseline Follow-up: 6 months	**LVEF ↑** LVEF baseline to follow-up: 28.5 ± 3.8 to 39.1 ± 7.1 ($P < .001$)

(*continued*)

TABLE 2-4 Clinical Trials for Primary Prevention of Cancer Therapy–Related Cardiotoxicity (*continued*)

Author (year/study design)	N	Cancer type/cardio-toxic chemotherapy	Cardioprotective intervention	Primary outcome/follow-up	Results
Statins					
Acar et al (2011/RCT)[25]	40	Lymphoma/multiple myeloma/leukemia Anthracyclines	Atorvastatin 40 mg daily (*n* = 20) Control group (*n* = 20)	LVEF <50% Follow-up: 6 months	**No LVEF ↓** • LVEF <50%- 1 (5%) in statin group/5 (25%) in control group (*P* = .18) • LVEF baseline to follow-up (*P* < .001): statin group: 61.3 ± 7.9 to 62.6 ± 9.3 • control group: 62.9 ± 7 to 55 ± 9.5
Seicean et al (2012/retrospective)[26]	628	Breast cancer Anthracyclines	Statin prescribed for other indication (*n* = 67) Propensity-matched controls (*n* = 134)	Incident HF events Follow-up: 5 years	**No HF ↑** Statin group-vs-placebo: 6%-vs-17.2% (*P* = .04)

ACEI, angiotensin-converting enzyme inhibitor; ARB, angiotensin receptor blocker; BNP, brain natriuretic peptide; CE, clinical event; CMR, cardiovascular magnetic resonance; CXR, chest X-ray; DOE, dyspnea on exertion; HF, heart failure; LVEDVI, left ventricular end-diastolic volume indexed; LVEF, left ventricular ejection fraction; MI, myocardial infarction; PND, paroxysmal nocturnal dyspnea; RCT, randomized controlled trial; TNI, Troponin-I.

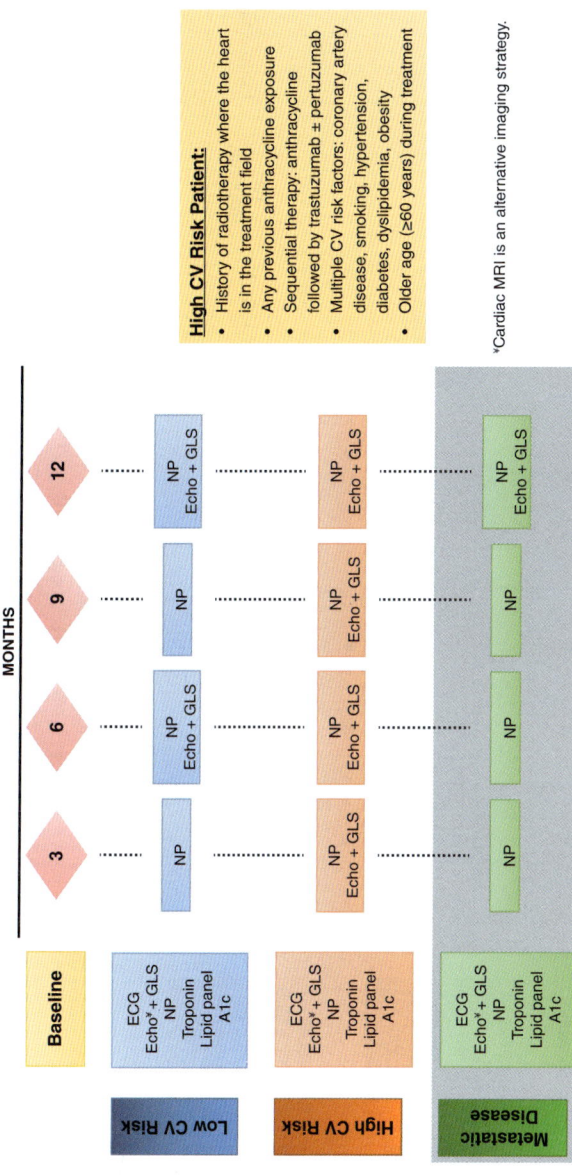

Figure 2-1. Surveillance strategy in patients receiving anthracyclines. A1c, hemoglobin A1c; CV, cardiovascular; ECG, electrocardiogram; GLS, global longitudinal strain; JVP, jugular venous pressure; NP, natriuretic peptide. (© Washington University School of Medicine in St. Louis.)

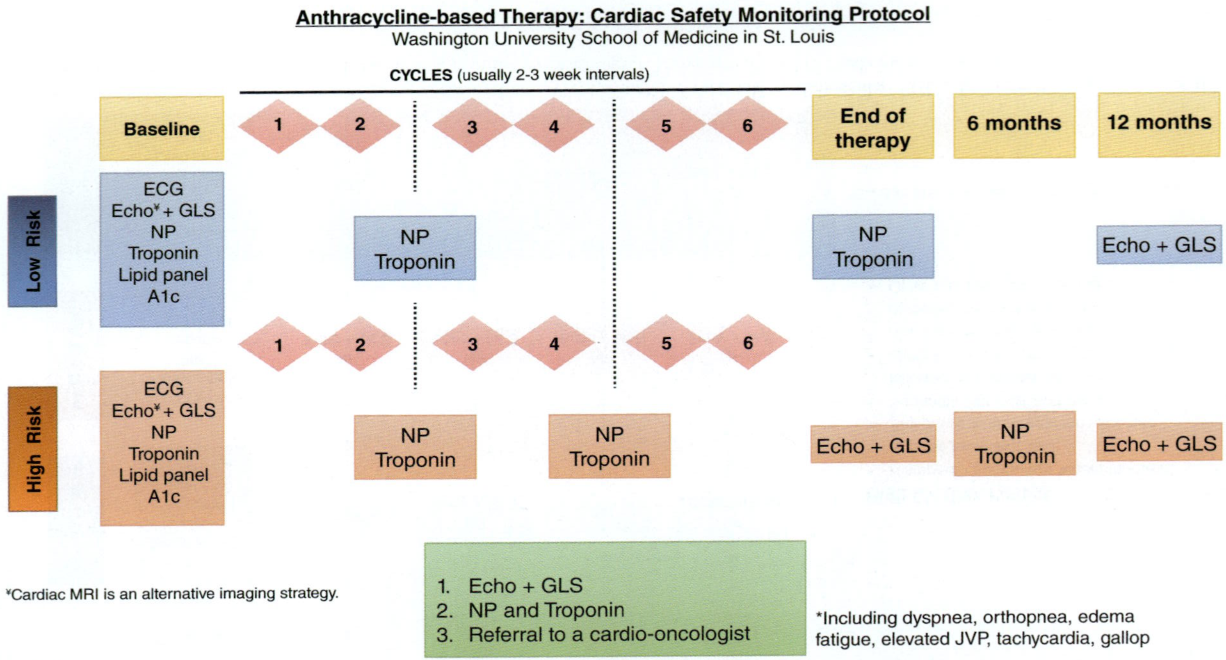

Anthracycline-based Therapy: Cardiac Safety Monitoring Protocol
Washington University School of Medicine in St. Louis

CYCLES (usually 2-3 week intervals)

Low Risk

Baseline:
- ECG
- Echo* + GLS
- NP
- Troponin
- Lipid panel
- A1c

Cycles: 1, 2, 3, 4, 5, 6

Between cycles 2-3: NP Troponin

End of therapy: NP Troponin

12 months: Echo + GLS

High Risk

Baseline:
- ECG
- Echo* + GLS
- NP
- Troponin
- Lipid panel
- A1c

Cycles: 1, 2, 3, 4, 5, 6

Between cycles 2-3: NP Troponin
Between cycles 4-5: NP Troponin

End of therapy: Echo + GLS

6 months: NP Troponin

12 months: Echo + GLS

*Cardiac MRI is an alternative imaging strategy.

*Including dyspnea, orthopnea, edema fatigue, elevated JVP, tachycardia, gallop

1. Echo + GLS
2. NP and Troponin
3. Referral to a cardio-oncologist

Figure 2-2. Surveillance strategy in patients receiving HER2 antagonists. A1c, hemoglobin A1c; ECG, electrocardiogram; GLS, global longitudinal strain; NP, natriuretic peptide. (© Washington University School of Medicine in St. Louis.)

therapy–related cardiac dysfunction. Careful review and integration of all measurements (2D LVEF, 3D LVEF, and GLS) should be performed prior to changing the cancer treatment plan. In difficult cases, CMR should be used to clarify the echocardiographic findings.
- Assessment of diastolic function (mitral inflow pulse wave Doppler, tissue Doppler) can help to guide fluid management in patients with preserved LVEF.

Cardiac Magnetic Resonance Imaging

- CMR is the gold standard for evaluation of LVEF and cardiac structure.[40] It is highly reproducible and also detects abnormalities in cardiac tissue (ie, myocardial edema, fibrosis) that are present in various stages of anthracycline-induced cardiotoxicity.[41]
- CMR strain analysis measures myocardial deformation in the longitudinal, radial, and circumferential dimensions and has demonstrated utility in the detection of early subclinical changes in patients receiving cardiotoxic chemotherapy.
- Accessibility is an important barrier to the use of CMR for surveillance.

Multigated Acquisition Angiogram

- Historically, multigated acquisition angiogram (MUGA) was used to screen for anthracycline-related cardiac dysfunction.
- Disadvantages of MUGA include radiation exposure and limited information on cardiac structure.
- Echocardiography and CMR are now the preferred modalities for cardiac imaging surveillance, but this modality can be used if echocardiographic evaluation or CMR cannot be done.

REFERENCES

1. Bloom MW, Hamo CE, Cardinale D, et al. Cancer therapy-related cardiac dysfunction and heart failure: part 1: definitions, pathophysiology, risk factors, and imaging. *Circ Hear Fail.* 2016;9(1):e002661.
2. Plana JC, Galderisi M, Barac A, et al. Expert consensus for multimodality imaging evaluation of adult patients during and after cancer therapy: a report from the American Society of Echocardiography and the European Association of Cardiovascular Imaging. *J Am Soc Echocardiogr.* 2014;27(9):911-939.
3. Zamorano JL, Lancellotti P, Rodriguez Muñoz D, et al. 2016 ESC Position Paper on cancer treatments and cardiovascular toxicity developed under the auspices of the ESC Committee for Practice Guidelines: The Task Force for cancer treatments and cardiovascular toxicity of the European Society of Cardiology (ESC). *Eur J Heart Fail.* 2017;19(1):9-42.
4. Henriksen PA. Anthracycline cardiotoxicity: an update on mechanisms, monitoring and prevention. *Heart.* 2018;104(12):971-977.
5. Zhang S, Liu X, Bawa-Khalfe T, et al. Identification of the molecular basis of doxorubicin-induced cardiotoxicity. *Nat Med.* 2012;18(11):1639-1642.
6. Curigliano G, Cardinale D, Dent S, et al. Cardiotoxicity of anticancer treatments: epidemiology, detection, and management. *CA Cancer J Clin.* 2016;66(4):309-325.
7. Cardinale D, Sandri MT, Martinoni A, et al. Left ventricular dysfunction predicted by early troponin I release after high-dose chemotherapy. *J Am Coll Cardiol.* 2000;36(2):517-522.
8. Mackey JR, Clemons M, Côté MA, et al. Cardiac management during adjuvant trastuzumab therapy: recommendations of the Canadian Trastuzumab Working Group. *Curr Oncol.* 2008;15(1):24-35.
9. Dhesi S, Chu M, Blevins G, et al. Cyclophosphamide-induced cardiomyopathy: a case report, review, and recommendations for management. *J Investig Med High Impact Case Rep.* 2013;1(1).
10. Aleman BMP, Van Den Belt-Dusebout AW, De Bruin ML, et al. Late cardiotoxicity after treatment for Hodgkin lymphoma. *Blood.* 2007;109(5):1878-1886.

11. Felker GM, Thompson RE, Hare JM, et al. Underlying causes and long-term survival in patients with initially unexplained cardiomyopathy. *N Engl J Med.* 2000;342(15):1077-1084.
12. Curigliano G, Lenihan D, Fradley M, et al. Management of cardiac disease in cancer patients throughout oncological treatment: ESMO consensus recommendations. *Ann Oncol.* 2020;31(2):171-190.
13. Jones LW, Courneya KS, Mackey JR, et al. Cardiopulmonary function and age-related decline across the breast cancer: survivorship continuum. *J Clin Oncol.* 2012;30(20):2530-2537.
14. van Dalen EC, Michiels EMC, Caron HN, Kremer LCM. Different anthracycline derivates for reducing cardiotoxicity in cancer patients. *Cochrane Database Syst Rev.* 2010;2010(5):CD005006.
15. Tebbi CK, London WB, Friedman D, et al. Dexrazoxane-associated risk for acute myeloid leukemia/myelodysplastic syndrome and other secondary malignancies in pediatric Hodgkin's disease. *J Clin Oncol.* 2007;25(5):493-500.
16. Macedo AVS, Hajjar LA, Lyon AR, et al. Efficacy of dexrazoxane in preventing anthracycline cardiotoxicity in breast cancer. *JACC CardioOncol.* 2019;1(1):68-79.
17. Van Tine BA, Hirbe AC, Oppelt P, et al. Interim analysis of the phase II study: Noninferiority study of doxorubicin with upfront dexrazoxane plus olaratumab for advanced or metastatic soft-tissue sarcoma. *Clin Cancer Res.* 2021;27(14):3854-3860.
18. Schmitz KH, Courneya KS, Matthews C, et al. American college of sports medicine roundtable on exercise guidelines for cancer survivors. *Med Sci Sports Exerc.* 2010;42(7):1409-1426.
19. Bosch X, Rovira M, Sitges M, et al. Enalapril and carvedilol for preventing chemotherapy-induced left ventricular systolic dysfunction in patients with malignant hemopathies: the OVERCOME trial (prevention of left ventricular dysfunction with enalapril and caRvedilol in patients submitted to intensive ChemOtherapy for the treatment of malignant hEmopathies). *J Am Coll Cardiol.* 2013;61(23):2355-2362.
20. Cardinale D, Colombo A, Sandri MT, et al. Prevention of high-dose chemotherapy-induced cardiotoxicity in high-risk patients by angiotensin-converting enzyme inhibition. *Circulation.* 2006;114(23):2474-2481.
21. Georgakopoulos P, Roussou P, Matsakas E, et al. Cardioprotective effect of metoprolol and enalapril in doxorubicin-treated lymphoma patients: a prospective, parallel-group, randomized, controlled study with 36-month follow-up. *Am J Hematol.* 2010;85(11):894-896.
22. Pituskin E, Mackey JR, Koshman S, et al. Multidisciplinary approach to novel therapies in cardio-oncology research (MANTICORE 101-Breast): a randomized trial for the prevention of trastuzumab-associated cardiotoxicity. *J Clin Oncol.* 2017;35(8):870-877.
23. Avila MS, Ayub-Ferreira SM, de Barros Wanderley MR, et al. Carvedilol for prevention of chemotherapy-related cardiotoxicity: the CECCY trial. *J Am Coll Cardiol.* 2018;71(20):2281-2290.
24. Gulati G, Heck SL, Ree AH, et al. Prevention of cardiac dysfunction during adjuvant breast cancer therapy (PRADA): a 2 × 2 factorial, randomized, placebo-controlled, double-blind clinical trial of candesartan and metoprolol. *Eur Heart J.* 2016;37(21):1671-1680.
25. Acar Z, Kale A, Turgut M, et al. Efficiency of atorvastatin in the protection of anthracycline-induced cardiomyopathy. *J Am Coll Cardiol.* 2011;58(9):988-999.
26. Seicean S, Seicean A, Plana JC, Budd GT, Marwick TH. Effect of statin therapy on the risk for incident heart failure in patients with breast cancer receiving anthracycline chemotherapy: an observational clinical cohort study. *J Am Coll Cardiol.* 2012;60(23):2384-2390.
27. Boekhout AH, Gietema JA, Kerklaan BM, et al. Angiotensin II Receptor inhibition with candesartan to prevent trastuzumab-related cardiotoxic effects in patients with early breast cancer a randomized clinical trial. *JAMA Oncol.* 2016;2(8):1030-1037.
28. Armenian SH, Lacchetti C, Barac A, et al. Prevention and monitoring of cardiac dysfunction in survivors of adult cancers: American Society of Clinical Oncology clinical practice guideline. *J Clin Oncol.* 2017;35(8):893-911.

29. Lancellotti P, Nkomo VT, Badano LP, et al. Expert Consensus for multi-modality imaging evaluation of cardiovascular complications of radiotherapy in adults: a report from the European association of cardiovascular imaging and the American society of echocardiography. *J Am Soc Echocardiogr*. 2013;26(9):1013-1032.
30. Thavendiranathan P, Grant AD, Negishi T, Plana JC, Popović ZB, Marwick TH. Reproducibility of echocardiographic techniques for sequential assessment of left ventricular ejection fraction and volumes: application to patients undergoing cancer chemotherapy. *J Am Coll Cardiol*. 2013;61(1):77-84.
31. Thavendiranathan P, Poulin F, Lim KD, Plana JC, Woo A, Marwick TH. Use of myocardial strain imaging by echocardiography for the early detection of cardiotoxicity in patients during and after cancer chemotherapy: a systematic review. *J Am Coll Cardiol*. 2014;63(25 Pt A):2751-2768.
32. Kalay N, Basar E, Ozdogru I, et al. Protective effects of carvedilol against anthracycline-induced cardiomyopathy. *J Am Coll Cardiol*. 2006;48(11):2258-2262.
33. Nabati M, Janbabai G, Baghyari S, Esmaili K, Yazdani J. Cardioprotective effects of carvedilol in inhibiting doxorubicin-induced cardiotoxicity. *J Cardiovasc Pharmacol*. 2017;69(5):279-285.
34. Janbabai G, Nabati M, Faghihinia M, Azizi S, Borhani S, Yazdani J. Effect of enalapril on preventing anthracycline-induced cardiomyopathy. *Cardiovasc Toxicol*. 2017;17(2):130-139.
35. Guglin M, Krischer J, Tamura R, et al. Randomized trial of lisinopril versus carvedilol to prevent trastuzumab cardiotoxicity in patients with breast cancer. *J Am Coll Cardiol*. 2019;73(22):2859-2868.
36. Leong DP, Cosman T, Alhussein MM, et al. Safety of continuing trastuzumab despite mild cardiotoxicity. *JACC CardioOncol*. 2019;1(1):1-10.
37. Lynce F, Barac A, Geng X, et al. Prospective evaluation of the cardiac safety of HER2-targeted therapies in patients with HER2-positive breast cancer and compromised heart function: the SAFE-HEaRt study. *Breast Cancer Res Treat*. 2019;175:595-603.
38. Akpek M, Ozdogru I, Sahin O, et al. Protective effects of spironolactone against anthracycline-induced cardiomyopathy. *Eur J Heart Fail*. 2015;17(1):81-89.
39. Singh JP, Solomon SD, Fradley MG, et al. Association of cardiac resynchronization therapy with change in left ventricular ejection fraction in patients with chemotherapy-induced cardiomyopathy. *JAMA*. 2019;322(18):1799-1805.
40. Møgelvang J, Stokholm KH, Saunämaki K, et al. Assessment of left ventricular volumes by magnetic resonance in comparison with radionuclide angiography, contrast angiography and echocardiography. *Eur Heart J*. 1992;13(12):1677-1683.
41. Galán-Arriola C, Lobo M, Vílchez-Tschischke JP, et al. Serial magnetic resonance imaging to identify early stages of anthracycline-induced cardiotoxicity. *J Am Coll Cardiol*. 2019;73(7):779-791.

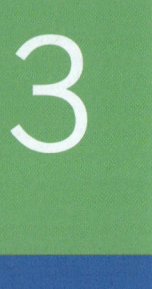

3 Cardiac Dysfunction: Small-Molecule Kinase Inhibitors, Immune-Based Therapies, and Proteasome Inhibitors

Jesus Jimenez and Jose A. Alvarez-Cardona

SMALL-MOLECULE KINASE INHIBITORS

DEFINITION

Small-molecule kinase inhibitors (SMKIs) **block downstream cell signaling** by directly inhibiting tyrosine kinases, kinase receptors, and/or other downstream substrates.[1]

ASSOCIATED DRUGS/THERAPIES

- ALK (anaplastic lymphoma kinase) inhibitor: alectinib, brigatinib, ceritinib, crizotinib, lorlatinib
- BCR/ABL (breakpoint cluster region-Abelson fusion protein) inhibitors: dasatinib, imatinib, nilotinib, ponatinib
- BRAF (B-Raf kinase) inhibitors: cobimetinib, dabrafenib, encorafenib, vemurafenib
- BTK (Bruton's tyrosine kinase) inhibitor: acalabrutinib, ibrutinib, zanubrutinib
- CDK (cyclin-dependent kinase) inhibitor: abemaciclib, ribociclib, palbociclib
- C-MET inhibitor: capmatinib
- EGFR (epidermal growth factor receptor) inhibitor: erlotinib, cetuximab, osimertinib
- HER2 (human epidermal growth factor receptor) inhibitor: lapatinib (see Chapter 2)
- MEK (mitogen-activated protein extracellular signal regulated kinase) inhibitors: binimetinib, trametinib
- Other inhibitors: copanlisib, entrectinib, erdafitinib, fedratinib, fostamatinib, gilteritinib, midostaurin, nintedanib
- VSP (vascular endothelial growth factor signaling pathway) inhibitors (see below): axitinib, cabozantinib, lenvatinib, pazopanib, regorafenib, sunitinib, sorafenib, vandetanib

EPIDEMIOLOGY

Primary Uses

- BCR/ABL inhibitors—chronic myeloid leukemia
- ALK and EGFR inhibitors—non–small cell lung cancer
- Combination of BRAF and MEK inhibitors—melanoma
- BTK inhibitors—mantle cell lymphoma

CARDIOTOXICITY

- SMKIs have been associated with cardiotoxicities including arterial or venous thromboembolism, edema, hypertension, arrhythmias, QT prolongation, myocardial ischemia, left ventricular (LV) dysfunction, and/or heart failure (HF).[1,2]
- Cardiotoxicities can often be a **class effect, related to the SMKI target**. HER2 antagonists, for instance, are associated with LV dysfunction. Other cardiotoxicities, though, such as pulmonary hypertension with dasatinib, are more specific to the drug itself.
- Tyrosine kinase inhibitors often have multiple targets that contribute to toxicity profiles. Osimertinib, for instance, is an EGFR antagonist that also has action against the HER2 receptor, which has been associated with increased cardiotoxicity (including arrhythmias and LV dysfunction) compared to other EGFR antagonists.
- C-MET inhibitors (capmatinib) have a 52% incidence of peripheral edema of unclear etiology. Edema was managed in the clinical trial with compression stockings, leg elevation, and dietary salt modification. The edema may or may not also be partially responsive to diuretics.
- VSP inhibitors have a significant association with hypertension (see below).
- See Table 3-1.

MONITORING

- Determine cardiovascular (CV) risk through comprehensive baseline history and physical examination including assessment of exercise tolerance. Obtain baseline electrocardiograph (ECG) and consider transthoracic echocardiogram (TTE) in patients at higher risk, patients with more cardiotoxic planned therapy, or patients with CV symptoms.
- Cardiotoxicities may require interrupting, reducing, or discontinuing treatment depending on recurrence/severity, although often these cardiotoxicities may be able to be appropriately managed while continuing therapy (see Chapter 20).
  - Vascular abnormalities:
    - Arterial or venous thromboembolism: monitor for evidence of thromboembolisms.
    - Edema: optimize fluid status if symptomatic.
    - Hypertension: blood pressure goal of generally <140/90 mm Hg.
- A lower goal of 130/80 mm Hg has not been specifically studied in patients on cancer therapy and the potential CV benefit of a lower goal must be weighed against the risk of hypotension in patients at risk for anorexia, nausea, vomiting, etc.
- Patient prognosis can also be considered, as the benefit of the lower treatment goal in the SPRINT trial (<120/80 mm Hg) showed benefit largely after 2 years.[3] Although patients on cancer treatment were not included in the SPRINT trial, it is reasonable to aim for a blood pressure goal of <120/80 mm Hg, if tolerated, and certainly in patients with higher CV risk.
  - Myocardial abnormalities:
    - Myocardial ischemia: manage clinically as indicated.
    - LV dysfunction: monitor for reduced ejection fraction on TTE.
    - HF: optimize volume status and implement guideline-directed medical therapy as tolerated.
  - Electrical abnormalities:
    - Arrhythmias: manage clinically as indicated.

TABLE 3-1 Small-Molecule Kinase Inhibitors

Drug class	Drug name	ATE	VTE	Edema	HTN	Arrhythmias	QT prolongation	Myocardial ischemia	LV dysfunction	HF
ALK	Alectinib[23]		•	•		•	•			
	Brigatinib[24]		•	•	•					
	Ceritinib[25]			•		•	•	•		
	Crizotinib[26]		•	•		•	•			
	Lorlatinib[27]	•	•	•	•					
BCR/ABL	Dasatinib[28]	•	•	•	•	•		•	•	•
	Imatinib[29]		•	•		•		•	•	•
	Nilotinib[30]	•		•	•	•	•	•		•
	Ponatinib[31]	•		•	•		•	•		•
BRAF	Cobimetinib[32]			•	•		•		•	•
	Dabrafenib[33]			•	•	•	•			
	Encorafenib[34]			•	•		•			
	Vemurafenib[35]			•		•	•			
BTK	Acalabrutinib[36]				•	•				
	Ibrutinib[37]				•	•		•	•	•
	Zanubrutinib[38]					•				
CDK	Abemaciclib[39]	•	•	•			•			
	Ribociclib[40]			•			•			

EGFR	Erlotinib[41]						•	•	
	Cetuximab[42]				•		•	•	•
	Osimertinib[43]				•		•	•	•
MEK	Binimetinib[44]				•		•		•
	Trametinib[45]				•				•
Other	Copanlisib[46]			•	•				
	Entrectinib[47]			•			•		•
	Erdafitinib[48]					•	•		
	Fedratinib[49]			•			•		•
	Fostamatinib[50]		•		•		•	•	•
	Gilteritinib[51]				•		•		
	Midostaurin[52]				•	•	•	•	•
	Nintedanib[53]	•							

•, any reported adverse event from package insert; ALK, anaplastic lymphoma kinase; ATE, arterial thromboembolism; BCR/ABL, breakpoint cluster region-Abelson fusion protein; BRAF, B-Raf kinase; BTK, Bruton's tyrosine kinase; CDK, cyclin-dependent kinase; EGFR, epidermal growth factor receptor; HF, heart failure; HTN, hypertension; LV, left ventricular; MEK, mitogen-activated protein extracellular signal regulated kinase; VTE, venous thromboembolism.

○ QTc prolongation: for QTc >500 msec or >60 msec change from baseline, dose adjustment or treatment discontinuation may be required, if clinically indicated after discussion with the oncology team, especially if associated with signs/symptoms of serious arrhythmias including torsades de pointes, polymorphic ventricular tachycardia, or unexplained syncope.

VASCULAR ENDOTHELIAL GROWTH FACTOR SIGNALING PATHWAY INHIBITORS

DEFINITION

- Vascular endothelial growth factor **(VEGF) signaling pathway** (VSP) inhibitors **block VSP** by inactivating or trapping the VEGF ligand as well as by directly inhibiting VEGF receptors or other off targets to prevent activation of cellular processes that promote angiogenesis.[2]

ASSOCIATED DRUGS/THERAPIES

- VEGFA monoclonal antibody (mAb): bevacizumab
- VEGF trap: aflibercept
- VEGFR2 (VEGF receptor 2) mAb: ramucirumab
- SMKIs with anti-VEGF activity: axitinib, cabozantinib, lenvatinib, pazopanib, regorafenib, sunitinib, sorafenib, vandetanib

EPIDEMIOLOGY

- VSP inhibitors are primarily used in advanced renal cell carcinoma, metastatic colon cancer, and metastatic gastric cancer.

CARDIOTOXICITY

- See Table 3-2.
- **Hypertension** is the **most common vascular abnormality** that develops in **almost all patients** undergoing treatment with VSPs.[2]
- In general, the incidence of thromboembolic events, hypertension, and/or LV dysfunction increases when VSPs are combined with another cancer treatment.[4]

MONITORING

- See Figure 3-1 for recommended monitoring approach.

IMMUNE CHECKPOINT INHIBITORS

DEFINITION

- Immune checkpoint inhibitors (ICIs) **block different costimulatory signaling molecules on T lymphocytes and antigen-presenting cells** including programmed

TABLE 3-2 Vascular Endothelial Growth Factor Signaling Pathway (VSP) Inhibitors

Drug name	Vascular abnormalities[a]	Myocardial abnormalities[a]	Electrical abnormalities[a]
Bevacizumab[54]	Hypertension (5%-18%), edema (15%), VTE (5%-11%), ATE (5%)	LV dysfunction (1%)	
Aflibercept[55]	Hypertension (19%), VTE (8%), ATE (1.8%)		
Ramucirumab[56]	Hypertension (6%-15%), edema (up to 2%), ATE (1%-2%)		
Axitinib[57]	Hypertension (16%), hypertensive crisis (<1%), VTE (3%), ATE (1%)		
Cabozantinib[58]	Hypertension (15%), VTE (7.3%), ATE (0.9%)		
Lenvatinib[59]	Hypertension (44%), edema (0.4%), VTE (%), ATE (3%)	LV dysfunction (2%)	QTc prolongation (2%)
Pazopanib[60]	Hypertension (4%-7%), edema (2%), VTE (up to 5%), ATE (up to 2%)	LV dysfunction (up to 11%), myocardial infarction (0.3%)	QTc prolongation (2%), torsades de pointes (<1%)
Regorafenib[61]	Hypertension (30%), hypertensive crisis (0.18%)	Myocardial infarction (1.2%)	
Sunitinib[62]	Hypertension (up to 13%), edema (up to 2%), VTE (2.2%)	LV dysfunction (up to 3%)	Torsades de pointes (<1%)
Sorafenib[63]	Hypertension (9.4%-16.9%)	Heart failure (1.1%-1.9%), myocardial infarction (2.7%-2.9%)	
Vandetanib[64]	Hypertension (9%)	Heart failure (0.9%)	QTc prolongation (8%)

ATE, arterial thromboembolism; LV, left ventricular; VTE, venous thromboembolism.
[a]Grade 3 or higher adverse reactions reported as % incidence.

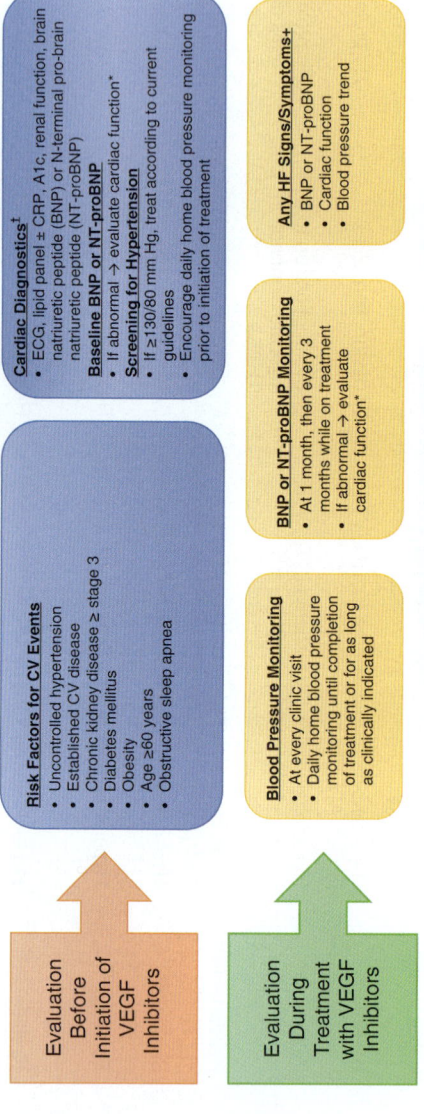

Figure 3-1. Cardiovascular monitoring before and during treatment with VEGF inhibitors. This figure depicts the cardiovascular evaluation before initiation and during treatment with VEGF inhibitors. It highlights the importance of establishing a patient's baseline cardiovascular risk and provides a guide for the implementation of screening and diagnostic tools in the care of these patients. CV, cardiovascular; HF, heart failure; JVP, jugular venous pressure; MRI, magnetic resonance imaging; TTE, transthoracic echocardiogram. (© Washington University School of Medicine in St. Louis.)

cell death protein (PD-1), programmed death-ligand 1 (PD-L1), and cytotoxic T-lymphocyte antigen 4 (CTLA-4) to break T-cell immune tolerance and attack cancer cells.[5]

ASSOCIATED DRUGS/THERAPIES

- Anti-PD-1: nivolumab, cemiplimab, pembrolizumab
- Anti-PD-L1: atezolizumab, avelumab, durvalumab
- Anti-CTLA-4: ipilimumab

EPIDEMIOLOGY

- ICIs are commonly used for metastatic, unresectable, relapsed, and/or progressive cancer such as melanoma, renal cell cancer, Hodgkin lymphoma, or non–small cell lung cancer.

CARDIOTOXICITY

- See Table 3-3.
- Life-threatening myocarditis occurs in <1% of patients, with a median time to onset of 30 days after initiation of ICI.[6] Confirmation of diagnosis can be difficult, though cardiac MRI can be helpful, and endomyocardial biopsy remains the gold standard.
- Relative to monotherapy, **combination** of **ICIs** has been associated with **increased incidence of myocarditis**.[7]
- Checkpoint inhibitor therapy has also been more commonly associated with **promoting accelerated atherosclerosis**, which likely predisposes patients to increased risk of myocardial infarction.[8]
- Increased CV events following ICI treatment have been noted in patients with baseline coronary and aortic calcification on computed tomographic (CT) imaging.[9] These patients may benefit from increased preventive therapy.
- Overall, though, checkpoint inhibitor therapy has a relatively low CV side-effect profile, and one study found no increased risk of CV events.[10]

MONITORING

- See Figure 3-2 for recommendations on monitoring.
- Although it may be helpful to monitor patients for cardiac biomarkers as a screen for checkpoint inhibitor–associated myocarditis, the risk that an otherwise asymptomatic patient with mildly elevated troponin will subsequently develop life-threatening myocarditis is unknown.
- Patients with troponin elevations with otherwise no signs of clinically significant myocarditis likely benefit from increased monitoring, but there are no data to suggest that cancer therapy has to be discontinued. Decisions regarding continuation or adjustment of cancer therapy should be made carefully with a multidisciplinary approach.

TABLE 3-3 Immune Checkpoint Inhibitors

Drug name	Vascular abnormalities[a]	Myocardial abnormalities[a]	Electrical abnormalities[a]
Nivolumab[65]	Vasculitis (<1%), edema (up to 1.5%)	Myocarditis (<1%)	Ventricular arrhythmia (<10%)
Cemiplimab[66]	Vasculitis (<1%)	Myocarditis (<1%), pericarditis (<1%)	
Pembrolizumab[67]	Vasculitis (1%), edema (1.1%)	Myocarditis (0.5%), myocardial infarction (2%), pericarditis (2%), pericardial effusion (2%), cardiac tamponade (2%)	Arrhythmia (4%)
Atezolizumab[68]	Vasculitis (<1%), edema (up to 2%)	Myocarditis, cardiac arrest, myocardial infarction (<1%)	
Avelumab[69]	Vasculitis (<1%), edema (up to 0.4%) myositis (<1%)	Myocarditis (<1%)	
Durvalumab[70]	Myositis (<1%), edema (2%), myositis (<1%)	Vasculitis (<1%), edema (2%), myositis (<1%)	
Ipilimumab[71]	Vasculitis (<1%)	Pericarditis (<1%), myocarditis (<1%)	

[a]Grade 3 or higher adverse reactions reported as % incidence.

CHIMERIC ANTIGEN RECEPTOR T-CELL THERAPY

DEFINITION

T cells are genetically engineered to produce **chimeric antigen receptors** to **target cancer cells**.[11]

ASSOCIATED DRUGS/THERAPIES

- Axicabtagene ciloleucel, tisagenlecleucel

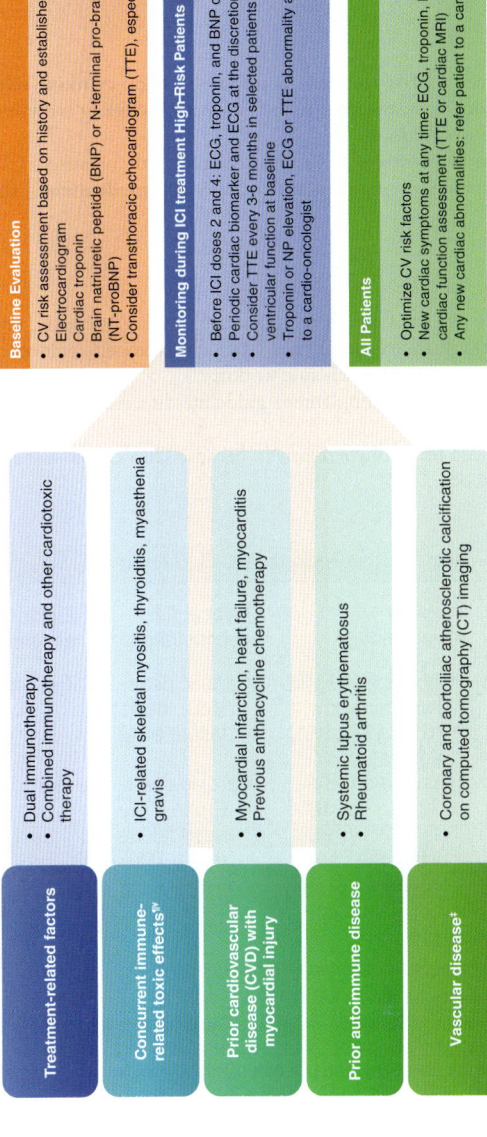

Figure 3-2. Cardiovascular monitoring during treatment with immune checkpoint inhibitors. This figure illustrates potential risk factors for immune checkpoint inhibitor–related cardiovascular toxicity based on treatment-related factors, presence of other immune-related adverse effects, prior cardiovascular disease with myocardial injury, history of autoimmune disease, and presence of vascular disease. It further provides a surveillance strategy based on the patient's baseline evaluation and risk for cardiovascular toxicity. MRI, magnetic resonance imaging; NP, natriuretic peptide. (© Washington University School of Medicine in St. Louis.)

EPIDEMIOLOGY

- Axicabtagene ciloleucel and tisagenlecleucel are indicated for the treatment of adult patients with relapsed or refractory large B-cell lymphoma.
- Tisagenlecleucel is also indicated for relapsed or refractory B-cell acute lymphoblastic leukemia in patients up to 25 years old.

CARDIOTOXICITY

- See Table 3-4.
- Up to 94% (any grade adverse reaction) of patients develop **cytokine release syndrome** (CRS),[12] which was associated with CV events including arrhythmias, HF, cardiogenic shock, and CV death.[11,13]
- **Troponin elevation** with severe CRS is associated with increased CV events, and early administration of interleukin-6 antagonist (**tocilizumab**) **should be considered**.[11,13]

MONITORING

- Because of the high risk for CRS that is associated with CV events, review past medical history and evaluate baseline ECG, TTE, and exercise tolerance.[11]
  - If abnormal screening, consider ischemic workup.
  - Optimize volume status and implement guideline-directed medical therapy as tolerated.
  - Closely monitor need for antihypertensives, because CRS can be associated with hypotension and shock.

TABLE 3-4 Chimeric Antigen Receptor T-Cell Therapy

Drug name	Vascular abnormalities[a]	Myocardial abnormalities[a,b]	Electrical abnormalities[a]
Axicabtagene ciloleucel[72]	Hypotension (15%), hypertension (6%), VTE (1%), edema (1%)	Cardiac death (6%), heart failure (4%)	Tachycardia (2%), arrhythmias (7%)[c]
Tisagenlecleucel[73]	Hypotension (8%-22%), hypertension (2%-6%), VTE (3%-7%), edema (1%-2%)	Cardiac death (up to 4%), heart failure (up to 7%)	Tachycardia (3%-4%), arrhythmias (up to 6%)[d]

VTE, venous thromboembolism.
[a]Grade 3 or higher adverse reactions reported as % incidence.
[b]Secondary to cytokine release syndrome (23%-49%).
[c]Includes sinus arrhythmia, atrial fibrillation, atrial flutter, atrioventricular block, right bundle branch block, QT prolongation, premature atrial and ventricular contractions, supraventricular tachycardia, ventricular tachycardia.
[d]Includes atrial fibrillation, premature ventricular contractions.

BISPECIFIC ANTIBODIES

DEFINITION

- Bispecific antibodies are **antibodies** with two or more antigen-binding sites that are engineered to recognize different antigens or epitopes with the goal of simultaneously **binding a cytotoxic cell** and a target like a tumor cell to be destroyed.[14]

ASSOCIATED DRUGS/THERAPIES

- Blinatumomab

EPIDEMIOLOGY

- Blinatumomab is only approved for acute lymphoblastic leukemia, but there are several ongoing clinical trials with other antibodies for solid tumors including triple-negative breast cancer, refractory lymphomas, advanced gastrointestinal cancer, and others.[15,16]

CARDIOTOXICITY

- See Table 3-5.
- Although edema and arrhythmias can be associated with treatment, severe myocardial abnormalities are typically secondary to **CRS**.[17,18]

MONITORING

- Because of the risk for CRS that is associated with CV events, review past medical history and evaluate baseline ECG, TTE, and exercise tolerance.[11]
  - If abnormal screening, consider ischemic workup.
  - Optimize volume status and implement guideline-directed medical therapy as tolerated.
  - Evaluate need for antihypertensives because CRS can be associated with hypotension and shock.

TABLE 3-5 Bispecific Antibodies

Drug name	Vascular abnormalities[a]	Myocardial abnormalities[a,b]	Electrical abnormalities[a,c]
Blinatumomab[74]	Edema (1%), hypotension (<1%)	Heart failure	Bradycardia, tachycardia, arrhythmias (2%)

[a]Grade 3 or higher adverse reactions reported as % incidence.
[b]Secondary to cytokine release syndrome (3%).
[c]Includes sinus arrhythmia, premature ventricular contractions.

PROTEASOME INHIBITORS

DEFINITION

- Proteasome inhibitors (PIs) prevent the **degradation of proteins within the cell**, which leads to cell apoptosis.

ASSOCIATED DRUGS/THERAPIES

- Reversible, nonselective inhibitor: bortezomib
- Reversible, selective inhibitor: ixazomib
- Irreversible, selective inhibitor: carfilzomib

EPIDEMIOLOGY

- PIs are used to treat multiple myeloma.
- Bortezomib is also used to treat AL (light chain) amyloidosis.

CARDIOTOXICITY

- PIs are associated with CV adverse events such as HF particularly within the first 3 months of treatment and are more commonly seen with carfilzomib.[19]
- Bortezomib[20]
  - HF (<1%)
- Ixazomib[21]
  - Edema (25%)
- Carfilzomib[22]
  - HF (7%)
  - Hypertension (14.3%)

MONITORING

- Determine CV risk by obtaining past medical history, baseline TTE, and exercise tolerance.
  - Vascular abnormalities:
    - Edema: optimize fluid status if symptomatic.
    - Hypertension: blood pressure goal of <140/90 mm Hg during treatment. A goal of <130/80 mm Hg can be considered if easily obtainable but should be balanced against risks of hypotension during therapy.
  - Myocardial abnormalities:
    - LV dysfunction: monitor for reduced ejection fraction and LV hypertrophy on TTE.
    - HF: optimize volume status and implement guideline-directed medical therapy as tolerated.
- See Figure 3-3 for recommendations on CV monitoring in patients receiving carfilzomib based on the PROTECT study.[19]

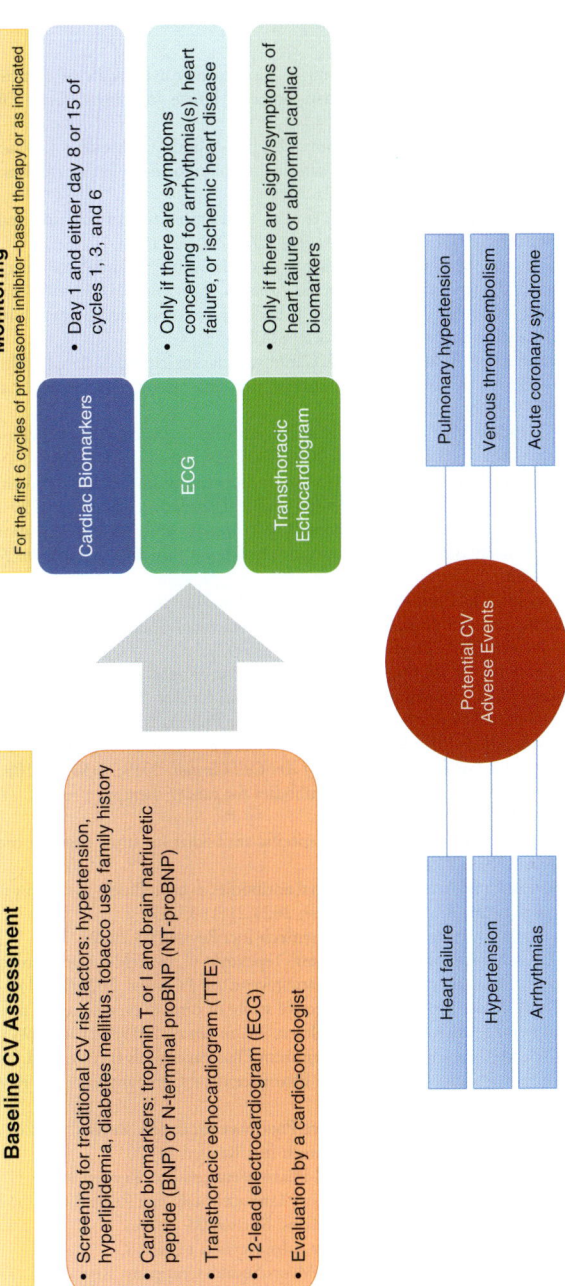

Figure 3-3. Cardiovascular monitoring during treatment with carfilzomib. Evaluating for cardiovascular risk factors or disease in patients that will receive carfilzomib is of utmost importance when considering the potential cardiovascular adverse events associated with this therapy. A surveillance strategy using cardiac biomarkers, electrocardiogram, and transthoracic echocardiogram can help clinicians identify patients at risk for cardiovascular adverse events. (From Cornell RF, Ky B, Weiss BM, et al. Prospective study of cardiac events during proteasome inhibitor therapy for relapsed multiple myeloma. *J Clin Oncol.* 2019;37:1946-1955.)

REFERENCES

1. Jin Y, Xu Z, Yan H, He Q, Yang X, Luo P. A comprehensive review of clinical cardiotoxicity incidence of FDA-approved small-molecule kinase inhibitors. *Front Pharmacol*. 2020;11:891.
2. Li W, Croce K, Steensma DP, McDermott DF, Ben-Yehuda O, Moslehi J. Vascular and metabolic implications of novel targeted cancer therapies: focus on kinase inhibitors. *J Am Coll Cardiol*. 2015;66:1160-1078.
3. Group SR, Wright JT Jr, Williamson JD, et al. A randomized trial of intensive versus standard blood-pressure control. *N Engl J Med*. 2015;373:2103-2116.
4. Touyz RM, Herrmann SMS, Herrmann J. Vascular toxicities with VEGF inhibitor therapies-focus on hypertension and arterial thrombotic events. *J Am Soc Hypertens*. 2018;12:409-425.
5. Lyon AR, Yousaf N, Battisti NML, Moslehi J, Larkin J. Immune checkpoint inhibitors and cardiovascular toxicity. *Lancet Oncol*. 2018;19:e447-e458.
6. Salem JE, Manouchehri A, Moey M, et al. Cardiovascular toxicities associated with immune checkpoint inhibitors: an observational, retrospective, pharmacovigilance study. *Lancet Oncol*. 2018;19:1579-1589.
7. Mahmood SS, Fradley MG, Cohen JV, et al. Myocarditis in patients treated with immune checkpoint inhibitors. *J Am Coll Cardiol*. 2018;71:1755-1764.
8. Drobni ZD, Alvi RM, Taron J, et al. Association between immune checkpoint inhibitors with cardiovascular events and atherosclerotic plaque. *Circulation*. 2020;142:2299-2311.
9. Schiffer WB, Deych E, Lenihan DJ, Zhang KW. Coronary and aortic calcification are associated with cardiovascular events on immune checkpoint inhibitor therapy. *Int J Cardiol*. 2021;322:177-182.
10. Zhang L, Reynolds KL, Lyon AR, Palaskas N, Neilan TG. The evolving immunotherapy landscape and the epidemiology, diagnosis, and management of cardiotoxicity: JACC: CardioOncology Primer. *JACC CardioOncol*. 2021;3:35-47.
11. Ganatra S, Carver JR, Hayek SS, Ky B, et al. Chimeric antigen receptor T-cell therapy for cancer and heart: JACC council perspectives. *J Am Coll Cardiol*. 2019;74:3153-3163.
12. Axicabtagene ciloleucel (Yescarta). Package insert. Kite Pharma Inc; Revised 05 2020.
13. Alvi RM, Frigault MJ, Fradley MG, et al. Cardiovascular events among adults treated with chimeric antigen receptor T-cells (CAR-T). *J Am Coll Cardiol*. 2019;74:3099-3108.
14. Krishnamurthy A, Jimeno A. Bispecific antibodies for cancer therapy: a review. *Pharmacol Ther*. 2018;185:122-134.
15. Dees S, Ganesan R, Singh S, Grewal IS. Bispecific antibodies for triple negative breast cancer. *Trends Cancer*. 2021;7(2):162-173.
16. Jullien M, Touzeau C, Moreau P. Monoclonal antibodies as an addition to current myeloma therapy strategies. *Expert Rev Anticancer Ther*. 2021;21(1):33-43.
17. Bevacizumab (Avastin). Package insert. Genentech Inc; Revised 05 2020.
18. Lobenwein D, Kocher F, Dobner S, Gollmann-Tepekoylu C, Holfeld J. Cardiotoxic mechanisms of cancer immunotherapy—a systematic review. *Int J Cardiol*. 2021;323:179-187.
19. Cornell RF, Ky B, Weiss BM, et al. Prospective study of cardiac events during proteasome inhibitor therapy for relapsed multiple myeloma. *J Clin Oncol*. 2019;37:1946-1955.
20. Bortezomib (Velcade). Package insert. Millennium Pharmaceuticals Inc; Revised 10, 2014.
21. Ixazomib (Ninlaro). Package insert. Takeda Pharmaceutical Company Limited; Revised 11, 2015.
22. Carfilzomib (Kyprolis). Package insert. Onyx Pharmaceuticals Inc; Revised 07, 2012.
23. Alectinib (Alecensa). Package insert. Genentech Inc; Revised 11, 2017.
24. Brigatinib (Alunbrig). Package insert. Ariad Pharmaceuticals Inc; Revised 04, 2017.
25. Ceritinib (Zykadia). Package insert. Novartis Pharmaceuticals Inc; Revised 05, 2017.
26. Crizotinib (Xalkori). Package insert. Pfizer Labs; Revised 03, 2016.
27. Lorlatinib (Lorbrena). Package insert. Pfizer Labs; Revised 11, 2018.
28. Dasatinib (Sprycel). Package insert. Bristol-Myers Squibb Company; Revised 11, 2017.
29. Imatinib (Gleevec). Package insert. Novartis Pharmaceuticals Corporation; Revised 08, 2020.

30. Nilotinib (Tasigna). Package insert. Novartis Pharmaceuticals Corporation; Revised 12, 2017.
31. Ponatinib (Iclusig). Package insert. Millennium Pharmaceuticals Inc; Revised 12, 2020.
32. Cobimetinib (Cotellic). Package insert. Genentech USA Inc; Revised 11, 2015.
33. Dabrafenib (Tafinlar). Package insert. Novartis Pharmaceuticals Corporation; Revised 04, 2018.
34. Encorafenib (Braftovi). Package insert. Array BioPharma Inc; Revised 06, 2018.
35. Vemurafenib (Zelboraf). Package insert. Genentech Inc; Revised 11, 2017.
36. Acalabrutinib (Calquence). Package insert. AstraZeneca Pharmaceuticals LP; Revised 10, 2017.
37. Ibrutinib (Imbruvica). Package insert. Pharmacyclics LLC; Revised 08, 2017.
38. Zanubrutinib (Brukinsa). Package insert. BeiGene USA Inc; Revised 11, 2019.
39. Abemaciclib (Verzenio). Package insert. Lilly USA LLC; Revised 02, 2018.
40. Ribociclib (Kisqali). Package insert. Novartis Pharmaceuticals Corporation; Revised 03, 2017.
41. Erlotinib (Tarceva). Package insert. Genentech USA Inc; Revised 10, 2016.
42. Cetuximab (Erbitux). Package insert. Eli Lilly and Company; Revised 04, 2019.
43. Osimertinib (Tagrisso). Package insert. AstraZeneca Pharmaceuticals LP; Revised 03, 2017.
44. Binimetinib (Mektovi). Package insert. Array BioPharma Inc; Revised 06, 2018.
45. Trametinib (Mekinist). Package insert. Novartis Pharmaceuticals Corporation; Revised 04, 2018.
46. Copanlisib (Aliqopa). Package insert. Bayer HealthCare Pharmaceuticals Inc; Revised 09, 2017.
47. Entrectinib (Rozlytrek). Package insert. Genentech USA Inc; Revised 08, 2019.
48. Erdafitinib (Balversa). Package insert. Janssen Products; Revised 04, 2019.
49. Fedratinib (Inrebic). Package insert. Celgene Corporation; Revised 08, 2019.
50. Fostamatinib (Tavalisse). Package insert. Rigel Pharmaceuticals; Revised 04, 2018.
51. Gilteritinib (Xospata). Package insert. Astellas Pharma US Inc; Revised 11, 2018.
52. Midostaurin (Rydapt). Package insert. Novartis Pharmaceuticals Corporation; Revised 04, 2017.
53. Nintedanib (Ofev). Package insert. Boehringer Ingelheim Pharmaceuticals Inc; Revised 09, 2019.
54. Bevacizumab (Avastin). Package insert. Genentech Inc; Revised 05, 2020.
55. Aflibercept (Zaltrap). Package insert. Sanofi-Aventis US LLC; Revised 06, 2020.
56. Ramucirumab (Cyramza). Package insert. Eli Lilly and Company; Revised 05, 2019.
57. Axitinib (Inlyta). Package insert. Pfizer Labs; Revised 01, 2012.
58. Cabozantinib (Cabometyx). Package insert. Exelixis Inc; Revised 04, 2016.
59. Lenvatinib (Lenvima). Package insert. Eisai Inc; Revised 02, 2015.
60. Pazopanib (Votrient). Package insert. GlaxoSmithKline; Revised 04, 2012.
61. Regorafenib (Stivarga). Package insert. Bayer HealthCare Pharmaceuticals; Revised 09, 2012.
62. Sunitinib (Sutent). Package insert. Pfizer Labs; Revised 11, 2017.
63. Sorafenib (Nexavar). Package insert. Bayer HealthCare Pharmaceuticals Inc; Revised 10, 2010.
64. Vandetanib (Caprelsa). Package insert. AstraZeneca Pharmaceuticals LP; Revised 03, 2014.
65. Nivolumab (Optivo). Package insert. Bristol-Myers Squibb Company; Revised 11, 2016.
66. Cemiplimab (Libtayo). Package insert. Regeneron Pharmaceuticals Inc; Revised 09, 2018.
67. Pembrolizumab (Keytruda). Package insert. Merck and Co Inc; Revised 04, 2019.
68. Atezolizumab (Tecentriq). Package insert. Genentech Inc; Revised 03, 2019.
69. Avelumab (Bavencio). Package insert. Pfizer Inc; Revised 05, 2019.
70. Durvalumab (Imfinzi). Package insert. AstraZeneca Pharmaceuticals LP; Revised 04, 2017.
71. Ipilimumab (Yervoy). Package insert. Bristol-Myers Squibb Company; Revised 07, 2018.
72. Axicabtagene ciloleucel (Yescarta). Package insert. Kita Pharma Inc; Revised 05, 2020.
73. Tisagenlecleucel (Kymriah). Package insert. Novartis Pharmaceuticals Corporation; Revised 05, 2018.
74. Blinatumomab (Blincyto). Package insert. Amgen Inc; Revised 03, 2020.

4. Valvular Heart Disease

Manuel Rivera Maza, Kathleen W. Zhang, and Nishath Quader

GENERAL PRINCIPLES

- As cancer survival improves with advances in cancer therapies, more patients with prior or ongoing cancer therapy are likely to seek consultation for the management of valvular heart disease (VHD). Attention to unique procedural risk factors related to cancer therapy is necessary for these patients.
- Radiation-induced valve disease and carcinoid heart disease are important primary causes of VHD in the cardio-oncology population that will be reviewed in this chapter. Nonbacterial thrombotic endocarditis (NBTE) is a potential complication of the prothrombotic state associated with active malignancy that will also be discussed.
- A multidisciplinary care team including cardiologists, cardiac surgeons, oncologists, and radiologists with experience caring for patients with cardiac complications of cancer therapy is optimal for the management of VHD in cancer patients.

APPROACH TO VALVULAR HEART DISEASE IN THE CANCER PATIENT

- In general, diagnosis and management of VHD in patients with prior or ongoing cancer treatment should follow standard clinical practice guidelines.[1]
- **In cardio-oncology patients, unique procedural risks related to prior or ongoing cancer therapy should be considered as part of the surgical risk assessment process.** These include:
  - **Cardiac dysfunction** because of cardiotoxic chemotherapy (see Chapters 2 and 3)
  - **Mediastinal fibrosis** because of prior thoracic radiation (see *Radiation-Induced Valvular Heart Disease* in the section that follows)
  - **Pulmonary disease** because of prior thoracic radiation and/or chemotherapy-induced pulmonary toxicity
  - **Anemia and/or thrombocytopenia** because of ongoing myelosuppressive cancer therapy
  - **Unfavorable performance status or increased frailty** in patients receiving cancer therapy
- In patients with active malignancy, the decision to proceed with surgical or transcatheter valvular intervention should be made in collaboration with the treating oncologist. In general, procedural intervention should be considered only when expected survival exceeds 1 year with acceptable quality of life.
- Transcatheter aortic or mitral valve replacement may be preferred over surgical valve replacement for patients with active malignancy. Among patients undergoing

transcatheter aortic valve replacement for severe aortic stenosis, those with an active malignancy had similar 30-day mortality but higher 1-year mortality (15%) as compared to those without cancer (9%). Long-term mortality was driven largely by cancer progression.[2]

RADIATION-INDUCED VALVULAR HEART DISEASE

GENERAL PRINCIPLES

- Thoracic radiation is an integral component of cancer therapy for several malignancies including Hodgkin lymphoma, breast cancer, esophageal cancer, and lung cancer. VHD is a late cardiac complication of thoracic radiation when the heart is in the radiation field.
- Contemporary radiation techniques optimize radiation delivery to the tumor while minimizing the total heart dose of radiation using techniques such as shielding, advanced respiratory gating techniques with deep inspiratory breath holds, and narrow tangential beams. Because of the late onset of radiation-induced VHD, which may occur several decades after radiation therapy, recognition and management of this condition remain highly relevant to current cardio-oncology practice.

Epidemiology/Risk Factors

- **Radiation-induced VHD primarily affects the aortic valve and mitral valve, and may cause valvular regurgitation and/or stenosis. Risk of VHD increases with total heart radiation dose (especially >30 Gy), concomitant anthracycline chemotherapy, and time from radiation therapy** (Table 4-1).[3-5]
- Among asymptomatic patients with Hodgkin lymphoma who received a median of 43 Gy of mantle radiation, there was a 34-fold increased risk of moderate or severe aortic regurgitation as compared to the general population. Incidence of moderate or severe aortic regurgitation increased from 2.3% at 11 to 20 years from cancer treatment to 15% at >20 years from cancer treatment.[5] Incidence of aortic stenosis was 16% at >20 years in this study.
- Among patients with lung cancer who received a median heart dose of 12 Gy, the incidence of VHD was 2.1% at 20 months follow-up.[6]
- Among women with breast cancer who received a mean heart dose of 2 to 6 Gy, the incidence ratio of VHD was 1.54 (95% confidence interval [CI] 1.11-2.13) as compared to women who did not receive radiation.[7]

TABLE 4-1 Risk Factors for Radiation-Induced Valvular Heart Disease

Risk factors
Higher total cardiac radiation dose (especially >30 Gy)
History of mantle chest radiation (ie, for lymphoma)
Concomitant anthracycline chemotherapy
Increased time from radiation therapy

- Older age and female gender appear to be additional risk factors for aortic regurgitation in patients who receive mantle radiation for the treatment of Hodgkin lymphoma.[5]
- Among survivors of childhood Hodgkin lymphoma, the hazard ratio for valvular abnormalities was 10.5 (95% CI 6.1-17.9) as compared to a sibling control group at 20 years of follow-up.[8] Valvular dysfunction was associated with age ≤14 years at diagnosis, treatment in the 1980s, higher radiation dose, and exposure to an anthracycline dose of 250 mg/m^2 or more.

Diagnosis
History
- Dyspnea on exertion, lower extremity edema, and orthopnea are classic symptoms of VHD. Exertional chest pain and/or syncope may be seen in patients with severe aortic stenosis.
- Patients with mild VHD are usually asymptomatic.

Physical Examination
- Classically, cardiac auscultation demonstrates a diastolic murmur at the left lower sternal border for aortic regurgitation; a harsh, systolic, crescendo–decrescendo murmur at the right upper sternal border for aortic stenosis; a blowing systolic murmur at the left ventricular apex for mitral regurgitation; and a systolic murmur at the left lower sternal border for tricuspid regurgitation.
- Among asymptomatic patients with prior mantle radiation, the sensitivity of a diastolic murmur was only 6% for aortic regurgitation, whereas the positive predictive value of a systolic murmur was only 23% for significant aortic stenosis, mitral regurgitation, or tricuspid regurgitation.[5]

Echocardiography
- **Transthoracic echocardiography is the preferred imaging modality for initial evaluation of radiation-induced VHD. Diagnostic evaluation includes the identification of anatomic valvular abnormalities, quantitative assessment of valvular dysfunction, and assessment of the functional consequences of valvular dysfunction on cardiac structure and function.**
- Characteristic findings of radiation-induced VHD on echocardiography include fibrosis and calcification of the aortic root, aortic valve annulus, aortic valve leaflets, aortic–mitral inter-valvular fibrosa, mitral valve annulus, and the base and mid-portions of the mitral valve leaflets (Fig. 4-1). The mitral valve tips and commissures are typically spared, in contrast with rheumatic valve disease.
- Three-dimensional echocardiography and/or transesophageal echocardiography may be helpful to delineate valvular anatomy.
- Severity of valvular regurgitation or stenosis should be graded according to the American Society of Echocardiography guidelines.[9,10]

Cardiac Magnetic Resonance Imaging and Cardiac Computed Tomography Imaging
- Cardiac magnetic resonance imaging (CMR) and cardiac computed tomography (CT) imaging can be useful in patients with inadequate echocardiographic image quality or for procedural planning purposes.
- In patients with suspected radiation-induced myocardial disease or pericardial disease, CMR complements echocardiography for the assessment of left and right ventricular function and volumes, myocardial fibrosis, and pericardial disease along with anatomic and dynamic evaluation of valvular abnormalities.

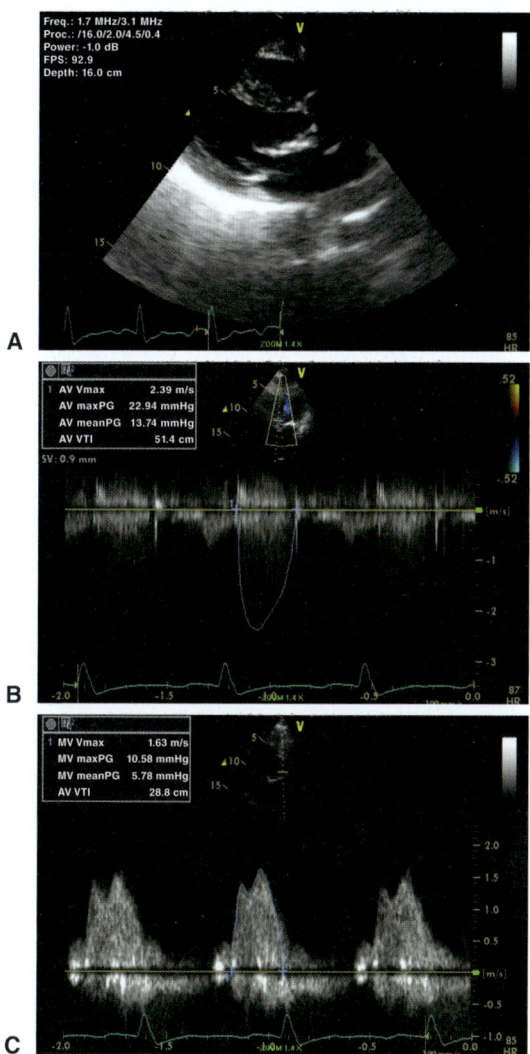

Figure 4-1. Echocardiographic findings of radiation-induced valvular heart disease. Calcified aortic and mitral valves and severe calcification of the aortomitral curtain (arrow) are classic findings (A). Increased continuous flow Doppler across aortic valve consistent with mild aortic stenosis (B). Increased continuous flow Doppler across mitral valve consistent wtih moderate mitral stenosis (C). (Images courtesy of Dr. Majesh Makan, Washington University in Saint Louis.)

- Cardiac CT provides high-resolution, cross-sectional imaging of valvular anatomy and is used routinely for procedural planning prior to transcatheter aortic and mitral valve replacement.

TREATMENT AND PROGNOSIS

- **Because of increased procedural complexity related to mediastinal fibrosis resulting from prior thoracic radiation, patients with radiation-induced VHD should seek treatment by a multidisciplinary care team at a comprehensive valve center.**
- In general, the management of radiation-induced VHD should follow standard clinical guidelines.[1]
  - Among 173 patients undergoing cardiac surgery with a history of thoracic radiation, there was an increased risk of all-cause mortality over 8 years of follow-up (55%) as compared to patients without a history of thoracic radiation (28%; hazard ratio 2.54 [95% CI 1.89-3.43]).[11]
  - Preoperative evaluation should include echocardiography, coronary angiography, cardiac CT imaging, and pulmonary function testing.[12]
  - Transcatheter, minimally invasive, and nonprocedural approaches may be preferable in patients with prior thoracic radiation.
- Among patients with prior mediastinal radiation and severe aortic stenosis, transcatheter aortic valve replacement appears to have superior short-term outcomes as compared to surgical aortic valve replacement.[13,14]
- The risk of reoperative cardiac surgery is particularly high in patients with prior thoracic radiation and should therefore be avoided.[15] A thorough evaluation for concomitant coronary artery disease and pericardial disease, both of which occur with increased frequency after thoracic radiation, is essential prior to cardiac surgery for radiation-induced VHD.
- Among patients undergoing cardiac surgery for radiation-induced VHD, increased aortomitral curtain thickness, higher preoperative surgical risk score, and lack of perioperative cardioprotective medications are associated with increased long-term mortality.[16]

PREVENTION AND SCREENING

- **Use of radiation protocols that minimize cardiac radiation exposure is the most important intervention to prevent radiation-induced VHD.**
- Contemporary thoracic radiation protocols aim to maximize radiation delivery to cancerous tissue while minimizing cardiac radiation exposure.[12] Specific techniques include:
  - Targeted radiation delivery as opposed to full mantle radiation for lymphoma (ie, involved field, involved site, and involved node radiation therapy)
  - Advanced delivery techniques such as deep inspiratory breath hold, which pulls the heart inferiorly and allows for unimpeded upper mediastinal treatment
  - Proton therapy, which protects normal tissue that is distal to the target of radiation
  - Three-dimensional conformal radiation and prone positioning for breast cancer
- **Expert consensus guidelines recommend that asymptomatic patients with a history of chest radiation undergo screening echocardiograms to monitor for**

radiation-induced cardiac disease, including VHD as well as heart failure, left ventricular dysfunction, and pericardial disease.[17] In particular, patients treated without cardioprotective radiation protocols should be screened. Screening should begin 10 years after completion of radiation therapy and be repeated every 5 years. Patients at high risk for radiation-induced VHD should begin screening 5 years after completion of therapy.[17]

CARCINOID HEART DISEASE

GENERAL PRINCIPLES

- Neuroendocrine tumors are rare, slow-growing malignancies that usually arise from the gastrointestinal tract and can cause carcinoid syndrome and/or carcinoid heart disease.
- Carcinoid syndrome is characterized by episodes of flushing, hypotension, diarrhea, and bronchospasm, and occurs in the presence of hepatic metastases whereby vasoactive substances produced by the tumor (ie, serotonin [5-hydroxytryptamine, 5-HT], bradykinin, histamine, and prostaglandins) access the systemic circulation via the hepatic vein.
- Carcinoid heart disease is thought to result from chronic cardiac exposure to vasoactive substances, especially 5-HT, and manifests as plaque-like fibrous tissue that deposits on the valve leaflets, subvalvular apparatus, papillary muscles, and/or endocardial surfaces.
- **The tricuspid and pulmonic valves are most commonly affected because the damaging vasoactive substances are inactivated in the pulmonary vasculature. Valvular regurgitation occurs more commonly than valvular stenosis.**[18] Left-sided cardiac valves may be involved in the setting of an intracardiac shunt (such as a patent foramen ovale), extensive liver metastasis, or bronchial carcinoid tumors.

Epidemiology/Risk Factors

- Neuroendocrine tumors occur rarely, with an estimated incidence of 1.2 to 2.1 cases per 100,000 of the general population. Approximately 30% to 40% of patients with neuroendocrine tumors develop carcinoid syndrome, and 20% to 50% of patients with carcinoid syndrome develop carcinoid heart disease.[18-20]
- Up to 20% of patients with carcinoid syndrome present with carcinoid heart disease at the time of diagnosis.[21]

Diagnosis

History and Physical Examination
- Many patients with carcinoid heart disease are asymptomatic at the time of presentation.
- Symptoms of significant tricuspid and/or pulmonic regurgitation include fatigue, lower extremity edema, and abdominal distension. Patients with significant mitral and/or aortic regurgitation may also present with dyspnea on exertion and orthopnea.
- Findings of tricuspid regurgitation on physical examination include a systolic murmur along the left lower sternal border that increases with inspiration, elevated jugular venous pressure with prominent V-wave, and (in severe cases) a pulsatile liver. Patients with right heart failure may also have abdominal distension and lower extremity edema.

Echocardiography

- **Classic findings of carcinoid heart disease are thickening, shortening, and retraction of the valve leaflets, resulting in incomplete coaptation and valvular regurgitation and/or stenosis. In some patients, the leaflets are rigid and fixed in a semi-open position.**
- The tricuspid and pulmonic valves are most commonly involved. Moderate or severe tricuspid regurgitation is seen in 53% to 90% of patients with carcinoid heart disease (Fig. 4-2). Moderate or severe pulmonic stenosis and/or pulmonic regurgitation is seen in approximately 20% of patients with carcinoid heart disease (Fig. 4-3).[18,20]
- Severe tricuspid regurgitation is associated with a dense, often triangular spectral profile on continuous-wave Doppler examination as well as systolic flow reversal in the hepatic vein. Severity of valvular regurgitation and stenosis should be quantified according to standard practice guidelines.[9,22]

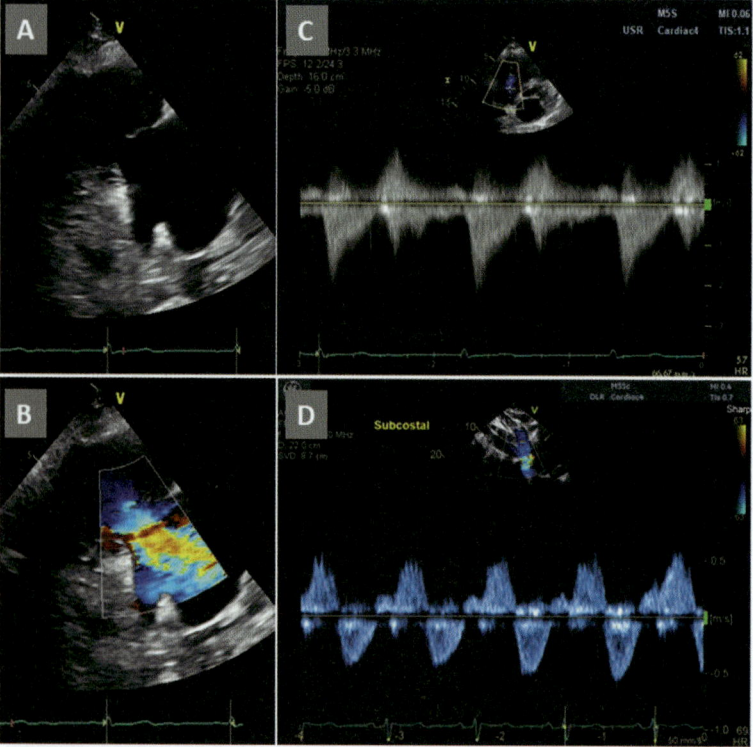

Figure 4-2. Echocardiographic findings of carcinoid heart disease: tricuspid regurgitation. Parasternal long-axis view of the tricuspid valve shows shortening and retraction of the valvular leaflets with fixed opening of the leaflet tips at end systole (A). Severe tricuspid regurgitation seen by color Doppler (B) and dense, triangular spectral profile on continuous-wave Doppler (C). Pulse wave Doppler of the hepatic vein shows systolic flow reversal, consistent with severe tricuspid regurgitation (D). (Images courtesy of Dr. Kathleen. W Zhang, Washington University in Saint Louis.)

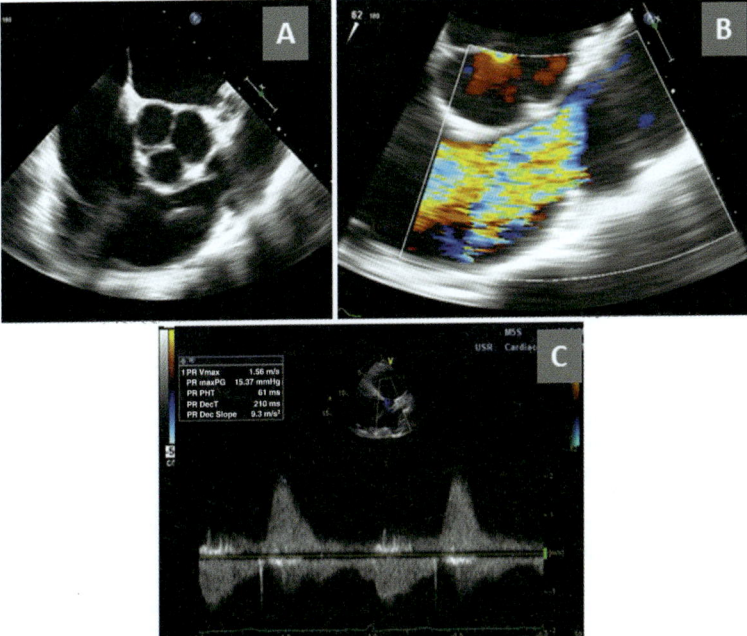

Figure 4-3. Echocardiographic findings of carcinoid heart disease: pulmonic regurgitation. Thickening and retraction of the pulmonic valve leaflets are seen on transesophageal echocardiography at end systole (A). Severe pulmonic regurgitation is seen by color Doppler (B) and continuous-wave Doppler (C). (Images courtesy of Dr. Kathleen W. Zhang, Washington University in Saint Louis.)

- Chronic, severe right-sided valvular regurgitation leads to right atrial and right ventricular enlargement, and eventually right ventricular dysfunction.

Cardiac Magnetic Resonance Imaging
- CMR is useful in patients with poor echocardiographic image quality or when accurate assessment of right ventricular function is needed. CMR can also help to quantify the severity of valvular dysfunction.

Laboratory Testing
- 24-hour urine 5-hydroxyindoleacetic acid (5-HIAA, a breakdown product of 5-HT) and plasma 5-HIAA levels are used to diagnose and monitor carcinoid syndrome. Diagnosis and management of patients with carcinoid syndrome should be performed in collaboration with a medical oncologist.
- Among patients with carcinoid syndrome, a 24-hour urine 5-HIAA level of >300 μmol is associated with a 2- to 3-fold increased risk of developing carcinoid heart disease.[23]
- N-terminal pro-brain natriuretic peptide (NT-proBNP) appears to be the best biomarker for screening patients with carcinoid syndrome for evidence of clinically

significant carcinoid heart disease. Among patients with carcinoid syndrome, an NT-proBNP cutoff level of 260 pg/mL had 92% sensitivity and 91% specificity for carcinoid heart disease.[24]

TREATMENT

- A multidisciplinary care team including cardiologists, cardiac surgeons, medical oncologists, and radiologists with experience in managing carcinoid heart disease is recommended for optimal clinical outcomes.
- Long-acting somatostatin analogs are the mainstay of therapy to reduce 5-HIAA levels and prevent development and/or progression of carcinoid heart disease. In refractory cases, adjunctive therapies include interferon alfa, peptide receptor radionuclide therapy, and transcatheter arterial embolization.
- In patients with symptomatic carcinoid heart disease, loop diuretics should be used to treat symptoms of right and/or left heart failure.
- **In patients with advanced carcinoid heart disease, valve surgery is the most effective treatment option. Valve replacement is recommended for tricuspid and pulmonic disease, whereas valve repair may be feasible for mitral and aortic disease.**
  - The optimal timing of valve surgery is not known. In general, valve surgery should be considered in patients with stable carcinoid syndrome and symptomatic valvular disease.
  - The optimal type of valve prosthesis for carcinoid heart disease is not known. Mechanical valves are durable but require chronic anticoagulation, which increases the risk of bleeding in patients with extensive liver disease. Bioprosthetic valves are susceptible to premature degeneration because of vasoactive peptides secreted by the carcinoid tumor, and optimization of medical therapy for carcinoid syndrome is particularly important after bioprosthetic valve replacement.
  - To prevent carcinoid crisis perioperatively, patients should be treated with a continuous octreotide infusion at a rate of 50 to 100 μg/hour. Patients receiving high doses of octreotide should be monitored for bradycardia.[25]

OUTCOME/PROGNOSIS

- **Carcinoid heart disease is the major cause of morbidity and mortality in patients with carcinoid syndrome. Prompt diagnosis and timely surgical intervention are essential for optimal clinical outcomes.**
- Median survival for patients with carcinoid heart disease improved from 1.5 years in the 1980s to 4.4 years in the late 1990s, largely because of increased rates of cardiac surgery. Among 32 patients undergoing cardiac surgery for carcinoid heart disease from 2005 to 2015, survival rates were 75% at 1 year and 69% at 2 years.[26]
- Although earlier studies showed high perioperative mortality rates (30%-60%) primarily because of postoperative bleeding and heart failure, surgical mortality rates have decreased to 10% to 13% in contemporary studies as a result of improved surgical technique and surgical experience.[26]
- Older age, tobacco use, worse New York Heart Association class, and right ventricular dilatation appear to be predictors of worse clinical outcomes in patients undergoing cardiac surgery for carcinoid heart disease.[26]

NONBACTERIAL THROMBOTIC ENDOCARDITIS

GENERAL PRINCIPLES

- **NBTE, also called marantic endocarditis, is a serious and potentially underdiagnosed condition associated with thrombophilia of malignancy. The most common malignancies associated with NBTE are lung, pancreatic, and gastric malignancies, as well as adenocarcinomas of unknown primary sites.**[27]
- NBTE is characterized by deposition of small (1-5 mm) sterile, loosely attached thrombi along the lines of valve closure, which are not associated with bacteremia or valvular destruction (Fig. 4-4).
- The main clinical manifestation of NBTE is systemic thromboembolism, particularly recurrent or multiple ischemic cerebrovascular strokes.
- A high index of suspicion is required for the diagnosis of NBTE. Patients with new cardiac murmurs or suspected cardioembolic stroke should be evaluated with transthoracic and/or transesophageal echocardiography for valvular vegetations. Transesophageal echocardiography has higher sensitivity for valvular vegetations and is the preferred diagnostic test when the pretest probability of disease is high. Infective endocarditis must be excluded.
- **Treatment of NBTE consists of therapy directed at the underlying malignancy as well as systemic anticoagulation. Unfractionated heparin and low-molecular-weight heparin are preferred anticoagulants; recurrent thromboembolic events have been reported on warfarin therapy and the efficacy of the novel oral anticoagulants for treatment of NBTE is not known.**[27]
- Cardiac surgery may be considered in carefully selected patients.

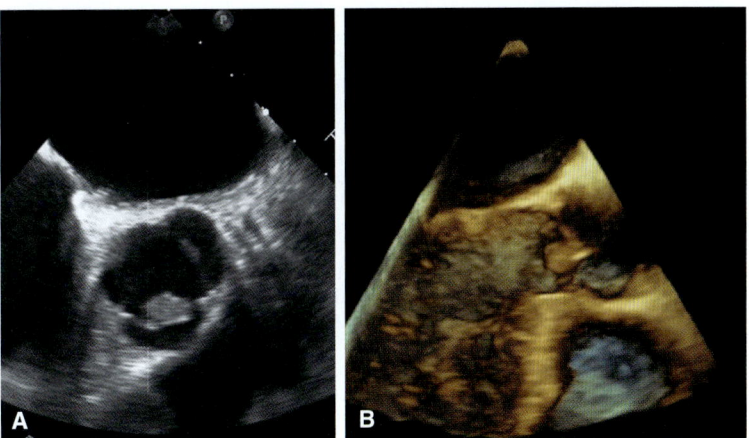

Figure 4-4. Echocardiographic findings of Nonbacterial Thrombotic Endocarditis (NBTE). Transesophageal echocardiogram from a patient with NBTE showing vegetation on right coronary cusp (A) as well as three-dimensional reconstruction (B). (Images courtesy of Dr. Kathleen W. Zhang, Washington University in Saint Louis.)

REFERENCES

1. Otto CM, Nishimura RA, Bonow RO, et al. 2020 ACC/AHA guideline for the management of patients with valvular heart disease: a report of the American College of Cardiology/American Heart Association Joint Committee on Clinical Practice Guidelines. *Circulation*. 2021;143(5):e72-e227. doi:10.1161/cir.0000000000000923
2. Landes U, Iakobishvili Z, Vronsky D, et al. Transcatheter aortic valve replacement in oncology patients with severe aortic stenosis. *JACC Cardiovasc Interv*. 2019;12(1):78-86. doi:10.1016/j.jcin.2018.10.026
3. Cella L, Liuzzi R, Conson M, et al. Dosimetric predictors of asymptomatic heart valvular dysfunction following mediastinal irradiation for Hodgkin's lymphoma. *Radiother Oncol*. 2011;101(2):316-321. doi:10.1016/j.radonc.2011.08.040
4. Cutter DJ, Schaapveld M, Darby SC, et al. Risk for valvular heart disease after treatment for hodgkin lymphoma. *J Natl Cancer Inst*. 2015;107(4):1-9. doi:10.1093/jnci/djv008
5. Heidenreich PA, Hancock SL, Lee BK, Mariscal CS, Schnittger I. Asymptomatic cardiac disease following mediastinal irradiation. *J Am Coll Cardiol*. 2003;42(4):743-749. doi:10.1016/S0735-1097(03)00759-9
6. Atkins KM, Rawal B, Chaunzwa TL, et al. Cardiac radiation dose, cardiac disease, and mortality in patients with lung cancer. *J Am Coll Cardiol*. 2019;73(23):2976-2987. doi:10.1016/j.jacc.2019.03.500
7. McGale P, Darby SC, Hall P, et al. Incidence of heart disease in 35,000 women treated with radiotherapy for breast cancer in Denmark and Sweden. *Radiother Oncol*. 2011;100(2):167-175. doi:10.1016/j.radonc.2011.06.016
8. Mulrooney DA, Yeazel MW, Kawashima T, et al. Cardiac outcomes in a cohort of adult survivors of childhood and adolescent cancer: retrospective analysis of the childhood cancer survivor study cohort. *BMJ*. 2009;339. doi:10.1136/bmj.b4606
9. Zoghbi WA, Adams D, Bonow RO, et al. Recommendations for noninvasive evaluation of native valvular regurgitation: a report from the American Society of Echocardiography developed in collaboration with the Society for Cardiovascular Magnetic Resonance. *J Am Soc Echocardiogr*. 2017;30(4):303-371. doi:10.1016/j.echo.2017.01.007
10. Baumgartner H, Hung J, Bermejo J, et al. Recommendations on the echocardiographic assessment of aortic valve stenosis: a focused update from the European Association of Cardiovascular Imaging and the American Society of Echocardiography. *J Am Soc Echocardiogr*. 2017;30(4):372-392. doi:10.1016/j.echo.2017.02.009
11. Wu W, Masri A, Popovic ZB, et al. Long-term survival of patients with radiation heart disease undergoing cardiac surgery: a cohort study. *Circulation*. 2013;127(14):1476-1484. doi:10.1161/CIRCULATIONAHA.113.001435
12. Desai MY, Windecker S, Lancellotti P, et al. Prevention, diagnosis, and management of radiation-associated cardiac disease: JACC Scientific Expert Panel. *J Am Coll Cardiol*. 2019;74(7):905-927. doi:10.1016/j.jacc.2019.07.006
13. Zhang D, Guo W, Al-Hijji MA, et al. Outcomes of patients with severe symptomatic aortic valve stenosis after chest radiation: transcatheter versus surgical aortic valve replacement. *J Am Heart Assoc*. 2019;8(10):e012110. doi:10.1161/JAHA.119.012110
14. Elbadawi A, Albaeni A, Elgendy IY, et al. Transcatheter versus surgical aortic valve replacement in patients with prior mediastinal radiation. *JACC Cardiovasc Interv*. 2020;13(22):2658-2666. doi:10.1016/j.jcin.2020.08.010
15. Ejiofor JI, Ramirez-Del Val F, Nohria A, et al. The risk of reoperative cardiac surgery in radiation-induced valvular disease. *J Thorac Cardiovasc Surg*. 2017;154(6):1883-1895. doi:10.1016/j.jtcvs.2017.07.033
16. Desai MY, Wu W, Masri A, et al. Increased aorto-mitral curtain thickness independently predicts mortality in patients with radiation-associated cardiac disease undergoing cardiac surgery. *Ann Thorac Surg*. 2014;97(4):1348-1355. doi:10.1016/j.athoracsur.2013.12.029
17. Lancellotti P, Nkomo VT, Badano LP, et al. Expert consensus for multi-modality imaging evaluation of cardiovascular complications of radiotherapy in adults: a report from the

European Association of Cardiovascular Imaging and the American Society of Echocardiography. *J Am Soc Echocardiogr*. 2013;26(9):1013-1032. doi:10.1016/j.echo.2013.07.005
18. Pellikka PA, Tajik AJ, Khandheria BK, et al. Carcinoid heart disease: clinical and echocardiographic spectrum in 74 patients. *Circulation*. 1993;87(4):1188-1196. doi:10.1161/01.cir.87.4.1188
19. Bernheim AM, Connolly HM, Hobday TJ, Abel MD, Pellikka PA. Carcinoid heart disease. *Prog Cardiovasc Dis*. 2007;49(6):439-451. doi:10.1016/j.pcad.2006.12.002
20. Bhattacharyya S, Toumpanakis C, Caplin ME, Davar J. Analysis of 150 patients with carcinoid syndrome seen in a single year at one institution in the first decade of the twenty-first century. *Am J Cardiol*. 2008;101(3):378-381. doi:10.1016/j.amjcard.2007.08.045
21. Bhattacharyya S, Davar J, Dreyfus G, Caplin ME. Carcinoid heart disease. *Circulation*. 2007;116(24):2860-2865. doi:10.1161/CIRCULATIONAHA.107.701367
22. Baumgartner H, Hung J, Bermejo J, et al. Echocardiographic assessment of valve stenosis: EAE/ASE recommendations for clinical practice. *J Am Soc Echocardiogr*. 2009;22(1):1-23. doi:10.1016/j.echo.2008.11.029
23. Bhattacharyya S, Toumpanakis C, Chilkunda D, Caplin ME, Davar J. Risk factors for the development and progression of carcinoid heart disease. *Am J Cardiol*. 2011;107(8):1221-1226. doi:10.1016/j.amjcard.2010.12.025
24. Bhattacharyya S, Toumpanakis C, Caplin ME, Davar J. Usefulness of N-terminal pro-brain natriuretic peptide as a biomarker of the presence of carcinoid heart disease. *Am J Cardiol*. 2008;102(7):938-942. doi:10.1016/j.amjcard.2008.05.047
25. Davar J, Connolly HM, Caplin ME, et al. Diagnosing and managing carcinoid heart disease in patients with neuroendocrine tumors: an expert statement. *J Am Coll Cardiol*. 2017;69(10):1288-1304. doi:10.1016/j.jacc.2016.12.030
26. Hassan SA, Banchs J, Iliescu C, Dasari A, Lopez-Mattei J, Yusuf SW. Carcinoid heart disease. *Heart*. 2017;103(19):1488-1495. doi:10.1136/heartjnl-2017-311261
27. El-Shami K, Griffiths E, Streiff M. Nonbacterial thrombotic endocarditis in cancer patients: pathogenesis, diagnosis, and treatment. *Oncologist*. 2007;12(5):518-523. doi:10.1634/theoncologist.12-5-518

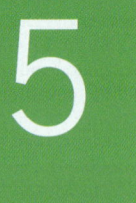

Vascular Disease in Cardio-Oncology

Prashanth D. Thakker and Ronald J. Krone

*This chapter discusses vascular pathologies associated with cancer or cancer therapy such as **superior vena cava (SVC) syndrome, coronary vasospasm, atherosclerosis,** and **acute coronary syndrome (ACS)** along with the management of these pathologies.*

GENERAL PRINCIPLES

- Patients with cancer are at increased risk for cardiovascular complications because of the effect of cancer therapy (both systemic therapy and radiation) and increased inflammation associated with the underlying malignancy. In addition, because cancer and atherosclerosis are prevalent in older populations, and may share risk factors, especially smoking, cancer patients may have a high incidence of occult cardiac or vascular disease.
- Interactions with the vascular system are common in patients with cancer, as the result of external compression on great vessels, chemotherapy-exacerbated endothelial injury, direct vessel injury, or accelerated atherosclerosis.
- Clinical management of ACS in a patient with cancer can be particularly challenging given the increased risk of both thrombosis and thrombocytopenia, as well as the need to balance intervention with the continued treatment of the malignancy, especially the need for curative cancer surgery.

SUPERIOR VENA CAVA SYNDROME

GENERAL PRINCIPLES

- **SVC syndrome** is a clinical sequela **of direct compression or occlusion** of the **SVC** with the production of elevated pressures in the veins draining the arms and head.
- Malignancy accounts for approximately 70% of cases of SVC obstruction, of which 50% are secondary to non–small cell lung cancer, 25% small cell lung cancer, and 25% secondary to lymphomas and other concerns.[1] Thrombosis because of indwelling catheters and devices accounts for the rest.
- Etiology of compression can vary and can be due to a right-sided mass, paratracheal or carinal lymph nodes.
- Obstruction without compression can be due to intravascular tumor, which is rare, or intravascular thrombus, which is more common.

DIAGNOSIS

Clinical Presentation and Initial Evaluation
- Obstruction of the SVC usually presents **with upper body swelling** involving the neck, the upper extremities, the face, or the chest. Dyspnea from **laryngeal edema** or neurologic symptoms is a major concern. Patients can at times present with more subtle changes along with sinus tachycardia and increased dyspnea on exertion and/or increased headaches or symptoms of head fullness (Table 5-1).
- In chronic cases, **dilated visible collateral vessels** can be seen over the right chest. In more severe cases, neurologic symptoms such as headaches, dizziness, confusion, obtundation, and mental status changes can manifest because of cerebral edema and constitute an emergent situation.[2]
- The appearance of laryngeal edema with stridor or mental symptoms is an emergency requiring prompt opening of the obstruction because coma and death are possible.[3,4]
- **Computed tomography (CT)** and **magnetic resonance imaging (MRI)** are the imaging modalities of choice for the evaluation of SVC syndrome.
- Contrast-enhanced CT imaging is helpful in distinguishing thrombus and the extent of venous obstruction as well as evaluating the lungs for cancer, and hence the most effective treatment modality (Fig. 5-1).
- MRI is useful in distinguishing thrombus from tumor or fibrosis but is not usually required if the distinction can be made in other ways.

TABLE 5-1　Kishi Score to Evaluate Superior Vena Cava Syndrome

Clinical signs	Score
Awareness disorders or coma	4
Visual disorders, headache, vertigo, or memory disorders	3
Mental disorders	2
Malaise	1
Orthopnea or laryngeal edema	3
Stridor, dysphagia, or dyspnea	2
Coughing or pleurisy	1
Lip edema, nasal obstruction, epistaxis	2
Facial edema	1
Neck, face, arm vessel dilation	1

More severe cases involving laryngeal edema, edema of face or lips, and mental disorders can develop, including headache, memory, or attention issues and in severe cases coma from cerebral edema. The appearance of laryngeal edema and stridor or mental symptoms can be considered an emergency requiring prompt opening of the obstruction. A score of 4 or higher is indicative of a need for urgent relief of obstructive symptoms or urgent lowering of venous pressure.

Derived from Kishi K, Sonomura T, Mitsuzane K, et al. Self-expandable metallic stent therapy for superior vena cava syndrome: clinical observations. *Radiology*. 1993;189:531-535.

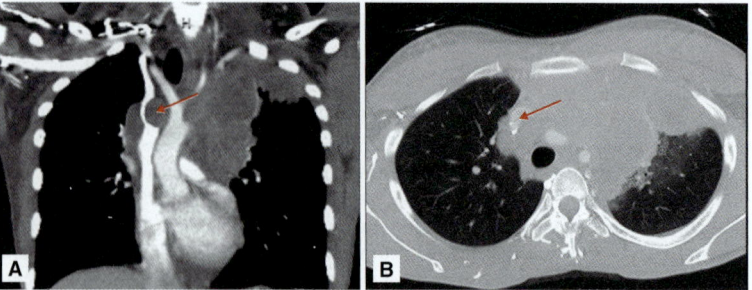

Figure 5-1. Superior vena cava (SVC) syndrome because of extrinsic compression and thrombus. An anterior mediastinal mass compresses the SVC with mass extension causing severe stenosis (A, red arrow). In addition to extrinsic compression, bland thrombus with a venous catheter is seen within the SVC (B, red arrow).

- The presence of an indwelling catheter in the SVC is usually a good presumption that thrombus may be the etiology of obstruction.

MANAGEMENT

- **Emergent symptom management** is crucial in patients with neurologic deterioration or respiratory compromise because of laryngeal edema.
- **Percutaneous intervention** with stent placement or catheter-directed thrombolytic therapy is often rapidly effective in relieving the obstruction. **Percutaneous thrombectomy** can also be considered in favorable cases. Adjunctive steroid therapy may be considered especially in the setting of laryngeal or cerebral edema.[2,5]
- If a device-related occlusion is identified, the lead or line must be removed and a subsequent stent placed to relieve the obstruction. If there is significant clot burden and concern for distal embolization, thrombectomy should be considered prior to line or lead removal.
- **Chemo-radiosensitive tumors may rapidly respond to appropriate treatment**, but biopsy should be obtained to confirm diagnosis prior to treatment if the obstruction is not life threatening.
- If a stent is placed, the patient will require aspirin, anticoagulation, and a P2Y12 inhibitor for a short time. Data guiding decision-making regarding duration of anticoagulation are limited and practice varies by institution.
- Management of SVC syndrome usually requires multispecialty consultation with radiologists to establish the etiology, an interventionalist to place the stent and consider thrombectomy, surgeons or interventional radiologists to deal with the biopsy, and the oncologist to define definitive treatment.

CORONARY VASOSPASM AND 5-FLUOROURACIL

GENERAL PRINCIPLES

- Vasospasm has been observed with 5-fluorouracil (5-FU) administration with clinical, biochemical, and electrocardiographic (ECG) findings consistent with myocardial ischemia in the absence of obstructive coronary disease.

- The incidence of 5-FU-induced vasospasm is variable, and studies have reported serious adverse effects to be around 1% to 5%.[6]
- The prevalence of silent ischemia in patients treated with 5-FU has been shown to be approximately 14%, with ACS seen in approximately 5% of patients.
- The mechanism of vasospasm is thought to originate with **endothelial dysfunction**, leading to **abnormal vasodilatory response and paradoxical vasoconstriction**. In addition to endothelial dysfunction, smooth muscle dysfunction has also been independently implicated in causing coronary vasoconstriction.[7] This also occurs with the administration of capecitabine, a prodrug that is converted through enzymatic action in the tumor to 5-FU.
- Microvascular dysfunction and direct cellular damage of the myocardium can play a concomitant role in 5-FU cardiac toxicity.[7]

DIAGNOSIS

Clinical Presentation

- Traditional cardiac risk factors have shown to play a role in potentiating **endothelial** and **smooth muscle dysfunction** in patients treated with 5-FU.
- Patients undergoing 5-FU infusion usually present with **angina** and may have associated **dyspnea** or **palpitations**. These symptoms can occur during rest or with exertion.
- Asymptomatic myocardial ischemia can often be demonstrated on ECG.
- Symptoms often appear during the first cycle of administration, manifesting during the infusion or within 72 hours of completion.
- Symptoms usually improve after discontinuation of 5-FU.[7]

MANAGEMENT AND CLINICAL FOLLOW-UP

- Prior to the initiation of 5-FU or capecitabine, an evaluation of cardiac risk factors is essential. **Hyperlipidemia, hypertension, diabetes**, and **smoking** should be evaluated and treated aggressively.
- **Low-dose aspirin**, if platelets permit, should be considered.
- In the setting of angina, it is important to determine if the patient has myocardial injury by obtaining an ECG and high-sensitivity troponin.
  - The infusion must be stopped to prevent further ischemia.
  - If there is a concern for underlying coronary disease, a **coronary angiogram** or **coronary CT angiogram** should be obtained to rule out severe, obstructive coronary artery disease and revascularization should be considered before proceeding with the chemotherapy.
  - If the patient has symptoms even without ECG findings or biomarkers, the infusion must be still stopped, and nitrates and/or **non-dihydropyridine calcium channel blockers (diltiazem or verapamil)** should be initiated before resuming therapy. Noninvasive testing with **CT angiography** or **stress testing** is recommended.
  - If there is evidence of myocardial injury, observation in a cardiac unit is advised for at least 24 hours.
- The decision to rechallenge with 5-FU depends on the importance of continuing with 5-FU and the severity of the coronary response.
  - **Vasodilators with nitrates** and **calcium channel blockers**, especially non-dihydropyridine, are recommended to pretreat patients in these instances.

- Historically, **recurrence of symptoms or cardiotoxicity is as high as 90% with a non-insignificant fatality rate in patients rechallenged with 5-FU**.[7] This must be considered when planning to proceed with a rechallenge, though rechallenging has increasingly been more successful with optimal management.[8]
- If rechallenging, consider bolus 5-FU, lowering the dose, or switching to capecitabine. Close monitoring (with ECG) and cessation of therapy with first signs of cardiotoxicity are key. Our approach to rechallenge is to **pretreat with a calcium blocker**, usually diltiazem, to a dose limited by heart rate and blood pressure prior to rechallenge. **Long-acting nitrates** are also usually used and sublingual nitroglycerine is used to promptly treat any anginal or ischemic symptoms. Close collaboration with the treating oncologist is essential, with availability to the patient during the infusion.
- These precautions are usually effective and permit completion of the treatment.

ACCELERATED ATHEROSCLEROSIS

GENERAL PRINCIPLES

- **Inflammatory processes** are associated with accelerated atherosclerosis. As such, oncologic processes and treatments portend a higher risk for atherosclerosis and establish the basis for careful cardiac evaluation and treatment for cardiac risk factors prior to the development of symptomatic disease.
- Treatments that specifically increase inflammation include **radiation therapy (RT), tyrosine kinase inhibitors (TKIs), vascular endothelial growth factor (VEGF) inhibitors, and immune checkpoint inhibitors (ICIs)**. Patients who have undergone **stem cell transplant** and **develop graft-versus-host disease (GVHD)** with ongoing inflammation also tend to have a higher risk of developing premature atherosclerosis.
- A careful evaluation for potential risk factors prior to chemotherapy, which includes **hyperlipidemia with a low-density lipoprotein (LDL) cholesterol >100, strong family history, hypertension, diabetes, and smoking history**, should be done. These factors need to be recognized and corrected. The target for cholesterol can be modified according to risk and in high-risk patients a **lower LDL target can be set, usually <70 mg/m^2**. In patients who have had a chest CT, calcification in the specific coronary arteries and thoracic and abdominal aorta can be used to evaluate risk. (This is often not included in the report, so the CT needs to be reviewed by the cardio-oncologist.)
- Patients who are prone to developing atherosclerosis are often asymptomatic, hence a high degree of clinical suspicion is key in identifying these patients early so that optimal therapy can be introduced and hopefully will reduce the likelihood of progression.

Radiation Therapy

- RT is used as a neoadjuvant or adjuvant treatment for multiple lung, breast, head, and neck malignancies in approximately 40% to 50% of patients undergoing treatment.[9]
- RT, mechanistically, is responsible for **promoting inflammation and causing accelerated atherosclerosis and endothelial dysfunction**, leading to micro- and macrovascular damage.[10]

- The effect on the coronary vasculature is related to the radiation dose, length of treatment, and proximity to the myocardium. Patients treated for breast cancer especially of the left breast, patients of younger age (<35 years) at the time of RT, and patients with increased volume of radiation (>30-35 Gy) seem to have a higher predisposition for promoting accelerated atherosclerosis.[11,12] Patients treated for Hodgkin disease with high-dose mediastinal radiation are at particularly high risk for these effects.[13]
- The impact of radiation-induced cardiovascular disease is not limited to the coronaries and can cause **severe valvulopathy** (usually thickened fibrotic and ultimately stenosis of the mitral, aortic, and tricuspid valve, or aortic valve fibrosis with regurgitation), pericardial disease, and affect the **mediastinal vasculature** (such as carotid and subclavian stenosis). Radiation to the chest also has implications for coronary surgery with damage to the internal mammary arteries plus concerns for sternal wound healing. Possible silent **subclavian stenosis** may limit flow down the internal mammary artery leading to coronary steal if this artery is used for revascularization and carotid stenosis needs to be evaluated before surgery (Fig. 5-2).
- Traditional risk factors such as **obesity, hypertension, tobacco use, diabetes mellitus, and hyperlipidemia** increase the risk of developing atherosclerosis.

Graft-Versus-Host Disease

- **GVHD** is a known complication of hematopoietic stem cell transplantation. GVHD is the result of immune activation of donor T cells on host tissues leading to a proinflammatory state resulting in tissue damage.[14] Fibrosis of the lungs, skin, and thickening of the bowel leading to malabsorption states are frequent.
- Cardiac involvement includes **bradyarrhythmia, cardiomyopathy**, and **coronary intimal hyperplasia**.[15]
- Coronary involvement in patients with GVHD has been thought to be the result of the inflammatory and immune-reactive mechanism of GVHD. Patients have been found to have significant coronary luminal narrowing with intimal proliferation as well as coronary artery disease with atheromatous plaque formation in more chronic forms of GVHD.[14,15]
- Symptoms of angina may not be present even with severe disease and so aggressive evaluation of coronary arteries with the development of symptoms of ischemia or new ECG findings or new heart failure is crucial. Noninvasive evaluation with **CT angiography** or **stress testing** with echocardiography or myocardial perfusion single-photon emission CT (SPECT) is a good approach in appropriate individuals. In patients with symptoms of ischemia or with ischemia on noninvasive tests, coronary angiography is more definitive and can determine need and potential for revascularization.

Nilotinib and other BCR-ABL Tyrosine Kinase Inhibitors

- **Nilotinib**, a second-generation Bcr-Abl TKI, the abnormal tyrosine kinase created by the Philadelphia chromosome abnormality in chronic myeloid leukemia (CML), is implicated to alter endothelial function by increasing expression of cell adhesion molecules (CAMs) leading to proatherogenic changes in the vessel wall.[16]
- Early studies revealed an increased incidence of **peripheral arterial disease** in patients undergoing treatment with nilotinib requiring early invasive therapy or

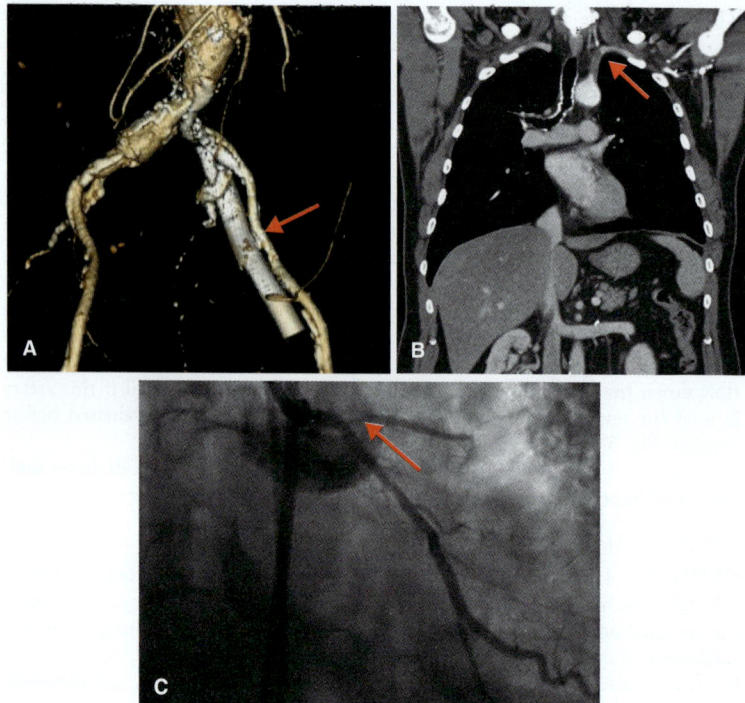

Figure 5-2. Radiation-induced vascular disease. Peripheral atherosclerosis and left iliac vein occlusion with stent placement because of pelvic radiation (A, red arrow). Chest radiation–induced left subclavian stenosis (B, red arrow). Subtotal occlusion of the left anterior descending artery in a young patient because of prior chest radiation and chronic graft-versus-host disease (C, red arrow).

amputation.[17] In addition, long-term follow-up of patients on nilotinib, as well as other second-generation Bcr-Abl TKIs, as compared to imatinib, a first-generation Bcr-Abl TKI, revealed a significantly higher risk of arterial ischemic events.[18] Close monitoring for peripheral and coronary vascular disease is thus important in this subset of patients as well as careful control of coronary risk factors, especially cholesterol.

Immune Checkpoint Inhibitors

- Approximately 44% of patients with cancer have an indication for ICIs and these indications are continually expanding. A recent retrospective study found a threefold higher risk of atherosclerotic cardiovascular events in patients treated with ICI with matched controls. An imaging substudy was notable for **accelerated atherosclerosis** as seen by an increase in the rate of progression of total aortic plaque volume in patients treated with ICI when compared to matched controls. In addition, these risks were higher in patients who were older and had diabetes, hypertension, and prior radiation treatment.[19]

- It is proposed that the cardiovascular implications for these therapies are mostly driven by inhibition of programmed cell death protein 1 (PD-1), programmed death-ligand 1 (PD-L1), and cytotoxic T-lymphocyte-associated protein 4 (CTLA-4), which act as negative regulators of atherosclerosis. The general inflammatory state promoted by this process occasionally leads to myocarditis and is presumably the mechanism for increased coronary events. **Myocarditis** because of an ICI is frequently extremely serious, with a case fatality rate approaching 50%. This is discussed in more detail elsewhere.

CLINICAL PRESENTATION

- Patients with a history of mediastinal radiation or therapies that potentiate atherosclerosis are at increased risk for coronary disease, so presurgical evaluation needs to keep this in mind and consider evaluation for silent severe disease.[20] Diagnostic workup may involve imaging, such as a **coronary CT angiography** or **functional studies** to assess for ischemia.
- Patients facing stressful therapy, especially high-risk surgery, require ischemic evaluation with coronary CT imaging or stress testing depending on their functional status and symptom profile.

  Coronary angiography may be needed if adequate noninvasive imaging is not possible. If ischemia is identified noninvasively, then coronary angiography is indicated. If the cancer or treatment involves thrombocytopenia, then a radial approach where hemostasis is better should be considered.

MANAGEMENT

- Aggressive risk factor modification and treatment of traditional risk factors with reduction of **LDL <70 mg/dL, smoking cessation, and appropriate blood pressure control** are essential. Selection of statins that are not metabolized by the CYP3A4 pathway (ie, rosuvastatin or pravastatin) is recommended if interaction with chemotherapy or direct oral anticoagulants (DOACs) is anticipated.
- Medical management with **lipid-lowering therapy, antianginals, and antiplatelets** is indicated. Coronary angiography with percutaneous intervention is appropriate in patients with symptoms refractory to medical therapy or with unstable symptoms. Surgical revascularization is necessary in selected situations, but usually this is restricted to severe ischemic disease untreatable percutaneously.
- Revascularization should be reserved for patients with symptoms refractory to medical management, severe left main disease, or multivessel disease with reduced ejection fraction.[21,22]

ACUTE CORONARY SYNDROME

GENERAL PRINCIPLES

- **ACS** in patients with active cancer presents unique challenges. In addition to baseline risk factors for coronary artery disease, various chemotherapeutic agents predispose patients to accelerated atherosclerosis and vasospasm.

Cisplatin and Platinum Compounds

Cisplatin and other platinum compounds, through **procoagulant and direct endothelial dysfunction, have been implicated to be thrombogenic**. Multiple studies have identified cisplatin as an agent that potentiates coronary artery disease in cancer survivors.[23,24] In a large retrospective analysis, 18.1% of patients had a thrombogenic event and of these 11.3% had arterial thrombi.[25] Approximately 2% of patients in this study had either myocardial or cerebrovascular ischemia.

Vascular Endothelial Growth Factor Inhibitors

- VEGF inhibitors, such as bevacizumab, lead to endothelial dysfunction and through various mechanisms promote thrombosis.[26]
- VEGF inhibitors increase the risk of **cardiac ischemia and ACS given the increased incidence of arterial thrombosis with these chemotherapeutic agents.**
- There was no dose-effect relationship seen with arterial thromboembolism as is seen with VEGF inhibitor–associated hypertension.[27,28]

CLINICAL MANAGEMENT CONSIDERATIONS IN PATIENTS WITH ACUTE CORONARY SYNDROME

- Patients presenting with **ST-elevation myocardial infarction (STEMI)** will require immediate **coronary angiography and percutaneous intervention** to the culprit vessel to salvage myocardium. High-risk non-STEMI ACS is best handled with early angiography and percutaneous intervention.
- Coronary intervention requires patients to be anticoagulated with **systemic heparin, low-molecular-weight heparin, or direct thrombin inhibitors** during the procedure. In addition, patients will need to remain on antiplatelet therapy for some period of time post–percutaneous intervention. Because of the high incidence of mortality and disability in patients with STEMIs, intervention should proceed unless contraindicated. In patients with non-STEMI ACS, consultation with the oncologist can be helpful in planning strategy (Fig. 5-3).

REVASCULARIZATION IN ACUTE CORONARY SYNDROME IN THE SETTING OF THROMBOCYTOPENIA

- **Thrombocytopenia** possesses a unique challenge in this patient population. The frequency of thrombocytopenia is 10% to 25% in patients with solid tumors on chemotherapy as well as with acute leukemia, lymphoma, myelodysplastic syndrome, and multiple myeloma.[29] The risk varies according to the type of cancer and anticipated therapy.
- Management strategy varies in patients based on platelet count and expected nadir (Table 5-2). Patients presenting with unstable coronary syndromes warrant coronary evaluation and consideration for percutaneous intervention (Fig. 5-3). A radial approach, if feasible, should be the access of choice to reduce the risk of bleeding and access site complications. Recently published retrospective data from MD Anderson Cancer Center revealed the safety of coronary angiography and percutaneous intervention in patients presenting with ACS.[30]
- **Intravascular imaging with percutaneous intervention** optimizes stent placement and can minimize the risk of **stent thrombosis (ST)**.[31] In addition, the stent architecture and drug coating can also influence the duration of **dual antiplatelet therapy** (DAPT).
- The stent **type and duration of DAPT** are more controversial and continue to evolve. Recently, multiple studies have demonstrated the efficacy of shorter duration

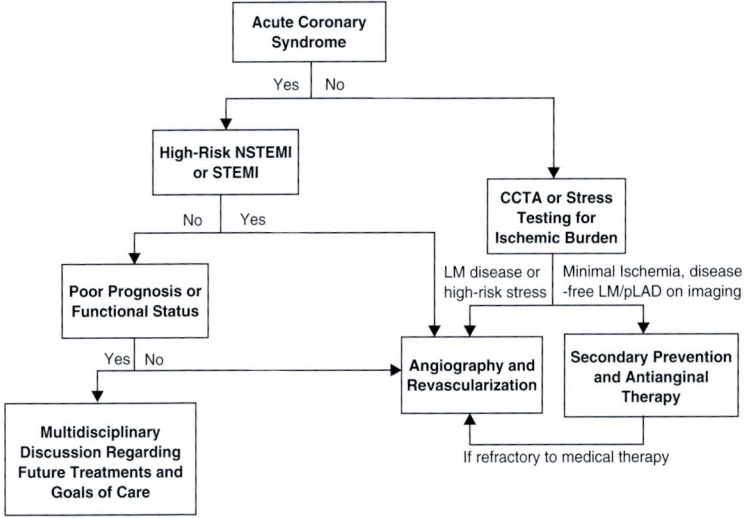

Figure 5-3. Management of cardio-oncology patients with symptoms concerning for coronary artery disease. CCTA, coronary computed tomography angiography; LM, left main coronary artery; NSTEMI, non–ST-segment elevation myocardial infarction; pLAD, proximal left anterior descending artery; STEMI, ST-elevation myocardial infarction.

of DAPT in patients receiving newer-generation drug-eluting stents such as Resolute, Xience, Synergy, or Ultimaster stents where 1 to 3 months of DAPT therapy may be adequate. In all cases, optimal stent placement using intravascular ultrasound is recommended. This renders the need for bare metal stents (BMSs) obsolete.[32-34] These newer stents and studies were developed after the guidelines for DAPT were rewritten and are not reflected in the guidelines.[35] If **there is no concern about thrombocytopenia, then at least 6 months of DAPT is recommended in the setting of stable angina or 12 months in the setting of ACS**.

- The risk of **ST** and the risk of bleeding dictate the length of DAPT. Long stented segments, bifurcation disease, inadequate spent expansion, and edge dissections are lesion- and stent-related factors for ST. The use of **intravascular imaging and newer-generation stents** reduces the risk of in-stent thrombosis or target vessel revascularization and hence makes short duration of DAPT safe. Clear discussions with the interventional cardiologist in determining the adequate length of DAPT is essential.
- The use of DAPT for a period of 4 weeks may be reasonable in patients with thrombocytopenia or with high bleeding risk post–percutaneous coronary intervention (PCI). Studies such as STOP-DAPT 2, ONYX One, and MASTER DAPT trials using the Xience, ONYX, or Ultimate stents, respectively, showed that one month of DAPT followed by monotherapy with clopidogrel (STOP-DAPT 2) or either aspirin or clopidogrel (ONYX ONE, MASTER DAPT) were non-inferior to longer therapy.[34,36]
- The **risks of cardiac events after noncardiac surgery are elevated after a stent**, regardless of the type of stent. The risk of these events is highest in the first month after stenting and decreases for 6 months when risk stabilizes regardless of the type of stent (BMS or DES). Current recommendations are to delay surgery optimally for

TABLE 5-2	Thrombocytopenia, Coronary Interventions, and Antiplatelet Management
Nadir platelet count	**Therapeutic management**
>10,000/μL	Monotherapy with aspirin for secondary prevention can be administered while monitoring for bleeding
>30,000/μL	DAPT with aspirin and clopidogrel can be continued for recent PCI
<50,000/μL	Multidisciplinary discussion regarding benefits of PCI and DAPT is warranted, low-dose heparin can be used for systemic anticoagulation (30-50 U/kg) when clinically indicated
>50,000/μL	DAPT and coronary interventions can be performed using bleeding avoidance strategies

DAPT, dual antiplatelet therapy; PCI, percutaneous coronary intervention.

Derived from Levine GN, Bates ER, Bittl JA, et al. 2016 ACC/AHA guideline focused update on duration of dual antiplatelet therapy in patients with coronary artery disease: a report of the American College of Cardiology/American Heart Association Task Force on Clinical Practice Guidelines. *J Am Coll Cardiol*. 2016;68:1082-1115; McCarthy CP, Steg G, Bhatt DL. The management of antiplatelet therapy in acute coronary syndrome patients with thrombocytopenia: a clinical conundrum. *Eur Heart J*. 2017;38:3488-3492; Schiffer CA, Bohlke K, Delaney M, et al. Platelet transfusion for patients with cancer: American Society of Clinical Oncology clinical practice guideline update. *J Clin Oncol*. 2018;36:283-299; Iliescu CA, Grines CL, Herrmann J, et al. SCAI expert consensus statement: evaluation, management, and special considerations of cardio-oncology patients in the cardiac catheterization laboratory (endorsed by the Cardiological Society of India, and Sociedad Latino Americana de Cardiologia Intervencionista). *Catheter Cardiovasc Interv*. 2016;87:E202-E223.

6 months after stenting. For cancer patients, this obviously means delaying possibly curative cancer surgery for 6 months if stenting is performed. Thus the recommendation for PCI, which requires delay of surgery, must be balanced against recommending coronary artery bypass graft (CABG) that has a shorter delay for curative surgery, which can be as short as 1 month post-CABG. In most cases, an exercise capacity >4 metabolic equivalents (METS) is acceptable for noncardiac surgery in patients with stable coronary disease.[20] Alternatively, in selected cases of stable coronary disease, revascularization can be postponed until after the cancer surgery or deferred until indicated by symptoms.[37] A multidisciplinary consultation is essential in planning the optimal strategy to treat both the coronary disease and the cancer.

REFERENCES

1. Friedman T, Quencer KB, Kishore SA, Winokur RS, Madoff DC. Malignant venous obstruction: superior vena cava syndrome and beyond. *Semin Intervent Radiol*. 2017;34:398-408.
2. Azizi AH, Shafi I, Shah N, et al. Superior vena cava syndrome. *JACC Cardiovasc Interv*. 2020;13:2896-2910.
3. Yu JB, Wilson LD, Detterbeck FC. Superior vena cava syndrome—a proposed classification system and algorithm for management. *J Thorac Oncol*. 2008;3:811-814.

4. Kishi K, Sonomura T, Mitsuzane K, et al. Self-expandable metallic stent therapy for superior vena cava syndrome: clinical observations. *Radiology.* 1993;189:531-535.
5. Straka C, Ying J, Kong FM, Willey CD, Kaminski J, Kim DW. Review of evolving etiologies, implications and treatment strategies for the superior vena cava syndrome. *Springerplus.* 2016;5:229.
6. Polk A, Vaage-Nilsen M, Vistisen K, Nielsen DL. Cardiotoxicity in cancer patients treated with 5-fluorouracil or capecitabine: a systematic review of incidence, manifestations and predisposing factors. *Cancer Treat Rev.* 2013;39:974-984.
7. Kanduri J, More LA, Godishala A, Asnani A. Fluoropyrimidine-associated cardiotoxicity. *Cardiol Clin.* 2019;37:399-405.
8. Padegimas A, Carver JR. How to diagnose and manage patients with fluoropyrimidine-induced chest pain. *JACC CardioOncol.* 2020;2:650-654.
9. Shoukat S, Zheng D, Yusuf SW. Cardiotoxicity related to radiation therapy. *Cardiol Clin.* 2019;37:449-458.
10. Raghunathan D, Khilji MI, Hassan SA, Yusuf SW. Radiation-induced cardiovascular disease. *Curr Atheroscler Rep.* 2017;19:22.
11. McGale P, Darby SC, Hall P, et al. Incidence of heart disease in 35,000 women treated with radiotherapy for breast cancer in Denmark and Sweden. *Radiother Oncol.* 2011;100:167-175.
12. Darby SC, Ewertz M, McGale P, et al. Risk of ischemic heart disease in women after radiotherapy for breast cancer. *N Engl J Med.* 2013;368:987-998.
13. Mulrooney DA, Nunnery SE, Armstrong GT, et al. Coronary artery disease detected by coronary computed tomography angiography in adult survivors of childhood Hodgkin lymphoma. *Cancer.* 2014;120:3536-3544.
14. Rackley C, Schultz KR, Goldman FD, et al. Cardiac manifestations of graft-versus-host disease. *Biol Blood Marrow Transplant.* 2005;11:773-780.
15. Dogan A, Dogdu O, Ozdogru I, et al. Cardiac effects of chronic graft-versus-host disease after stem cell transplantation. *Tex Heart Inst J.* 2013;40:428-434.
16. Manouchehri A, Kanu E, Mauro MJ, Aday AW, Lindner JR, Moslehi J. Tyrosine kinase inhibitors in leukemia and cardiovascular events: from mechanism to patient care. *Arterioscler Thromb Vasc Biol.* 2020;40:301-308.
17. Le Coutre P, Rea D, Abruzzese E, et al. Severe peripheral arterial disease during nilotinib therapy. *J Natl Cancer Inst.* 2011;103:1347-1348.
18. Moslehi JJ, Deininger M. Tyrosine kinase inhibitor-associated cardiovascular toxicity in chronic myeloid leukemia. *J Clin Oncol.* 2015;33:4210-4218.
19. Drobni ZD, Alvi RM, Taron J, et al. Association between immune checkpoint inhibitors with cardiovascular events and atherosclerotic plaque. *Circulation.* 2020;142:2299-2311.
20. Patel AY, Eagle KA, Vaishnava P. Cardiac risk of noncardiac surgery. *J Am Coll Cardiol.* 2015;66:2140-2148.
21. Al-Lamee R, Thompson D, Dehbi HM, et al. Percutaneous coronary intervention in stable angina (ORBITA): a double-blind, randomised controlled trial. *Lancet.* 2018;391:31-40.
22. Maron DJ, Hochman JS, Reynolds HR, et al. Initial invasive or conservative strategy for stable coronary disease. *N Engl J Med.* 2020;382:1395-1407.
23. Haugnes HS, Wethal T, Aass N, et al. Cardiovascular risk factors and morbidity in long-term survivors of testicular cancer: a 20-year follow-up study. *J Clin Oncol.* 2010;28:4649-4657.
24. Huddart RA, Norman A, Shahidi M, et al. Cardiovascular disease as a long-term complication of treatment for testicular cancer. *J Clin Oncol.* 2003;21:1513-1523.
25. Moore RA, Adel N, Riedel E, et al. High incidence of thromboembolic events in patients treated with cisplatin-based chemotherapy: a large retrospective analysis. *J Clin Oncol.* 2011;29:3466-3473.
26. Economopoulou P, Kotsakis A, Kapiris I, Kentepozidis N. Cancer therapy and cardiovascular risk: focus on bevacizumab. *Cancer Manag Res.* 2015;7:133-143.
27. Scappaticci FA, Skillings JR, Holden SN, et al. Arterial thromboembolic events in patients with metastatic carcinoma treated with chemotherapy and bevacizumab. *J Natl Cancer Inst.* 2007;99:1232-1239.

28. Ranpura V, Hapani S, Chuang J, Wu S. Risk of cardiac ischemia and arterial thromboembolic events with the angiogenesis inhibitor bevacizumab in cancer patients: a meta-analysis of randomized controlled trials. *Acta Oncol.* 2010;49:287-297.
29. Elting LS, Rubenstein EB, Martin CG, et al. Incidence, cost, and outcomes of bleeding and chemotherapy dose modification among solid tumor patients with chemotherapy-induced thrombocytopenia. *J Clin Oncol.* 2001;19:1137-1146.
30. Iliescu C, Balanescu DV, Donisan T, et al. Safety of diagnostic and therapeutic cardiac catheterization in cancer patients with acute coronary syndrome and chronic thrombocytopenia. *Am J Cardiol.* 2018;122:1465-1470.
31. Ong DS, Jang IK. Causes, assessment, and treatment of stent thrombosis—intravascular imaging insights. *Nat Rev Cardiol.* 2015;12:325-336.
32. Watanabe H, Domei T, Morimoto T, et al. Effect of 1-month dual antiplatelet therapy followed by clopidogrel vs 12-month dual antiplatelet therapy on cardiovascular and bleeding events in patients receiving PCI: the STOPDAPT-2 Randomized Clinical Trial. *JAMA.* 2019;321:2414-2427.
33. Varenne O, Cook S, Sideris G, et al. Drug-eluting stents in elderly patients with coronary artery disease (SENIOR): a randomised single-blind trial. *Lancet.* 2018;391:41-50.
34. Windecker S, Latib A, Kedhi E, et al. Polymer-based or polymer-free stents in patients at high bleeding risk. *N Engl J Med.* 2020;382:1208-1218.
35. Levine GN, Bates ER, Bittl JA, et al. 2016 ACC/AHA guideline focused update on duration of dual antiplatelet therapy in patients with coronary artery disease: a report of the American College of Cardiology/American Heart Association Task Force on Clinical Practice Guidelines. *J Am Coll Cardiol.* 2016;68:1082-1115.
36. Watanabe H, Domei T, Morimoto T, et al. Very short dual antiplatelet therapy after drug-eluting stent implantation in patients with high bleeding risk: insight from the STOPDAPT-2 trial. *Circulation.* 2019;140:1957-1959.
37. McFalls EO, Ward HB, Moritz TE, et al. Coronary-artery revascularization before elective major vascular surgery. *N Engl J Med.* 2004;351:2795-2804.
38. Iliescu CA, Grines CL, Herrmann J, et al. SCAI Expert consensus statement: evaluation, management, and special considerations of cardio-oncology patients in the cardiac catheterization laboratory (endorsed by the Cardiological Society of India, and Sociedad Latino Americana de Cardiologia Intervencionista). *Catheter Cardiovasc Interv.* 2016;87:E202-E223.
39. McCarthy CP, Steg G, Bhatt DL. The management of antiplatelet therapy in acute coronary syndrome patients with thrombocytopenia: a clinical conundrum. *Eur Heart J.* 2017;38:3488-3492.
40. Schiffer CA, Bohlke K, Delaney M, et al. Platelet transfusion for patients with cancer: American Society of Clinical Oncology clinical practice guideline update. *J Clin Oncol.* 2018;36:283-299.

6 Evaluation for Ischemic Heart Disease in Cardio-Oncology

Arick Park and Joshua D. Mitchell

GENERAL PRINCIPLES

- **Cancer patients are at increased risk for coronary artery disease (CAD) because of shared risk factors as well as cardiotoxic effects of their cancer therapy.**
- All patients with cancer should undergo a comprehensive baseline cardiovascular history and physical examination. Consideration for ischemic heart disease **begins with prevention** by identifying and optimizing cardiovascular risk factors as well as identifying asymptomatic CAD, such as with incidental **coronary artery calcifications (CACs) on computed tomography (CT)**.
- Cancer patients often have existing chest CT scans for either screening or surveillance, which provide important opportunities to simultaneously screen for CAC and help target preventive therapy (Fig. 6-1).
- Further evaluation for and management of ischemic heart disease should be done with **consideration for the patient's treatment** (prior, ongoing, and anticipated), **risk for bone marrow suppression**, **acuity of presentation**, and **cancer prognosis**.
- The evaluation and management of a patient with suspected or confirmed ischemic heart disease during cancer therapy should always be **multidisciplinary** in nature, with close **collaboration between oncology and cardiology**. The ultimate goal is to improve the quality of life and survival of the patient while minimizing interruptions in cancer treatment.

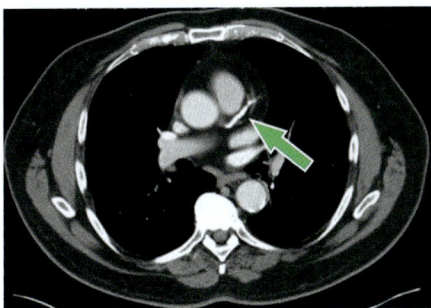

Figure 6-1. Extensive coronary artery calcification (arrow) is noted in the left anterior descending artery on a staging computed tomography scan in a patient with newly diagnosed prostate cancer. The patient eventually underwent three-vessel coronary artery bypass surgery after later developing unstable angina.

- The diagnosis of ischemic heart disease should never in itself be a contraindication to continuing life-prolonging cancer therapy, although cancer regimens with reduced cardiovascular toxicity and similar efficacy should be considered when available.

Definition

- Ischemic heart disease refers to the conditions arising from **coronary hypoperfusion** of myocardial tissue.
- The symptom of angina pectoris is the result of **myocardial oxygen demand exceeding supply** with the result of chest discomfort.
- Acute coronary syndrome (ACS), a subset of ischemic heart disease, is a medical emergency and is discussed in Chapter 5.

Classification

- Cardiac ischemia in cancer patients can be classified in a similar manner to cardiac ischemia in noncancer patients.
- Patients with ACS should be distinguished from those with stable or **chronic coronary syndrome (CCS)** and should be treated with respect to their oncologic history.
- Traditionally, patients presenting with ACS have ST elevation myocardial infarction (MI), non–ST elevation MI, or unstable angina. The evaluation and treatment of ACS is discussed in Chapter 5.
- Patients with stable coronary syndrome can have **obstructive CAD** or **myocardial ischemia and no obstructive coronary artery disease (INOCA)**.
- Examples of INOCA include **coronary artery vasospasm** and **coronary microvascular dysfunction**.
- **Angina can be classified as typical, atypical, or noncardiac chest discomfort.** Typical cardiac chest pain is generally marked by chest pain that is substernal, worse with exercise, and relieved with rest or nitroglycerin. Noncardiac pain is chest discomfort that harbors none of the typical features.

Epidemiology

- Approximately 50% of deaths in the United States are from either heart disease or cancers.[1]
- Among patients with cancer, greater than one-third die from malignancy and one-tenth die from heart disease, with **cardiovascular disease being the leading competing cause of morbidity and mortality**. Overall, cancer patients have a 2- to 6-fold higher risk of cardiovascular disease when compared to the general population.[2]

Etiology

- Cancers disproportionately affect older patients, and as a result this patient population typically has more traditional risk factors for developing coronary atherosclerosis, the predominant etiology for myocardial ischemia.
- Certain **cancer therapies can also accelerate or exacerbate coronary hypoperfusion through atherosclerosis, vasospasm, endothelial dysfunction, or thrombogenesis** (see section that follows).
- Obstructive coronary disease is predominantly caused by **coronary arteriosclerosis**, which presents either chronically (stable angina) or acutely (ACS). ACS is the result of coronary plaque rupture, erosion, or coronary thromboembolization. This is discussed further in Chapter 5.

- **Demand ischemia** is a common phenomenon of coronary supply-demand mismatch leading to subendomyocardial ischemia and often troponin biomarker elevation.

Risk Factors

- In addition to **traditional cardiovascular risk factors** (eg, smoking, hypertension, hyperlipidemia, diabetes mellitus), patients with cancers are exposed to therapies that can accelerate atherosclerotic disease.
- Common examples of known proatherosclerotic cancer therapies include chest radiation, **small molecule kinase inhibitors** (eg, nilotinib, sorafenib, ponatinib), and **immune checkpoint inhibitors**.[3,4]
- Certain cancer therapies have also been associated with **vasospasm** (sorafenib, 5-fluorouracil [5-FU], paclitaxel, gemcitabine) and **coronary thrombosis** (cisplatin) in the absence of atherosclerosis.[4] In these settings, the patient often presents with ACS (see Chapter 5).
- Survivors of **Hodgkin lymphoma are 3.8-fold more likely to develop CAD** after receiving mediastinal radiation alone. Patients that receive both radiation and anthracycline therapy have a 4.5-fold increased risk of coronary disease. These patients also have an increased risk of anthracycline-induced cardiomyopathy.[5]
- Patients with **breast cancer** who are treated with **left-sided radiation have a 2.7-fold increased risk of coronary disease** when compared to those receiving right-sided radiation. They are also 2.1-fold more likely to experience chest pain and 3.1-fold more likely to develop MI.[6]
- As cancer therapies are continually evolving, the clinician should maintain a high index of suspicion for potential cardiovascular toxicity in new and emerging agents.
- Patients with cancer are also especially susceptible to **coronary supply-demand mismatch**. For example, patients often have **anemia** from chronic disease, chemotherapy bone **marrow suppression**, or invasive bone marrow infiltration and are also at significantly increased risk for infections and **tachyarrhythmias** associated with cancer therapy.

DIAGNOSIS

Clinical History

- Patients with cancer should be screened for ischemic heart disease through detailed history and physical examination. Asymptomatic patients may also be identified through recognition of CAC on available CT imaging.
- Symptomatic chest pain history should be further qualified **as typical, atypical, or noncardiac chest pain**. Certain descriptors of chest pain can raise or lower the likelihood of having ACS, which can also help risk-stratify patients with CCSs from noncardiac chest pain. **Typical chest pain is reproducible pain or discomfort that is substernal, worse with exertion, and relieved with rest**, although only some factors may be present in patients with CCS. Symptoms that reduce the likelihood of cardiac chest pain include a pleuritic or positional nature, nonexertional pain, or pain reproducible with palpitation, based on a study of patients presenting with ACS (Table 6-1).
- **Anginal or ischemic equivalent** symptoms include progressive dyspnea and fatigue.
- Exertional dyspnea, lower extremity edema, orthopnea, and paroxysmal nocturnal dyspnea are suggestive **symptoms of heart failure**. Patients with cancer are at

TABLE 6-1 Chest Pain History and Acute Coronary Syndrome

Association decreases likelihood

Chest pain descriptor	LR
Pleuritic	0.2
Positional	0.3
Sharp	0.3
Reproducible with palpation	0.3
Inframammary location	0.8
Nonexertional	0.8

LR, likelihood ratio. Reproduced from Swap CJ, Nagurney JT. Value and limitations of chest pain history in the evaluation of patients with suspected acute coronary syndromes. *JAMA*. 2005;294:2623-2629.

increased risk for both nonischemic and ischemic cardiomyopathies, although an appropriate evaluation for potential underlying obstructive CAD is appropriate in all patients with cancer presenting with cardiomyopathy (angiography vs. noninvasive testing).
- Classification of ischemic chest pain often relies on gathering accurate history and symptomatology. However, the evaluation of ischemic heart disease symptoms in patients with cancers can be challenging and **requires gathering a detailed oncologic history**. Cancer-related symptoms can often mask or mimic cardiac symptoms including metastatic bone pain, pulmonary pathology, and cancer or cancer therapy–related fatigue.

Laboratory Evaluation
Chronic Coronary Syndrome
- **Lipid panel**
- **Hemoglobin A1c**
- **C-reactive protein** is used more often in Europe and has limited data in patients with cancer, who were excluded from the JUPITER trial as they were more likely to have elevated baseline proinflammatory biomarkers.
- **Brain natriuretic peptide (BNP)** or NT-proBNP may be useful in screening for underlying ischemic cardiomyopathy.
- **Troponins** can be elevated in ischemia as well as infiltrative cardiomyopathies.
- Guideline-appropriate screening for chronic diseases (eg, human immunodeficiency virus [HIV]) that have increased risk for coronary disease
- **Antiphospholipid antibody**, **lupus anticoagulant**, and **Factor V Leiden** if there is concern for thromboembolic coronary disease

Approach to Diagnostic Testing
- In addition to invasive coronary angiography (ICA), there are multiple noninvasive modalities to evaluate for cardiac ischemia and CAD. **Choosing the optimal test will depend on the patient's overall pretest probability for disease** (risk factors,

symptoms), additional useful information that can be obtained by the test (such as left ventricular function), indications or contraindications for revascularization if obstructive CAD is diagnosed, and the patient's cancer treatment and prognosis.
- **In patients with ACS, ICA is the gold standard** and generally the desired choice in the absence of absolute contraindications.
- ICA may also be appropriate in patients with cardiomyopathy or significantly symptomatic patients with high pretest probability for CAD for whom revascularization would be a viable option.
- In other patients, noninvasive testing is often preferred first.
- In asymptomatic survivors of **mediastinal radiation therapy**, screening for underlying CAD and/or ischemia is recommended beginning 5 years after completion of therapy and every 3 to 5 years thereafter.[7]
- **Functional stress testing** (treadmill, stress echocardiogram, myocardial perfusion imaging [MPI]) gives additional information on the clinical significance and potential flow-limiting nature of any underlying CAD but cannot, by design, diagnose nonobstructive CAD. **Anatomic testing** (CAC, coronary CT angiography [CCTA]) allows for the identification of nonobstructive CAD to target preventive therapy.
- Whenever diagnostic stress testing is performed, **exercise stress test is preferred over pharmacologic-induced stress when possible**.
  - Stress test with exercise allows (a) evaluating ischemia under more physiologic conditions, (b) correlation of ischemia symptoms with certain metrics of exertion, (c) functional assessment of cardiovascular health, and (d) assessment of chronotropic incompetence in select patients.
  - Patients with cancer may be particularly frail or have other cancer-related physical limitations, in which **exercise stress testing may not be feasible, and pharmacologic stress would be more appropriate.**
- The addition of imaging, either echocardiogram or nuclear perfusion, to stress electrocardiogram (ECG) improves the sensitivity for detecting coronary disease.
- Stress ECGs are also of limited utility in patients with resting left bundle branch block (**LBBB**) or significant **ST-T abnormalities**, and additional testing with stress echocardiogram or nuclear perfusion imaging should be done. **In patients with underlying LBBB undergoing nuclear perfusion imaging, pharmacologic-induced stress with agents such as adenosine or regadenoson is preferred** to exercise and dobutamine, which have been associated with false-positive tests.
- Patient anatomy, including body habitus, lung disease, or thoracic malignancies, may limit certain imaging modalities including echocardiography and nuclear perfusion imaging.
- Ultimately, **a diagnosis of CAD and/or stress-induced cardiac ischemia does not itself necessitate percutaneous coronary intervention (PCI) or a delay in cancer therapies.** An initial strategy of PCI and medical therapy compared to medical therapy alone does not improve patient survival or prevent MI in the general population.[8] (These studies notably did not prevent crossover to PCI if patients were not fully responding to medical therapy, and patients with left main disease were generally excluded.)
- Revascularization should be considered in patients with concern for **high-grade left main disease, severe multivessel coronary disease, ischemic cardiomyopathy with systolic dysfunction**, or stable coronary disease refractory toward optimal medical therapy.

Approach to Patients Prior to Noncardiac Surgery
- Similar principles apply to patients prior to **noncardiac surgery** including cancer resection.
- **Stress testing can be useful to help risk-stratify patients** to surgery, but presence of ischemia **does not necessitate revascularization** in patients with stable coronary symptoms.
- The **Coronary Artery Revascularization Prophylaxis (CARP) trial** enrolled patients with stable CAD undergoing elective vascular surgery and compared prophylactic coronary artery revascularization (via PCI or coronary artery bypass graft [CABG]) to no revascularization. There was no mortality benefit to prophylactic coronary revascularization.[9]
- Revascularization may still be considered in patients with high-risk lesions depending on the patients' overall expected treatment course. These decisions are best made in a **multidisciplinary** manner.

Noninvasive Imaging
Coronary Artery Calcification
Basic Principles
- Patients with cancer often have prior CT chest imaging that may have been performed for cancer screening, cancer staging, radiation therapy planning, or another indication (such as for prior concern of pulmonary embolism).
- The **evaluation of prior noncontrasted or contrasted CT chest imaging for CAC** provides a readily available opportunity to more accurately prognosticate a patient's risk for atherosclerotic cardiovascular disease (ASCVD) outcomes. The presence of CAC increases the pretest probability that a patient's chest pain may be cardiac in nature.
- In breast cancer survivors, the **presence and severity of CAC on surveillance CT, but not the Framingham risk score, was associated with a composite endpoint of all-cause mortality and cardiac events**.[10]
- Notably, **non-ECG-triggered CT scans** (ie, CT scans performed for indications other than coronary assessment) do have a notable 9% false-negative rate and are unable to fully rule out CAC. Although lack of coronary calcification on a non-ECG-gated scan lowers a patient's pretest probability for CAD, it cannot negate it.
- Compared to nongated noncontrast CT chest radiographs, formal CAC evaluation provides greater resolution via thickness of imaging slices and ECG-triggered gating, further enhancing calcium detection sensitivity.[11]
- Formal CAC assessment and scoring can be considered in patients without known CAD in whom diagnosis of CAC would change management (ie, patients not already on preventive therapy).

Indications
- In all patients with available chest CT imaging, the chest CT should be reviewed for presence and severity of CAC to help estimate cardiovascular risk and target preventive therapy.
- In agreement with American College of Cardiology/American Heart Association (ACC/AHA) guidelines, formal CAC scoring in asymptomatic patients without known CAD who are at borderline to intermediate risk for CAD **may help guide initiation of statin therapy**.[12]

- CAC scoring traditionally has reduced utility in patients with either low (<5% 10-year risk), who are less likely to benefit from statin therapy, or high (>20% 10-year risk) CAD probability, who should generally be treated with statins regardless of CAC assessment. However, it should be noted that 10-year risk scores markedly underestimate the cardiovascular risk in radiation survivors,[13] and **patients with cancer also have a significantly greater risk of developing coronary disease when compared to the general population.**[2]
- The presence and severity of CAC is directly related to a patient's underlying atherosclerotic burden and can be used to essentially reclassify the risk for cardiovascular events of patients whose cancer diagnoses would have otherwise been excluded from traditional 10-year risk scores.
- In patients with symptomatic chest pain, CAC scoring can help in determining the pretest probability for a cardiac etiology for the pain. However, it should not be used as a routine screening modality in symptomatic patients because of the false-negative rate and inability to rule out noncalcified plaque.

Interpretation
- **CAC is highly sensitive (91%)** and moderately specific (49%) for coronary artery stenosis >50%.[14]
- In asymptomatic patients, a **CAC score of zero confers little near-future risk of major adverse cardiac event (MACE), and statin therapy is unlikely to provide benefit in this low-risk population.**[15]
- **Long-term statin**-based therapies have been shown to be efficacious in reducing MACE in patients with **CAC scores >100** (Table 6-2) in the general population.[15]
- Given the proatherogenic nature of many patients with cancer, it is unclear if a lower threshold of CAC for initiation of statin therapy in this population would be more appropriate.

Coronary Computed Tomography Angiography

Basic Principles
- CCTA provides one of the **most accurate noninvasive diagnostic** imaging modalities for detecting coronary obstruction, >50% stenosis, with a **sensitivity >95% and specificity 60% to 80%.**[16,17] CCTA has an advantage over CAC of being able to evaluate for both calcified and noncalcified plaque.
- CCTA is generally a safe and quick diagnostic procedure. Patients must be able to follow directions, including breath holds.

TABLE 6-2	Interpretation of Coronary Artery Calcium Scoring			
Agatston units	**Coronary disease burden**	**aSHR**	**NNT**	***P*-value**
0	None identified	1.01	–	–
1-100	Mild	0.75	100	0.095
100+	Moderate to severe	0.38	12	<0.0001

aSHR, adjusted subhazard ratio; NNT, number needed to treat. Adapted from Mitchell JD, Fergestrom N, Gage BF, et al. Impact of statins on cardiovascular outcomes following coronary artery calcium scoring. *J Am Coll Cardiol*. 2018;72:3233-3242.

- CCTA is an ECG-gated imaging modality, which works best with patients in **normal sinus rhythm**. Tachyarrhythmias and atrial fibrillation affect test performance, although diagnostic evaluations are possible with rate-controlled atrial fibrillation.
- Contraindications include patients with severe **contrast allergies** and severe **renal dysfunction**, typically estimated glomerular filtration rate (eGFR) <30. In patients with cancer, there should be special consideration to preexisting renal disease as further impairment could potentially preclude cancer therapies.
- CCTA is a useful tool for **ruling out significant disease** in those patients with chest pain who are otherwise of low-to-intermediate risk of ASCVD.
- In the SCOT-HEART trial, the use of CCTA in patients with stable chest pain syndrome resulted in decreased incidence of cardiac death or nonfatal MI at 5 years.[18] As patients found to have noncardiac chest pain derived similar benefit, the detection of nonobstructive CAD and increased use of preventive therapy was likely a major driver of the improved clinical outcomes.

Indication
- In patients with **intermediate risk** of ASCVD, CCTA is a powerful diagnostic modality to rule out significant coronary disease because of its high sensitivity and exceptional **negative predictive value, approximating 100%**.
- Because of its moderate specificity, CCTA may prove **less useful in high-risk patients**. Some patients with obstructive lesions by CCTA will be found to have nonobstructive CAD by invasive angiography. If clinically useful, functional testing (stress echo, perfusion imaging, fractional flow reserve [FFR]) can evaluate the clinical significance of the CAD.
- Patients with cancer, who are otherwise asymptomatic, may have falsely abnormal MPI. Patients with abnormal MPI who are either at high risk for complications or have contraindications toward ICA should be considered for CCTA. **Approximately half of patients with abnormal MPI have nonobstructive disease by CCTA.**[19]
- Similar to formal CAC imaging, **CCTA can provide valuable prognostic information** and help guide primary prevention medical therapy.

Interpretation
- CCTA in intermediate-risk patients with **undetected coronary disease provides at least a 2-year warranty period** in those with acute chest pain and greater in those with stable chest symptoms.[20]
- Patients with >**50% stenosis should be considered for further ischemic evaluation**, which may include MPI or ICA. The choice of the next diagnostic evaluation should be tailored to the individual patient and regarding the status of their malignancy (Fig. 6-2).

Myocardial Perfusion Imaging

Basic Principles
- Myocardial uptake of radionuclide tracers at rest and stress allows the evaluation of **perfusion mismatch (ischemia)** and also evaluation for **viability or infarction** (Fig. 6-3).
- Compared to CTA and CCTA, perfusion imaging is a functional assessment of myocardial function. It can assess the clinical significance of underlying obstructive CAD but **cannot evaluate for nonobstructive CAD**.

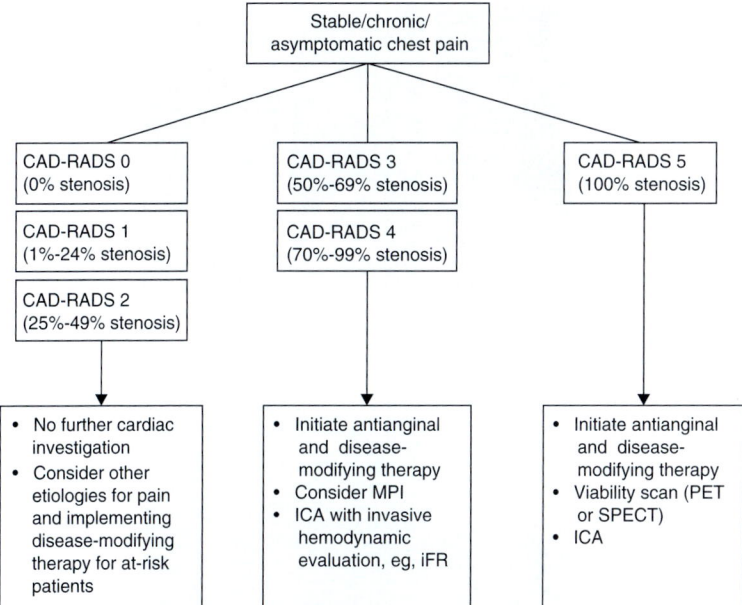

Figure 6-2. Interpretation of coronary computed tomography angiography results in patients with stable symptoms. CAD-RADS, coronary artery disease—reporting and data system; ICA, invasive coronary angiography; iFR, instantaneous wave-free ratio; MPI, myocardial perfusion imaging; PET, positron emission tomography; SPECT, single-photon emission computed tomography. (Modified from Cury RC, Abbara S, Achenbach S, et al. CAD-RADS: coronary artery disease—reporting and data system: an expert consensus document of the Society of Cardiovascular Computed Tomography (SCCT), the American College of Radiology (ACR) and the North American Society for Cardiovascular Imaging (NASCI). Endorsed by the American College of Cardiology. *J Am Coll Radiol.* 2016;13:1458-1466.e1459.)

- There are multiple modalities to induce stress, including dobutamine, regadenoson, adenosine, and exercise, each with advantages and disadvantages. **Exercise treadmill test provides the most valuable information as it most closely resembles physiologic stress**. However, many patients with cancer are often frail, limiting their ability to reach goal heart rates.
- Utility of perfusion imaging may be limited in patients with malignancies of the chest, which may be hypermetabolic creating attenuation artifact that suppresses relative myocardial signal.
- The sensitivity of MPI with **SPECT (single-photon emission computed tomography)** is approximately 80% and specificity is 70% in the general population.[21]

Indication

- Nuclear perfusion imaging is a relatively safe modality to evaluate for coronary ischemia in patients with **intermediate risk** for ASCVD.

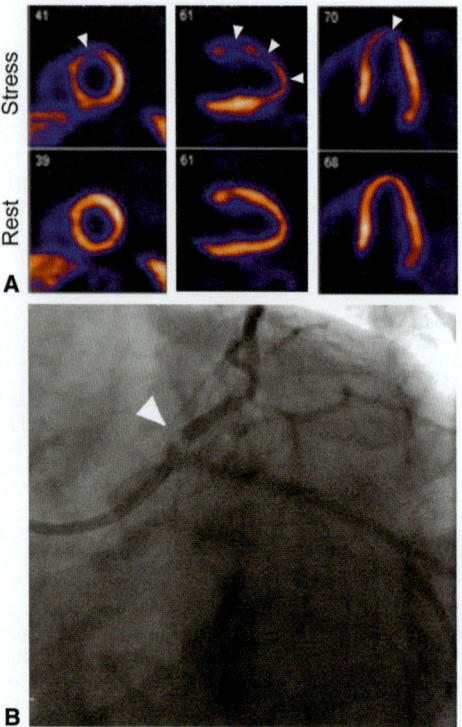

Figure 6-3. Regadenoson myocardial perfusion imaging showing decreased radiotracer uptake with stress when compared to rest in the anterior and apical walls suggestive of left anterior descending (LAD) distribution ischemia (A). Patient subsequently underwent coronary angiogram and was found to have 90% in-stent restenosis of an ostial LAD stent (arrowhead, B).

- In patients with high-risk features for ASCVD or with known obstructive CAD, perfusion imaging may help determine the area and severity of ischemia as well as identify areas of viability.
- The test is contraindicated in patients with ACS.

Interpretation

- **Cancer patients with positive nuclear perfusion imaging for ischemia or viability (in the setting of known coronary disease) should be evaluated by a cardiologist** to determine the extent of ischemia, symptoms, and systolic heart function and help determine the appropriate clinical course, whether it includes medical optimization, revascularization, or further testing.
- Abnormal MPI is quite common in patients with breast cancer treated with radiation therapy, approximately a 50% to 70% incidence after treatment,[22] and may be a result of CAD progression or direct myocardial damage. As stated previously, approximately half of patients with abnormal MPI have nonobstructive disease by CCTA.[19]

Stress Echocardiogram

Basic Principles
- Stress echocardiogram is a noninvasive imaging modality allowing for evaluation of **regional wall motion abnormalities** at rest and stress.
- The test provides additional clinically useful information, including quantification of **left ventricular function, evaluation for structural heart disease (valvular, pericardial, etc.), and chronotropic response to exercise**.
- Compared to nuclear SPECT perfusion imaging, stress echocardiogram provides similar accuracy with higher specificity at the cost of lower sensitivity.
- Echocardiographic **assessment of wall motion abnormalities may be enhanced with the use of contrast**.
- Exercise is the preferred stress modality. Dobutamine, or similar agent, can be used in patients with contraindication or inability to exercise.

Indications
- Stress echocardiogram is a generally well-tolerated procedure to assess for wall motion abnormalities in the detection of ischemia and infarction. It does not require the use of radiation or iodinated contrast.
- The presence of LBBB has historically felt to be a relative contraindication to stress echocardiogram because of difficulty in evaluating the septum. However, further studies have shown that exercise and pharmacologic stress echocardiogram have good specificity and prognostic value in patients with LBBB (https://www.asecho.org/wp-content/uploads/2019/11/Stress2019.pdf, page 22e).
- **β-Blocker therapy** can limit the test's sensitivity and is **often discontinued 24 to 48 hours prior to testing**.
- Stress echocardiogram is contraindicated in patients with ACS.

Interpretation
- Results of regional wall dysfunction (**hypokinesis, akinesis, or aneurysmal**) and subsequent management decisions should involve shared decision-making with the patient, oncologist, and cardiologist.
- Increasing concentrations of stress or dobutamine may help to determine the etiology of regional wall dysfunction (Table 6-3).
- Regional wall dysfunction can also occur in the setting of demand ischemia resulting from a hypertensive response to exercise. These patients will benefit from optimization of their blood pressure control.

TABLE 6-3 Regional Wall Motion Abnormalities in Response to Dobutamine

Etiology of akinesis	Low-dose dobutamine	Peak-dose dobutamine	Viable myocardium
Infarction	No △	No △	No
Hibernating myocardium	⇑	⇓	Yes
Nonischemic cardiomyopathy	⇑	⇓	Yes

Modified from Quader N, Makan M, Perez J. *The Washington Manual of Echocardiography.* 2nd ed. Wolters Kluwer; 2017.

INVASIVE IMAGING AND THERAPEUTICS

Invasive Coronary Angiogram
- ICA is the **gold standard** for detecting ischemic heart disease.
- Many patients with cancers are at higher **bleeding risk** because of underlying **thrombocytopenia**. These patients should undergo coronary angiogram by experienced operators with consideration for **radial access to reduce bleeding risks.**
- Femoral over radial access may be preferred in patients on dialysis (to preserve potential fistula sites) and with bilateral breast cancer (because of lymphedema).
- Etiologies of **INOCA** can also be further evaluated by ICA. For example, coronary vasospasm can be detected or induced, and microvascular disease can be evaluated by **coronary blood flow reserve (CFR).**
- **FFR** allows for hemodynamic evaluation of coronary lesions. This may prevent unwarranted revascularization in cases where lesions by CCTA or ICA appear more severe than determined by FFR.
- **ICA uses less iodinated contrast** when compared to CCTA and may be considered in patients who have significant renal dysfunction.

Medical Therapy for Coronary Disease
- All patients diagnosed with coronary disease should receive **optimal medical therapy including consideration for aspirin 81 mg and statin therapy.** In patients with prior MI or left ventricular dysfunction, β-blocker and angiotensin-converting enzyme inhibitor (ACE-I)/angiotensin receptor blocker (ARB)/angiotensin receptor neprilysin inhibitor (ARNI) may also be indicated.
- Even patients with **subclinical or asymptomatic disease should benefit from statin therapy for primary prevention of cardiovascular events.**[15]
- A diagnosis of **stable coronary disease with or without stress-induced ischemia does not necessitate prohibiting or delaying disease-modifying and -prolonging cancer therapies.** Patients initially treated with PCI + medical therapy compared to medical therapy alone had no significant differences in mortality outcomes.

Percutaneous Coronary Intervention
- In patients undergoing cancer therapy, discussions regarding **coronary revascularization and its timing should involve the multidisciplinary care team** (cardiologist, oncologist, etc.) and the patient.
- In patients with symptoms of stable angina, **PCI does not necessarily improve angina when compared to medical therapy alone.**[23] Additionally, in patients with stable angina and findings of moderate to severe ischemia, an initial strategy for PCI did not reduce MACEs at 3 years.[24]
- However, prior studies comparing PCI to optimal medical therapy do allow for crossover to PCI in patients with refractory symptoms. PCI can therefore be more readily considered in patients with **refractory angina to medical therapy**. Patients with more significant coronary obstruction by **FFR** are also more likely to benefit from PCI.
- Patients with ischemic coronary disease and **left ventricular systolic function ≤35% should be considered for CABG if a patient's cancer prognosis is at least ≥5 years.** CABG with medical therapy compared to medical therapy alone has no effect on all-cause mortality at 5 years.[25]
- Coronary stenting requires **dual antiplatelet therapy (DAPT)** and therefore consideration of stent placement requires specific consideration of a patient's risk for

future thrombocytopenia and bleeding with cancer treatment, planned or anticipated surgeries, and the urgency of such interventions as they relate the urgency of revascularization. In general, patients require **at least 1 month DAPT after bare metal stent (BMS) and at least 3 months DAPT after drug-eluting stent (DES).** Studies continue to investigate shorter DAPT intervals in newer DESs.
- In patients with thrombocytopenia, the following guidelines were recommended for antiplatelet use by the Society for Cardiovascular Angiography and Interventions:
  - Aspirin: platelet count >10,000
  - DAPT with clopidogrel: platelet count 30,000 to 50,000 (do not use prasugrel, ticagrelor, or IIB-IIIA inhibitors)
- In patients who also require anticoagulation, common practice is to treat with triple therapy for 1 month (anticoagulant, aspirin, and clopidogrel) and then to treat with clopidogrel and the anticoagulant for 1 year. The patient would continue on aspirin and the anticoagulant following 1 year after stent placement.

REFERENCES

1. Xu J, Murphy SL, Kockanek KD, Arias E. Mortality in the United States, 2018. *NCHS Data Brief.* 2020;(355):1-8. https://www.ncbi.nlm.nih.gov/pubmed/32487294
2. Sturgeon KM, Deng L, Bluethmann SM, et al. A population-based study of cardiovascular disease mortality risk in US cancer patients. *Eur Heart J.* 2019;40(48):3889-3897. doi:10.1093/eurheartj/ehz766
3. Drobni ZD, Alvi RM, Taron J, et al. Association between immune checkpoint inhibitors with cardiovascular events and atherosclerotic plaque. *Circulation.* 2020;142(24):2299-2311. doi:10.1161/CIRCULATIONAHA.120.049981
4. Herrmann J, Yang EH, Iliescu CA, et al. Vascular toxicities of cancer therapies: the old and the new—an evolving avenue. *Circulation.* 2016;133(13):1272-1289. doi:10.1161/CIRCULATIONAHA.115.018347
5. van Nimwegen FA, Schaapveld M, Janus CP, et al. Cardiovascular disease after Hodgkin lymphoma treatment: 40-year disease risk. *JAMA Intern Med.* 2015;175(6):1007-1017. doi:10.1001/jamainternmed.2015.1180
6. Harris EE, Correa C, Hwang WT, et al. Late cardiac mortality and morbidity in early-stage breast cancer patients after breast-conservation treatment. *J Clin Oncol.* 2006;24(25):4100-4106. doi:10.1200/JCO.2005.05.1037
7. Curigliano G, Lenihan D, Fradley M, et al. Management of cardiac disease in cancer patients throughout oncological treatment: ESMO consensus recommendations. *Ann Oncol.* 2020;31(2):171-190. doi:10.1016/j.annonc.2019.10.023
8. Mitchell JD, Brown DL. Harmonizing the paradigm with the data in stable coronary artery disease: a review and viewpoint. *J Am Heart Assoc.* 2017;6(11). doi:10.1161/JAHA.117.007006
9. McFalls EO, Ward HB, Moritz TE, et al. Coronary-artery revascularization before elective major vascular surgery. *N Engl J Med.* 2004;351(27):2795-2804. doi:10.1056/NEJMoa041905
10. Phillips WJ, Johnson C, Law A, et al. Comparison of Framingham risk score and chest-CT identified coronary artery calcification in breast cancer patients to predict cardiovascular events. *Int J Cardiol.* 2019;289:138-143. doi:10.1016/j.ijcard.2019.01.056
11. Hecht HS, Cronin P, Blaha MJ, et al. Erratum to "2016 SCCT/STR guidelines for coronary artery calcium scoring of noncontrast noncardiac chest CT scans a report of the society of Cardiovascular Computed Tomography and Society of Thoracic Radiology" [*J Cardiovasc Comput Tomogr.* 11 (2017) 74-84]. *J Cardiovasc Comput Tomogr.* 2017;11(2):170. doi:10.1016/j.jcct.2017.02.011
12. Arnett DK, Blumenthal RS, Albert MA, et al. 2019 ACC/AHA guideline on the primary prevention of cardiovascular disease: a report of the American College of Cardiology/American

Heart Association Task Force on clinical practice guidelines. *Circulation.* 2019;140(11):e596-e646. doi:10.1161/CIR.0000000000000678
13. Addison D, Spahillari A, Rokicki A, et al. The pooled cohort risk equation markedly underestimates the risk of atherosclerotic cardiovascular events after radiation therapy. *J Am Coll Cardiol.* 2018;71(suppl 11):A1862.
14. O'Rourke RA, Brundage BH, Froelicher VF, et al. American College of Cardiology/American Heart Association Expert Consensus Document on electron-beam computed tomography for the diagnosis and prognosis of coronary artery disease. *J Am Coll Cardiol.* 2000;36(1):326-340. doi:10.1016/s0735-1097(00)00831-7
15. Mitchell JD, Fergestrom N, Gage BF, et al. Impact of statins on cardiovascular outcomes following coronary artery calcium scoring. *J Am Coll Cardiol.* 2018;72(25):3233-3242. doi:10.1016/j.jacc.2018.09.051
16. Budoff MJ, Dowe D, Jollis JG, et al. Diagnostic performance of 64-multidetector row coronary computed tomographic angiography for evaluation of coronary artery stenosis in individuals without known coronary artery disease: results from the prospective multicenter ACCURACY (Assessment by Coronary Computed Tomographic Angiography of Individuals Undergoing Invasive Coronary Angiography) trial. *J Am Coll Cardiol.* 2008;52(21):1724-1732. doi:10.1016/j.jacc.2008.07.031
17. Meijboom WB, Meijs MF, Schuijf JD, et al. Diagnostic accuracy of 64-slice computed tomography coronary angiography: a prospective, multicenter, multivendor study. *J Am Coll Cardiol.* 2008;52(25):2135-2144. doi:10.1016/j.jacc.2008.08.058
18. Newby DE, Adamson PD, Berry C, et al. Coronary CT angiography and 5-year risk of myocardial infarction. *N Engl J Med.* 2018;379(10):924-933. doi:10.1056/NEJMoa1805971
19. Meinel FG, Schoepf UJ, Townsend JC, et al. Diagnostic yield and accuracy of coronary CT angiography after abnormal nuclear myocardial perfusion imaging. *Sci Rep.* 2018;8(1):9228. doi:10.1038/s41598-018-27347-8
20. Schlett CL, Banerji D, Siegel E, et al. Prognostic value of CT angiography for major adverse cardiac events in patients with acute chest pain from the emergency department: 2-year outcomes of the ROMICAT trial. *JACC Cardiovasc Imaging.* 2011;4(5):481-491. doi:10.1016/j.jcmg.2010.12.008
21. Loong CY, Anagnostopoulos C. Diagnosis of coronary artery disease by radionuclide myocardial perfusion imaging. *Heart.* 2004;90(suppl 5):v2-v9. doi:10.1136/hrt.2003.013581
22. Prosnitz RG, Hubbs JL, Evans ES, et al. Prospective assessment of radiotherapy-associated cardiac toxicity in breast cancer patients: analysis of data 3 to 6 years after treatment. *Cancer.* 2007;110(8):1840-1850. doi:10.1002/cncr.22965
23. Al-Lamee R, Thompson D, Dehbi HM, et al. Percutaneous coronary intervention in stable angina (ORBITA): a double-blind, randomised controlled trial. *Lancet.* 2018;391(10115):31-40. doi:10.1016/S0140-6736(17)32714-9
24. Maron DJ, Hochman JS, Reynolds HR, et al. Initial invasive or conservative strategy for stable coronary disease. *N Engl J Med.* 2020;382(15):1395-1407. doi:10.1056/NEJMoa1915922
25. Petrie MC, Jhund PS, She L, et al. Ten-year outcomes after coronary artery bypass grafting according to age in patients with heart failure and left ventricular systolic dysfunction: an analysis of the extended follow-up of the STICH Trial (Surgical Treatment for Ischemic Heart Failure). *Circulation.* 2016;134(18):1314-1324. doi:10.1161/CIRCULATIONAHA.116.024800

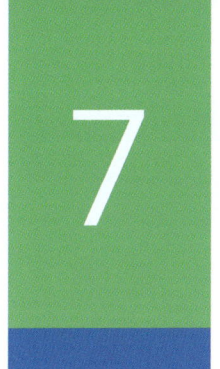

Pericardial Diseases in Malignancy

Rahul A. Chhana and Joshua D. Mitchell

GENERAL PRINCIPLES

- **Pericardial disease is highly prevalent in patients with malignancy.**
- Pericardial disease in patients with cancer may be directly related to the primary tumor or metastases, may be related to the patient's cancer therapy, or may be idiopathic in nature.
- Complications of pericardial disease, especially pericardial tamponade, can be fatal; recognition and timely management are important.
- In the majority of cases, cancer therapy does not need to be changed, especially in the setting of an incidental mild-to-moderate pericardial effusion.
- Alternative therapies can be considered in the setting of clinically significant pericardial disease in a patient on cancer therapy known to be associated with adverse pericardial side effects.

ANATOMY OF THE PERICARDIUM

- The pericardium is an elastic fibrous sac that encircles the heart.
- The pericardial space is the space between the pericardium and the myocardium and contains 10 to 50 mL of physiologic pericardial fluid that functions as a lubricant.
- **The elasticity of the pericardium allows it to expand and contract with the cardiac cycles.**

ACUTE PERICARDITIS

Definition

- **Pericarditis is defined broadly as inflammation of the pericardium.**

Etiology

- As with most inflammatory processes, the etiology of pericarditis can be infectious or noninfectious (Table 7-1).[1]
- Infectious:
  - Viral and bacterial infections (including tuberculosis)
- Noninfectious:
  - Idiopathic
  - Autoimmune disease
  - Systemic disease such as uremia, volume overload, and severe hypothyroidism
  - Cardiac injury from cardiac interventions (cardiac surgery, coronary interventions), myocardial infarction (Dressler syndrome), or direct trauma

TABLE 7-1 Etiology of Pericardial Disease in Malignancy

Chemotherapy and radiation

Checkpoint inhibitors (nivolumab and ipilimumab)

Cyclophosphamide

Docetaxel

Dasatinib

Anthracyclines (doxorubicin and daunorubicin)

Radiation therapy

Malignancy

Metastasis (breast, lung, Hodgkin lymphoma, and mesothelioma are most common)

Primary tumor of the heart (rhabdomyosarcomas, fibromas, lipomas, angiomas, leiomyomas, and teratomas)

Virtually any tumor can cause pericardial effusions.

- Oncology specific:
  - Checkpoint inhibitors[2,3]
    - **Pericardial disease can be seen in 7% to 13% of patients undergoing treatment with checkpoint inhibitors.**
    - **Incidence is higher in patients using combination therapy (nivolumab with ipilimumab).**
  - Metastatic malignancies and pericardial tumor invasion can be seen. Breast cancer, lung cancer, Hodgkin lymphoma, and mesothelioma are the most common malignancies affecting the pericardium.
  - Injury from radiation therapy
  - Other chemotherapies that can affect the pericardium include cyclophosphamide, docetaxel, dasatinib, and anthracyclines.[4]

Diagnosis

Clinical Signs and Symptoms
- **Patients often present with chest pain, usually described as pleuritic in nature.**
- Nonspecific inflammatory signs and symptoms such as fevers, chills, and leukocytosis are often present.
- Physical examination may demonstrate a pericardial friction rub.
- Asymptomatic pericarditis is at times implied by imaging in the absence of clear symptoms (pericardial thickening and effusion on computed tomography [CT]). The management of these patients is not well defined.

Diagnostic Testing
- Laboratory studies
- Inflammatory biomarkers, specifically erythrocyte sedimentation rate (ESR) and C-reactive protein (CRP), are often elevated.
- Markers for myocardial damage such as troponin levels may be elevated (which suggests myopericarditis vs concomitant myocardial infarction).

- **Evaluation of viral and bacterial infections (including evaluation for tuberculous infections) if infectious causes are suspected.**
  - Rheumatologic laboratory studies such as antinuclear antibody (ANA) may be helpful.
- Electrocardiogram (ECG) may show diffuse ST segment elevation with PR segment depressions (Fig. 7-1).
  - Patients with chest pain and ST segment elevations should be carefully and rapidly evaluated for myocardial infarction.
  - **All patients who present with chest pain should be evaluated for other life-threatening causes of chest pain (pulmonary embolism, acute myocardial infarction, pneumothorax, and aortic dissection).**

Imaging
- Magnetic resonance imaging (MRI) or CT can be helpful in select cases.
- Pericardial enhancement, diagnostic of pericardial inflammation, may be seen.
- Lymphadenopathy, signs of **malignancy**, pleural thickening, and granulomas are findings that could help lead to the etiology.

Pericardial Biopsy
- Extremely invasive and rarely indicated as part of the initial diagnostic workup
- If surgical pericardiectomy is performed for therapeutic purposes, tissue samples are generally sent for pathology.

Management
- Treat underlying etiology as indicated (such as antibiotics for bacterial infections, volume removal for volume overload).
- The purpose of treatment is to decrease patient discomfort and minimize inflammation. There are no clinical trials to support treatment in the setting of asymptomatic pericarditis, although experts have recommended consideration of treatment based on basic science evidence.
- **Colchicine and high-dose nonsteroidal anti-inflammatory drugs (NSAIDs) are the mainstay of treatment unless contraindicated.**

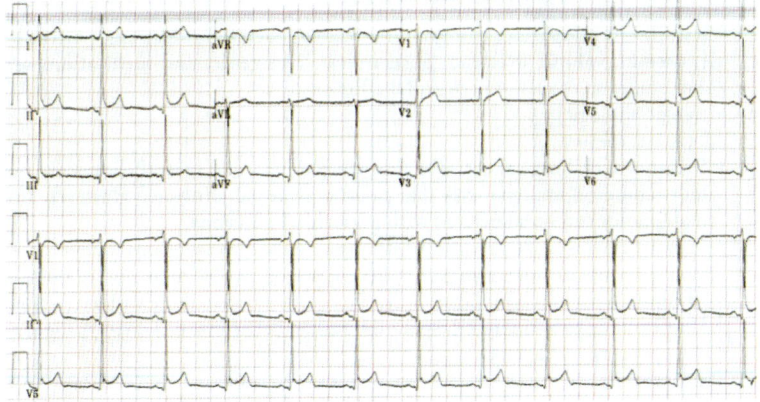

Figure 7-1. ECG findings in acute pericarditis. Diffuse ST segment elevation with PR segment depression. ECG, electrocardiogram.

- Steroids are reserved for patients who cannot tolerate colchicine or NSAIDs (eg, owing to renal dysfunction).
- Most patients with a low-risk profile can be treated as an outpatient.
- **Patients who are immunosuppressed, have high-risk findings (such as elevated troponin levels), are thought to have bacterial infections, or have large pericardial effusions should be hospitalized for close monitoring.**
- Treatment duration is guided by resolution of symptoms or normalization of inflammatory markers (CRP).
- NSAIDs are generally tapered gradually.

Consequences

- Pericardial effusions may develop and, depending on the volume and rate of accumulation, may cause heart failure symptoms or cardiac tamponade that could be potentially fatal (see Section "Pericardial Effusions").
- Chronic inflammation may lead to fibrosis of the pericardium, resulting in constrictive pericarditis (see Section "Constrictive Pericarditis").

PERICARDIAL EFFUSIONS

- Any process that affects the pericardium can cause pericardial fluid accumulation.
- An excess of pericardial volume can cause ventricular independence, where the hemodynamics of one ventricle is affected by changes in the other.
- Hemodynamically insignificant effusions are usually found incidentally by echocardiogram or other imaging modalities.
- Patients may present with signs of heart failure, such as worsening dyspnea or volume overload.
- ECG may show low-voltage QRS complexes or electrical alternans (beat-to-beat variation of the QRS complex amplitude as a result of the mechanical swinging of the heart in the pericardial fluid).

Etiology

- Any etiology that can cause pericarditis can lead to pericardial effusions (see Section "Acute Pericarditis") (Table 7-1).
  - **Viral illness, idiopathic, autoimmune-related, bacterial infections, pericarditis, uremia, volume overload, postsurgical, iatrogenic, and medications are other common causes of pericardial effusions.**[5,6]
- Oncologic etiologies
  - Metastatic tumors
    - **Breast cancer, lung cancer, Hodgkin lymphomas, and mesothelioma are the most common malignancies that cause pericardial effusions. However, any malignancy can be associated with pericardial effusions.**
    - In patients with cancer, pericardial effusions can be directly related to cancer metastasis (positive cytology on pericardiocentesis) or may be idiopathic. Idiopathic effusions in patients with cancer are still more common in those with metastases.
    - Direct tumor invasion into the pericardium can be seen with primary malignancies or metastatic lesions.
  - Primary tumors
    - Although very rare, primary tumors of the heart can be associated with pericardial effusions.

- These include rhabdomyosarcomas, fibromas, lipomas, angiomas, leiomyomas, and teratomas (see Chapter 9).
- Radiation and chemotherapy
  - **Acute pericarditis can happen early after radiation therapy, especially at higher doses. More than 50% of patients who received over 30 Gy developed pericarditis in one review.**
  - High-dose cyclophosphamide has been associated with as high as a 33% incidence of pericardial effusion, but incidence rates are lower with modern treatment. Pathognomonically, cyclophosphamide can cause hemorrhagic myopericarditis that can be fatal. It usually occurs <10 days after administration.
  - Anthracyclines such as doxorubicin and daunorubicin have also been associated with pericardial effusions.
  - Dasatinib can cause severe pericardial effusion in <1% of patients.
- Hemorrhagic effusions
  - Pericardial effusions with a mix of fibrin and blood products are typically diagnosed with pericardiocentesis.
  - The most common etiologies are iatrogenic from invasive cardiac procedures, tuberculous, and malignancies.
  - A high index of suspicion for occult malignancy should be considered for patients with hemorrhagic effusions.
  - For patients with known metastatic disease, advanced imaging such as MRI and CT can be considered to evaluate for tumors invading the pericardium.[7]

Diagnosis

Echocardiogram

- Transthoracic echocardiogram (TTE) is the initial imaging modality of choice to determine the size and location of the effusion and determine hemodynamic significance of the effusion (Fig. 7-2).
- All patients with suspected pericardial disease should have a TTE.[8]
- Effusions are determined to be small if <1 cm, moderate if 1 to 2 cm, and large if >2 cm.
- See Section "Pericardial Tamponade" for echocardiographic criteria of tamponade.

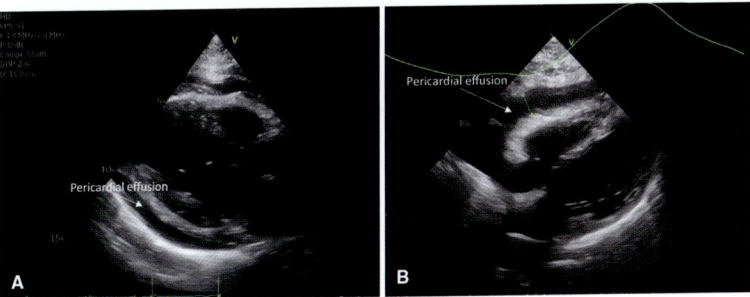

Figure 7-2. Pleural effusion as seen on echocardiogram on the parasternal long-axis view (**A**) and subcostal view (**B**).

Laboratory studies
- Laboratory studies looking for secondary causes of pericardial effusions should be obtained.
- Inflammatory biomarkers (autoimmune, inflammatory), troponin level (myopericarditis), thyroid hormone levels, blood urea nitrogen (uremia), blood cultures (bacterial, fungal infections), and viral panels (pericarditis) can help assist in diagnosing the etiology depending on the clinical scenario.

Imaging
- Chest radiography may show an enlarged cardiac silhouette in large effusions.
- Effusions are easily seen on MRI and CT and may be picked up during imaging for other concerns. They may be helpful if TTE or transesophageal echocardiography (TEE) are nondiagnostic and the index of suspicion is high.
- **MRI and CT can be useful for patients with known malignancies to evaluate for pericardial tumor invasion and staging as appropriate.**

Pericardiocentesis
- Pericardiocentesis is a percutaneous catheter–based intervention that involves obtaining pericardial fluid usually with echocardiographic or fluoroscopic guidance under conscious sedation.
- Complications include cardiac perforation, bleeding, pain, and infection.
- **Diagnostic pericardiocentesis can also be considered when the etiology is unknown. However, it is rarely required and should only be reserved for patients where infectious or malignant effusions are suspected and diagnosis will affect management.**[9]
- Pericardial fluid can be sent for bacterial culture, viral polymerase chain reaction (PCR), and cytology.

Management
Medical Management
- Pericardiocentesis or pericardial window is indicated in the setting of pericardial tamponade.
- **Patients with large effusions that are asymptomatic and with no evidence of tamponade can be monitored, although patients with significantly large effusions, even in the absence of clear tamponade, may have symptomatic benefit from drainage.**
- Surveillance echocardiogram should be performed to ensure stability.
- Avoid excessive diuretics and volume depletion.
- Treat underlying etiology.

Definitive Treatment
- Long-term prognosis should be considered for patients with malignancy before invasive pericardial procedures are performed.
- If the patient's prognosis is poor, palliative care with symptomatic management and medical management as described earlier may be more appropriate.

Pericardiocentesis
- Hemodynamically stable patients do not need drainage, except for diagnostic purposes if indicated.
- Pericardiocentesis is indicated for immediate treatment of all patients with tamponade.

- Usually, a pericardial drain is left in the pericardial space until drainage is negligible (24-48 hours). Follow-up limited echocardiogram can be performed to rule out reaccumulation of fluid.
- Importantly, although pericardiocentesis improves cardiac hemodynamics and may alleviate symptoms, recurrence of pericardial effusion after pericardiocentesis in patients with cancer is very high.[10]
- Other interventions as listed later may be associated with lower chances of recurrence.

Surgical Pericardial Window
- Surgical incision of the pericardium or pericardiectomy can be considered for patients with recurrent hemodynamic or symptomatic effusions despite pericardiocentesis and treatment of the underlying process.
- Surgery can also be considered for effusions felt to be unsafe for percutaneous pericardial drainage.
- Although at most centers this is not the initial choice of drainage owing to invasiveness of the procedure, some studies have demonstrated surgery via a subxiphoid approach as a reasonable treatment option for malignant pericardial effusions.[10,11]
- Subxiphoid approach was associated with minimal mortality and morbidity and a lower chance of pericardial effusion recurrence.

Infusion Therapy
- Owing to the high rate of recurrence of malignant pericardial effusions, alternative intrapericardial infusion of sclerosing agents or cytotoxic agents can be considered to help control recurrence in patients with advanced cancer as a palliative approach.[12]
- These include mitomycin, tetracycline, bleomycin, cisplatin, and carboplatin (off-label use).
- Our center utilizes mitomycin C 2 mg/20 mL in normal saline administered as a onetime dose through a pericardial drain.
- Careful patient selection and appropriate patient counseling should be done prior to this treatment because of the concern and risk of developing constrictive pericarditis.

PERICARDIAL TAMPONADE

Pathophysiology
- Tamponade is a low cardiac output syndrome that results from intrapericardial pressures that supersede intraventricular pressure caused by a large pericardial effusion.[13]
- Slower fluid accumulation allows the pericardium time to accommodate, whereas faster accumulation of pathologic pericardial effusion allows less time for the pericardium to accommodate.
- **When intrapericardial pressure exceeds intraventricular pressure, hemodynamic compromise can occur because the left ventricle is unable to adequately fill owing to intraventricular independence.**
- Pericardium that has had time to accommodate will take longer and sometimes require larger volumes of fluid to develop tamponade than pericardium that has not had time to accommodate.
- Pericardial tamponade, by definition, occurs when cardiac function is impaired and there are clinical signs of heart failure or shock.

Diagnosis

- Tamponade is a clinical diagnosis, often consisting of hypotension, distant heart sounds, and elevated jugular venous pressure (Table 7-2).
- **Patients almost always have some evidence of respiratory distress (new oxygen requirement, tachypnea, or pulmonary edema).**
- Measurement of pulsus paradoxus (decrease in systolic blood pressure during inspiration >10 mm Hg) is important in establishing a diagnosis of suspected tamponade.
- Signs of tamponade on TTE include[8]:
  - Right atrial collapse and right ventricle collapse
  - An increase in tricuspid inflow by 40% on the first beat of inspiration and a drop in mitral valve inflow velocity of 25% on the first beat of inspiration (respiratory variation)
  - Tricuspid variation can also be seen with noncardiac pulmonary disease.
  - Dilated inferior vena cava with <50% inspiratory collapse is highly sensitive (Fig. 7-3).
- **Septal bounce suggests ventricular independence (worse prognosis).**

CONSTRICTIVE PERICARDITIS

- The elastic properties of the normal pericardium allow the heart to expand and contract.
- **Fibrosis reduces the elasticity of the pericardium, thereby impairing diastolic filling as the ventricles are unable to expand.**
- This leads to ventricular interdependence, which could result in reduced cardiac output.

Etiology

- Similar etiologies as those of acute pericarditis and pleural effusions (Table 7-1)
- These include infectious (viral and bacterial), idiopathic, neoplastic, drug and toxin, and postprocedural.

TABLE 7-2	Accuracy of Clinical Signs and Symptoms for Tamponade
Echocardiogram findings	**History and physical**
Right atrial collapse (55% sensitivity; 68% specificity)	JVD (61% sensitivity)
IVC plethora (92%-97% sensitivity; 40% specificity)	Pulsus paradoxus (98% sensitivity; 83% specificity)
Right ventricular collapse (48% and 84%)	Dyspnea (88% sensitivity)

IVC, inferior vena cava; JVD, jugular venous distention.
From Himelman RB, Kircher B, Rockey DC, Schiller NB. Inferior vena cava plethora with blunted respiratory response: a sensitive echocardiographic sign of cardiac tamponade. *J Am Coll Cardiol.* 1988;12(6):1470-1477. doi:10.1016/s0735-1097(88)80011-1; Roy CL, Minor MA, Brookhart MA, Choudhry NK. Does this patient with a pericardial effusion have cardiac tamponade? *JAMA.* 2007;297(16):1810-1818. doi:10.1001/jama.297.16.1810

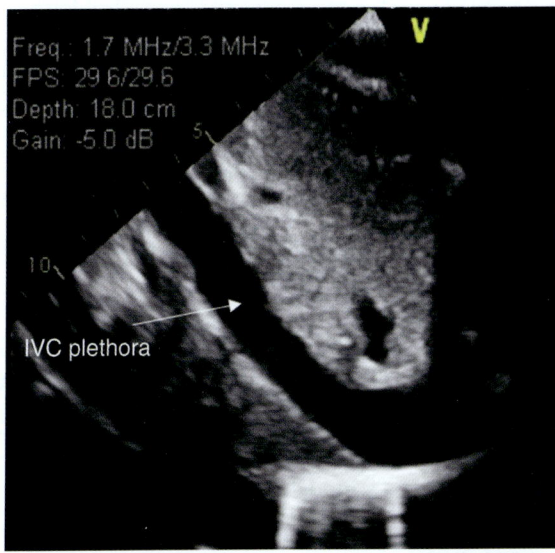

Figure 7-3. IVC plethora. Dilated IVC seen in patient with tamponade. IVC, inferior vena cava.

Diagnosis

Clinical Signs and Symptoms
- **Patients often present with signs and symptoms of heart failure (volume overload and dyspnea).**
- **Low-output symptoms including failure to thrive and fatigue may be present in patients with significant intraventricular dependence.**
- Cardiac cirrhosis could be a manifestation of long-standing hepatic congestion (jaundice, anasarca, and varices).
- Physical examination may demonstrate edema, elevated jugular venous pressure, pericardial knock, pulsus paradoxus, cachexia, and hepatomegaly.

Laboratory studies
- Diagnostic workup is similar to that of acute pericarditis and pericardial effusions.
- Elevated bilirubin, liver enzymes, and B-type natriuretic peptide (BNP) may be seen in patients with heart failure.

Echocardiography
- TTE should be performed on all patients in whom constrictive pericarditis is suspected.
- Findings include dilated inferior vena cava (IVC) with minimal respiratory variation, septal bounce, and evidence of abnormal diastolic filling on Doppler.
- Respiratory variation of the tricuspid and mitral valve inflow velocities is similar to those seen in pericardial tamponade when ventricular interdependence is present.

Imaging
- CT or MRI should be performed for further anatomic detail.
- **Pericardial calcification is suggestive of constrictive pericarditis but is not always present.**
- Other findings include pericardial thickening and scaring.

Cardiac Catheterization
- Invasive hemodynamic evaluation is appropriate when constriction is suspected to determine appropriate next steps in management.
- Constrictive pericarditis is often difficult to distinguish from restrictive cardiomyopathies, and the management between the two differs.

Management
Medical Management
- An extended course of NSAIDs and colchicine is indicated for patients with evidence of inflammation (including symptoms of pericarditis).[14]
- **Patients can be reevaluated for constrictive pericarditis to determine the duration of therapy and timing to wean anti-inflammatory medications.**

Surgical Management
- Patients with chronic constrictive pericarditis and evidence of heart failure may benefit from pericardiectomy.
- Pericardiectomy carries a high surgical mortality risk and should be reserved for patients with significant symptoms that are otherwise unable to be treated medically.
- Establishing the correct diagnosis with invasive hemodynamics is important when considering surgical intervention because patients with restrictive cardiomyopathy do not benefit from pericardiectomy.

Palliation
- **In patients with end-stage constrictive pericarditis who are deemed not to be surgical candidates, palliative care is appropriate.**
- Symptom management with diuretics can ease signs of volume overload.

Complications
- **Prolonged hepatic congestion from right heart failure can cause cardiac cirrhosis and its associated complications.**
- **Effusive constrictive pericarditis is defined as constrictive pericarditis with an associated effusion.**
  - **The effusion is generally not well tolerated as the ventricles are already hemodynamically impaired from the constrictive pericarditis.**

REFERENCES

1. Imazio M, Gaita F, LeWinter M. Evaluation and treatment of pericarditis: a systematic review. *JAMA*. 2015;314(14):1498-1506. doi:10.1001/jama.2015.12763. Erratum in: *JAMA*. 2015;314(18):1978. Erratum in: *JAMA*. 2016;315(1):90. Dosage error in article text.
2. Michot JM, Bigenwald C, Champiat S, et al. Immune-related adverse events with immune checkpoint blockade: a comprehensive review. *Eur J Cancer*. 2016;54:139-148. doi:10.1016/j.ejca.2015.11.016

3. Ala CK, Klein AL, Moslehi JJ. Cancer treatment-associated pericardial disease: epidemiology, clinical presentation, diagnosis, and management. *Curr Cardiol Rep.* 2019;21(12):156. doi:10.1007/s11886-019-1225-6
4. Chang HM, Okwuosa TM, Scarabelli T, Moudgil R, Yeh ETH. Cardiovascular complications of cancer therapy: best practices in diagnosis, prevention, and management: part 2. *J Am Coll Cardiol.* 2017;70(20):2552-2565. doi:10.1016/j.jacc.2017.09.1095
5. Levy PY, Corey R, Berger P, et al. Etiologic diagnosis of 204 pericardial effusions. *Medicine (Baltimore).* 2003;82(6):385-391. doi:10.1097/01.md.0000101574.54295.73
6. Corey GR, Campbell PT, Van Trigt P, et al. Etiology of large pericardial effusions. *Am J Med.* 1993;95(2):209-213. doi:10.1016/0002-9343(93)90262-n
7. Atar S, Chiu J, Forrester JS, Siegel RJ. Bloody pericardial effusion in patients with cardiac tamponade: is the cause cancerous, tuberculous, or iatrogenic in the 1990s? *Chest.* 1999;116(6):1564-1569. doi:10.1378/chest.116.6.1564
8. Klein AL, Abbara S, Agler DA, et al. American Society of Echocardiography clinical recommendations for multimodality cardiovascular imaging of patients with pericardial disease: endorsed by the Society for Cardiovascular Magnetic Resonance and Society of Cardiovascular Computed Tomography. *J Am Soc Echocardiogr.* 2013;26(9):965-1012.e15. doi:10.1016/j.echo.2013.06.023
9. Adler Y, Charron P, Imazio M, et al. 2015 ESC Guidelines for the diagnosis and management of pericardial diseases: The Task Force for the Diagnosis and Management of Pericardial Diseases of the European Society of Cardiology (ESC). Endorsed by: The European Association for Cardio-Thoracic Surgery (EACTS). *Eur Heart J.* 2015;36(42):2921-2964. doi:10.1093/eurheartj/ehv318
10. Virk SA, Chandrakumar D, Villanueva C, Wolfenden H, Liou K, Cao C. Systematic review of percutaneous interventions for malignant pericardial effusion. *Heart.* 2015;101(20):1619-1626. doi:10.1136/heartjnl-2015-307907
11. Hankins JR, Satterfield JR, Aisner J, Wiernik PH, McLaughlin JS. Pericardial window for malignant pericardial effusion. *Ann Thorac Surg.* 1980;30(5):465-471. doi:10.1016/s0003-4975(10)61298-2
12. Kaira K, Takise A, Kobayashi G, et al. Management of malignant pericardial effusion with instillation of mitomycin C in non-small cell lung cancer. *Jpn J Clin Oncol.* 2005;35(2):57-60. doi:10.1093/jjco/hyi019
13. Strobbe A, Adriaenssens T, Bennett J, et al. Etiology and long-term outcome of patients undergoing pericardiocentesis. *J Am Heart Assoc.* 2017;6(12):e007598. doi:10.1161/JAHA.117.007598
14. Welch TD. Constrictive pericarditis: diagnosis, management and clinical outcomes. *Heart.* 2018;104(9):725-731. doi:10.1136/heartjnl-2017-311683

8 Cancer-Associated Thrombosis and Embolism

Fahrettin Covut, Daniel J. Lenihan, and Kristen Sanfilippo

GENERAL PRINCIPLES

Definition
- **Cancer-associated thrombosis (CAT) is defined as an arterial or venous thromboembolic event occurring in a patient with active cancer**, excluding squamous or basal cell carcinoma of the skin.
- Cancer is considered active if a patient was diagnosed with cancer in the 6 months prior to thrombosis, received cancer-related treatment within the 6 months prior to thrombosis, or has recurrent or metastatic disease.

Epidemiology
- **Patients with cancer have a 4- to 7-fold increased risk of venous thromboembolism (VTE),** have an annual VTE incidence of 0.5%, **and represent 17% to 29% of all VTE cases.**[1] In a population-based study, the 6-month cumulative **incidence of arterial thromboembolism (ATE) was 4.7% in patients with cancer**, compared to 2.2% in the matched control cohort.[2] The occurrence of VTE and ATE is associated with up to 2- and 5-fold increased risk of mortality in patients with cancer, respectively.[3] **Overall, thromboembolism is the second leading cause of death in patients with cancer, after the underlying malignancy**.[4]
- The risk of thrombosis in cancer varies based on **patient-specific, disease-specific, and treatment-specific risk factors** (Table 8-1). Patient-specific risk factors for thrombosis include older age, female gender, black race, prior history of thromboembolism, inherited thrombophilia, prolonged immobilization, recent surgery, systemic infection, and other comorbidities such as renal and pulmonary disease. Disease-specific risk factors include certain primary sites and histologic features, distant metastasis, and time since diagnosis given that the incidence of thrombosis decreases over time.[5] Primary cancers of the brain, pancreas, stomach, ovary, kidney, and lung and patients with multiple myeloma (MM) have higher risk of thrombosis compared to other cancers.[5,6] Mucin-producing adenocarcinomas and higher grade tumors are associated with increased risk of VTE in certain cancers.[5] In a population-based study, adjusted relative risks of VTE for patients with stage I, II, III, and IV cancer were 2.9, 2.9, 7.5, and 17.1, respectively.[7]
- **The incidence of CAT has been increasing over the years, in part because of development of novel therapies with thrombogenic effects.** These drugs are discussed in the next section. Other treatment-specific risk factors for CAT include use of central venous catheter, steroid, and erythropoietin-stimulating agents.[6]

TABLE 8-1	Risk Factors for Thrombosis in Patients With Cancer	
Patient related	**Disease related**	**Therapy related**
• Previous VTE	• Primary site of malignancy	• Immunomodulatory drugs
• Older age	- Brain	• Tyrosine kinase inhibitors
• Obesity	- Pancreas	• VEGF inhibitors
• Surgery	- Stomach	• EGFR inhibitors
• Immobilization	- Ovary	• Chemotherapy
• Pacemaker	- Kidney	• Erythropoietin
• Inherited thrombophilia	- Multiple myeloma	• Steroid
• Comorbidities	• Histologic features	• Central venous catheter
- Cardiac disease	- Mucinous adenocarcinoma	
- Renal disease	- High grade	
- Hypertension	• Cancer burden	
- Diabetes mellitus	• Recent diagnosis	
- Acute infection		

EGFR, epidermal growth factor receptor; VEGF, vascular endothelial growth factor, VTE, venous thromboembolism.

ASSOCIATED DRUGS/THERAPIES

Table 8-2 summarizes the absolute increase in incidence of VTE and ATE with different therapeutic agents in patients with cancer.

Immunomodulatory Drugs
- Thalidomide, lenalidomide, and pomalidomide are first-, second-, and third-generation immunomodulatory drugs (IMiDs), respectively. IMiDs have direct antitumor effects, stimulate T cells, and interfere with the tumor microenvironment with their antiangiogenic and anti-inflammatory properties. All IMiDs have been Food and Drug Administration (FDA)-approved and are commonly used for the treatment of MM. In addition, thalidomide is FDA-approved for erythema nodosum leprosum and lenalidomide is FDA-approved for a subset of patients with myelodysplastic syndromes and mantle cell lymphoma.
- **IMiDs significantly increase the risk of thromboembolism**, possibly via the following underlying mechanisms:
  - Transient decrease in thrombomodulin, which inhibits procoagulant functions of thrombin

TABLE 8-2	The Absolute Increase in Incidence of VTE and ATE With Different Therapeutic Agents in Patients With Cancer	
Medication	**VTE**	**ATE**
IMiDs		
Thalidomide, Lenalidomide, Pomalidomide	↑↑	↑↑
Combination with other agents	↑↑↑	↑↑↑
TKIs targeting BCR-ABL		
Ponatinib	↑↑↑	↑↑↑
Nilotinib	↑	↑↑↑
Dasatinib, Bosutinib, Imatinib	Not increased	Not increased
TKIs targeting VEGFR		
Cabozantinib	Not increased	↑↑↑
Sunitinib, Pazopanib, Axitinib	Not increased	↑↑
Sorafenib	Not increased	↑
TKIs targeting BRAF and MEK		
Dabrafenib plus Trametinib	↑↑	Not increased
Vemurafenib plus Cobimetinib	↑↑	Not increased
Encorafenib plus Binimetinib	↑↑	Not increased
TKIs targeting CDK 4/6		
Abemaciclib	↑↑	Not increased
Palbociclib, Ribociclib	Not increased	Not increased
TKIs targeting EGFR		
Erlotinib, Gefitinib	Not increased	Not increased
VEGF inhibitors		
Bevacizumab	↑	↑
Aflibercept	↑	↑
Ramucirumab	Not increased	Not increased
EGFR inhibitors		
Cetuximab, Panitumumab, Necitumumab	↑	Not increased
Chemotherapy	↑↑↑	↑↑↑

↑: <2% increase, ↑↑: 2%-5% increase, ↑↑↑: >5% increase

ATE, arterial thromboembolism; EGFR, epidermal growth factor receptor; IMiD, immunomodulatory drug; TKI, tyrosine kinase inhibitor; VEGFR, vascular endothelial growth factor receptor; VTE, venous thromboembolism.

- Increased levels of von Willebrand factor antigen and factor VIII
- Enhanced expression of tissue factor
- Acquired activated protein C resistance
- High levels of cathepsin G, a platelet function agonist[8]
- **IMiDs are associated with higher VTE rates in newly diagnosed MM,** compared to relapsed refractory MM, **and when combined with other thrombogenic agents such as dexamethasone and cytotoxic chemotherapy** (Table 8-3). The incidence of VTE without routine thromboprophylaxis in newly diagnosed MM was 3% to 4% with thalidomide alone, 14% to 26% with thalidomide plus dexamethasone, 8% to 75% with lenalidomide plus dexamethasone, 10% to 20% with thalidomide plus melphalan, 10% to 27% with thalidomide plus doxorubicin, and 16% to 34% with thalidomide plus multiagent chemotherapies.[9] **Pomalidomide appears to be less thrombogenic compared to lenalidomide, in part because of mandatory VTE prophylaxis in clinical trials of pomalidomide.** The incidence of VTE with aspirin prophylaxis in relapsed refractory MM was 4% with pomalidomide plus dexamethasone.[10] The incidence of deep vein thrombosis (DVT) and pulmonary embolism (PE) in relapsed refractory MM was 8.4% and 6.6% with carfilzomib, lenalidomide, and dexamethasone, compared to 4.9% and 4.6% with lenalidomide and dexamethasone in a randomized clinical trial, respectively.[11]
- **The vast majority of VTE events occur within 6 months of treatment in newly diagnosed MM.** Prior VTE prophylaxis guidelines, published by the International Myeloma Working Group (IMWG) in 2008, were based on expert opinion.[9] However, only 55% of patients with MM participating in a randomized clinical trial who had been identified as high risk by the IMWG guidelines developed VTE, and the rate of VTE in the trial exceeded 10% at 6 months.[12] **More recently, two new risk prediction models, IMPEDE VTE and the SAVED score, were developed and validated to predict VTE risk in patients with newly diagnosed MM starting therapy.**[6,13,14] Future studies will determine the optimal prophylaxis strategies for patients identified at high risk of VTE using these validated scores.
- Although less common compared to VTE, IMiDs are also associated with higher risk of ATE. The rate of ATE in patients with MM treated with lenalidomide plus dexamethasone was 5.4% without thromboprophylaxis and 2.9% with aspirin prophylaxis.[15]

TABLE 8-3 Incidence of Venous Thromboembolism Without Routine Thromboprophylaxis in Clinical Trials of Newly Diagnosed Multiple Myeloma

Treatment	Venous thromboembolism incidence (%)
Thalidomide	3-4
Thalidomide + Dexamethasone	14-26
Thalidomide + Melphalan	10-20
Thalidomide + Doxorubicin	10-27
Thalidomide + Multiagent chemotherapies	16-34
Lenalidomide + Dexamethasone	8-75

Tyrosine Kinase Inhibitors

- Ponatinib and nilotinib are third- and second-generation BCR-ABL tyrosine kinase inhibitors (TKIs) that are associated with a 1.4- and 1.3-fold increased likelihood of thromboembolism according to the FDA analysis of the adverse event reporting system database.[16] Other second (dasatinib and bosutinib)- and first (imatinib)-generation BCR-ABL TKIs do not significantly increase the risk of thromboembolism. **In a phase 2 study of chronic myeloid and acute lymphoblastic leukemia patients treated with ponatinib, the rates of ATE and VTE were 25% and 6% after 5 years of follow-up**, respectively.[16] The 5-year update of a randomized clinical trial showed ATE rates of 13% versus 2% and VTE rates of 1.8% versus 0% in nilotinib versus imatinib arms, respectively.[17]
- The **vascular endothelial growth factor receptor (VEGFR) TKIs are associated with significantly increased risk of ATE, but not VTE**.[18] The incidence of ATE in patients with renal cell carcinoma treated with VEGFR TKIs was around 2.9% in phase II and III clinical trials.[19] **The rates of ATE were 11.5% with cabozantinib, 2.6% with sunitinib and pazopanib, 2.1% with axitinib, and 0.8% with tivozanib**.[19] Single-agent sorafenib and sunitinib were associated with a 3-fold increased risk of ATE (1.4% incidence), with no increase in the risk of VTE, compared to control arms in a meta-analysis of clinical trials.[20]
- A meta-analysis of randomized clinical trials showed that the use of B rapidly accelerated fibrosarcoma (BRAF) TKIs (vemurafenib, encorafenib, and dabrafenib) and MEK TKIs (binimetinib, cobimetinib, and trametinib) in melanoma was associated with a 4.4-fold increased risk of PE.[21] The rates of PE were 2.2% and 0.4% with combination of BRAF TKIs with MEK TKIs and BRAF TKIs alone, respectively.[21]
- In a meta-analysis of CDK 4/6 TKI clinical trials, **abemaciclib was associated with a 6-fold increase in the risk of VTE compared to control cohort**, with incidence of 3.3% versus 0.5%, respectively. Other CDK 4/6 TKIs such as palbociclib and ribociclib did not increase the risk of VTE compared to control arm.[22] The anaplastic lymphoma kinase (ALK) rearrangement was found to be an independent risk factor for ATE (3-fold increased risk) and VTE (4-fold increased risk) in lung cancer, but the contribution of ALK TKIs to the increased risk of thromboembolism is less clear.[23]

Vascular Endothelial Growth Factor Inhibitors

- Bevacizumab, a monoclonal antibody against vascular endothelial growth factor (VEGF), was associated with a 1.2- and 1.6-fold increased risk of VTE and ATE compared to the control arm in a meta-analysis of 22 colorectal cancer clinical trials, respectively. The addition of bevacizumab to the chemotherapy increased VTE rate from 6.5% to 8% and ATE rate from 1.1% to 2.3% in this analysis, with a follow-up duration ranging from 12 to 60 months in clinical trials.[24] **Multiple other meta-analyses including different advanced tumors also showed increased risk of ATE with bevacizumab**, but similar risk of VTE, compared to the control arm.[25]
- Aflibercept is a recombinant fusion protein that exhibits a stronger inhibition of VEGF pathway by binding to circulating VEGFs. A meta-analysis of three placebo-controlled clinical trials in different cancers did not show any increased risk of grade 3 or 4 VTE with aflibercept compared to the control arm. Addition of aflibercept to a chemotherapy regimen in a phase 3 clinical trial was associated with increase in all grade ATE from 0.5% to 1.8% and all grade VTE from 6.3% to 7.9% in patients with metastatic colorectal cancer.[25]

- Ramucirumab is a monoclonal antibody against VEGFR-2. In a meta-analysis of six phase three clinical trials, ramucirumab was not associated with increased risk of ATE or VTE compared to control arm. Notably, patients in the ramucirumab arm had lower VTE rates compared to control arm in four of these clinical trials.[25]

Epidermal Growth Factor Receptor Inhibitors
- Cetuximab and panitumumab are monoclonal antibodies against epidermal growth factor receptor (EGFR) and are used in the treatment of colorectal and head and neck cancers.
- In a meta-analysis of clinical trials, cetuximab and panitumumab were associated with a **1.3-fold increased risk of VTE without any increase in the risk of ATE**.[26] Necitumumab is a recombinant monoclonal antibody against the ligand-binding site of EGFR and was associated with a 1.6- to 1.7-fold increased risk of VTE in randomized clinical trials, compared to the control arm.[25]

Chemotherapy
- In a population-based study, chemotherapy was associated with a **6.5-fold increased risk of VTE compared to patients without cancer**.[27] The underlying mechanisms of chemotherapy-induced thrombosis include endothelial damage, increased expression and activity of tissue factor, and decline in natural anticoagulant proteins by direct hepatotoxicity.[5] **The Khorana score has been developed and validated extensively as a risk prediction tool for chemotherapy-associated thromboembolism.**[28] **The risk of thrombosis varies with different chemotherapy agents.**
- In a meta-analysis of 38 clinical trials, **cisplatin-based regimens were associated with a 1.7-fold increased risk of VTE** compared to non-cisplatin-based regimens in solid tumors. The risk of VTE was as high as 2.7-fold when a weekly equivalent cisplatin dose of >30 mg/m^2 was used.[29] In the PROTECHT trial, the risk of symptomatic thromboembolism was higher with cisplatin (7%), compared to other platinum agents such as carboplatin (5%) and oxaliplatin (1%) without thromboprophylaxis.[27]
- Gemcitabine is an antimetabolite drug that is used in different solid tumors. Although not statistically significant, gemcitabine-based therapy has a tendency to increase the risk of thromboembolism compared to non-gemcitabine-based therapy in a meta-analysis of clinical trials. The rates of VTE and ATE in the gemcitabine cohorts were 2.1% and 2.2%, respectively.[25]
- **Anthracycline-based chemotherapies increase the risk of thromboembolism and are associated with a 3.5-fold increased risk of VTE in patients with lymphoma and 7% thromboembolism rate in patients** with breast cancer.[25] Retrospective studies also noted increased risk of thromboembolism for patients treated with fluorouracil and irinotecan.[25]

DIAGNOSIS

Clinical Presentation
The signs and symptoms of thrombosis are nonspecific. **Extremity DVT usually manifests with unilateral swelling, tenderness, erythema, or warmth**. Presentation of visceral DVT varies based on the involved organ. The classical symptoms of **PE are acute unexplained pleuritic chest pain and dyspnea.**

Diagnosis

- The initial approach to suspected DVT or PE depends on the clinical pretest probability.
- **Compressive duplex ultrasonography and computed tomography pulmonary angiogram are the initial imaging tests of choice to diagnose extremity DVT and PE, respectively.**
- Wells score is one of the best studied prediction tools to stratify patients into low, moderate, and high probability.
- In patients with low to moderate pretest probability and D-dimer of <500 ng/mL, no further testing is needed.
- The D-dimer of >500 ng/mL requires further evaluation with an imaging test in these patients.
- D-dimer should not be ordered if expected to be high for another medical condition such as malignancy, sepsis, renal failure, or recent surgery.
- **Patients with high pretest probability require imaging study, given that D-dimer cannot reliably exclude DVT or PE in this setting**.

TREATMENT

Table 8-4 summarizes anticoagulant agents used for outpatient treatment of thromboembolism.

Initial Treatment of CAT

- The American Society of Clinical Oncology (ASCO) Clinical Practice Guidelines for Treatment of CAT recommend initial anticoagulation with **unfractionated heparin (UFH) drip, low-molecular-weight heparin (LMWH), fondaparinux, or rivaroxaban.**[30]
- Given the ease of use, and ability to administer in the outpatient setting, **LMWH may be preferred over UFH**.
- A subgroup analysis of patients with cancer enrolled in a study comparing initial therapy with once-daily (1.5 mg/kg) versus twice-daily (1 mg/kg) enoxaparin found higher rates of recurrent VTE in the once-daily arm (12.2% vs. 6.4% respectively).[31]
- Although limited data exist in patients with cancer, fondaparinux may be considered in special circumstances such as in patients with heparin-induced thrombocytopenia.
- Rivaroxaban in the treatment of CAT is discussed in the next section.

Long-Term Treatment of CAT

- When compared to patients without cancer, **patients with CAT have a 4-fold increased risk of VTE recurrence and a 2-fold increased risk of anticoagulant-associated major bleeding on oral vitamin K antagonists (VKA)**.[32] This may in part be secondary to the numerous food and medication interactions associated with VKAs, as well as the slow onset and offset of action. The CLOT trial was a randomized controlled trial comparing long-term treatment with VKA versus dalteparin (LMWH) following diagnosis of a first, symptomatic CAT.[33] **LMWH was associated with a 52% reduction in the risk of recurrent VTE at 6 months with no significant increase in the risk of major bleeding.** A subsequent systematic review and meta-analysis including 1908 patients with CAT found a significant reduction in the risk of recurrent CAT (hazard ratio [HR] 0.47; 95% confidence interval [CI] 0.32-0.71)

TABLE 8-4 Anticoagulant Agents for Outpatient Treatment of Thromboembolism

Anticoagulants	Route	Needs bridging	Long-term dosing	Half-life	Cost	Major bleeding risk compared to warfarin
Vitamin K antagonist						
Warfarin	Oral	Yes	Variable per INR	40 h	$	—
Low-molecular-weight heparin						
Enoxaparin	Subq	No	Fixed, twice daily	3-5 h	$$$	Lower risk
Fondaparinux	Subq	No	Fixed, once daily	17-21 h	$$$$$	
Direct factor Xa inhibitors						
Apixaban	Oral	No	Fixed, twice daily	12 h	$$$	Lower risk[a]
Rivaroxaban	Oral	No	Fixed, once daily	5-9 h	$$$	
Edoxaban	Oral	Yes	Fixed, once daily	10-14 h	$$$	
Direct thrombin inhibitor						
Dabigatran	Oral	Yes	Fixed, twice daily	12-14 h	$$$	Similar risk

INR, international normalized ratio; Subq, subcutaneous.
[a] Rivaroxaban and edoxaban might be associated with higher risk of gastrointestinal bleeding compared to low-molecular-weight heparin.

with LMWH versus VKA, and no difference in rates of major bleeding (relative risk [RR] 1.05; 95% CI 0.53-2.10). **These findings shifted recommendations in favor of LMWH for long-term treatment of VTE in patients with cancer.**
- However, with the introduction of direct oral anticoagulants (DOACs) and the morbidity associated with LMWH (subcutaneous injections, cost), recent randomized trials have focused on DOAC as long-term treatment for CAT. **The benefits of DOACs in patients with CAT include oral administration, limited drug–drug interactions, short half-life, and absence of the need for monitoring. Recently, three randomized controlled trials have compared DOACs with LMWH in patients with CAT.**
- In the Hokusai VTE Cancer trial, edoxaban (following initial treatment with LMWH for at least 5 days) was compared with dalteparin in 1050 patients with CAT.[34] The primary efficacy composite outcome (recurrent VTE or major bleeding) at 12 months of follow-up found edoxaban to be noninferior to dalteparin (12.8% vs. 13.5%; $P < .001$ noninferiority). However, **edoxaban was associated with a significantly higher risk of major bleeding (6.9% vs. 4%, $P = .04$). The higher risk of major bleeding was predominately noted in patients with gastrointestinal tumors.**
- The Select-D trial, a pilot study in 406 patients with CAT, compared initial therapy with rivaroxaban (15 mg twice daily for 21 days followed by long-term therapy with 20 mg daily) versus dalteparin over 6 months.[35] The primary outcome of 6-month recurrent VTE was significantly reduced with rivaroxaban compared to dalteparin (4% vs. 11%, HR 0.43; 95% CI 0.19-0.99). **Although there was no significant difference in the rate of major bleeding with rivaroxaban versus dalteparin (HR 1.83; 95% CI 0.68-4.96), there was a higher rate of clinically relevant nonmajor bleeding associated with rivaroxaban (HR 3.76; 95% CI 1.63-8.69).** As with Hokusai Cancer trial, higher rates of bleeding were noted in patients with gastrointestinal malignancies.
- CARAVAGGIO randomized 1155 patients with cancer-associated symptomatic or incidental acute proximal DVT or PE to treatment with apixaban (10 mg twice daily for 7 days followed by long-term treatment with 5 mg twice daily) versus dalteparin for a total of 6 months.[36] The primary objective outcome of recurrent VTE occurred in 5.6% of patients receiving apixaban compared to 7.9% receiving dalteparin (HR 0.63; 95% CI 0.37-1.07; $P < .001$ for noninferiority). There was no significant difference in the risk of major bleeding with apixaban compared to dalteparin (HR 0.82; 95% CI 0.40-1.69).
- Subsequently, these findings were analyzed in a systematic review and meta-analysis involving four randomized studies comparing DOACs versus LMWH for the treatment of CAT.[37] The primary efficacy outcome was recurrent VTE and the primary safety outcome major bleeding. Of the 2607 patients included in the meta-analysis, the **risk of recurrent VTE was lower with DOACs compared to LMWH; however, this finding was nonsignificant (RR 0.68; 95% CI 0.39-1.17). The risk of major bleeding was higher with DOACs compared to LMWH; however, this finding was also not statistically significant (RR 1.36; 95% CI 0.55-3.35).**
- Although guidelines have yet to be updated to include analyses of apixaban for treatment of CAT, the ASCO and the International Society for Thrombosis and Haemostasis recommend use of LMWH or DOACs over VKAs for treatment of VTE in patients with cancer after special consideration of individual bleeding risks.[30,38] When considering long-term treatment with a DOAC, caution is recommended for patients with an estimated high risk of bleeding, gastrointestinal tumors, or genitourinary tumors.

REFERENCES

1. Timp JF, Braekkan SK, Versteeg HH, Cannegieter SC. Epidemiology of cancer-associated venous thrombosis. *Blood.* 2013;122(10):1712-1723.
2. Navi BB, Reiner AS, Kamel H, et al. Risk of arterial thromboembolism in patients with cancer. *J Am Coll Cardiol.* 2017;70(8):926-938.
3. Khorana AA, Francis CW, Culakova E, Fisher RI, Kuderer NM, Lyman GH. Thromboembolism in hospitalized neutropenic cancer patients. *J Clin Oncol.* 2006;24(3):484-490.
4. Khorana AA, Francis CW, Culakova E, Kuderer NM, Lyman GH. Thromboembolism is a leading cause of death in cancer patients receiving outpatient chemotherapy. *J Thromb Haemost.* 2007;5(3):632-634.
5. Abdol Razak NB, Jones G, Bhandari M, Berndt MC, Metharom P. Cancer-associated thrombosis: an overview of mechanisms, risk factors, and treatment. *Cancers (Basel).* 2018;10(10):380.
6. Sanfilippo KM, Luo S, Wang TF, et al. Predicting venous thromboembolism in multiple myeloma: development and validation of the IMPEDE VTE score. *Am J Hematol.* 2019;94(11):1176-1184.
7. Cronin-Fenton DP, Sondergaard F, Pedersen LA, et al. Hospitalisation for venous thromboembolism in cancer patients and the general population: a population-based cohort study in Denmark, 1997–2006. *Br J Cancer.* 2010;103(7):947-953.
8. Palumbo A, Palladino C. Venous and arterial thrombotic risks with thalidomide: evidence and practical guidance. *Ther Adv Drug Saf.* 2012;3(5):255-266.
9. Palumbo A, Rajkumar SV, Dimopoulos MA, et al. Prevention of thalidomide and lenalidomide-associated thrombosis in myeloma. *Leukemia.* 2008;22(2):414-423.
10. Leleu X, Attal M, Arnulf B, et al. Pomalidomide plus low-dose dexamethasone is active and well tolerated in bortezomib and lenalidomide-refractory multiple myeloma: Intergroupe Francophone du Myelome 2009–02. *Blood.* 2013;121(11):1968-1975.
11. Stewart AK, Rajkumar SV, Dimopoulos MA, et al. Carfilzomib, lenalidomide, and dexamethasone for relapsed multiple myeloma. *N Engl J Med.* 2015;372(2):142-152.
12. Bradbury CA, Craig Z, Cook G, et al. Thrombosis in patients with myeloma treated in the Myeloma IX and Myeloma XI phase 3 randomized controlled trials. *Blood.* 2020;136(9):1091-1104.
13. Covut F, Ahmed R, Chawla S, et al. Validation of the IMPEDE VTE score for prediction of venous thromboembolism in multiple myeloma: a retrospective cohort study. *Br J Haematol.* 2021;193(6):1213-1219.
14. Li A, Wu Q, Luo S, et al. Derivation and validation of a risk assessment model for immunomodulatory drug-associated thrombosis among patients with multiple myeloma. *J Natl Compr Canc Netw.* 2019;17(7):840-847.
15. Maharaj S, Chang S, Seegobin K, Serrano-Santiago I, Zuberi L. Increased risk of arterial thromboembolic events with combination lenalidomide/dexamethasone therapy for multiple myeloma. *Expert Rev Anticancer Ther.* 2017;17(7):585-591.
16. Zeng P, Schmaier A. Ponatinib and other CML tyrosine kinase inhibitors in thrombosis. *Int J Mol Sci.* 2020;21(18):6556.
17. Hochhaus A, Saglio G, Hughes TP, et al. Long-term benefits and risks of frontline nilotinib vs imatinib for chronic myeloid leukemia in chronic phase: 5-year update of the randomized ENESTnd trial. *Leukemia.* 2016;30(5):1044-1054.
18. Qi WX, Min DL, Shen Z, et al. Risk of venous thromboembolic events associated with VEGFR-TKIs: a systematic review and meta-analysis. *Int J Cancer.* 2013;132(12):2967-2974.
19. Farooq MZ, Mathew J, Malik S, et al. Risk of arterial thromboembolic events (ATEs) with tyrosine kinase inhibitors (TKIs) used in renal cell carcinoma: a systematic review and meta-analysis. *J Clin Oncol.* 2019;37(suppl 15):e13119-e13119.
20. Sonpavde G, Bellmunt J, Schutz F, Choueiri TK. The double edged sword of bleeding and clotting from VEGF inhibition in renal cancer patients. *Curr Oncol Rep.* 2012;14(4):295-306.
21. Mincu RI, Mahabadi AA, Michel L, et al. Cardiovascular adverse events associated with BRAF and MEK inhibitors: a systematic review and meta-analysis. *JAMA Netw Open.* 2019;2(8):e198890.

22. Thein K, Ball S, Zaw M, et al. Abstract P1-16-04: Risk of venous thromboembolism with abemaciclib based regimen versus other CDK 4/6 inhibitor containing regimens in patients with hormone receptor-positive HER2-negative metastatic breast cancer. *Cancer Res.* 2019;79(suppl 4):P1-16-04-P11-16-04.
23. Al-Samkari H, Leiva O, Dagogo-Jack I, et al. Impact of ALK rearrangement on venous and arterial thrombotic risk in NSCLC. *J Thorac Oncol.* 2020;15(9):1497-1506.
24. Alahmari AK, Almalki ZS, Alahmari AK, Guo JJ. Thromboembolic events associated with bevacizumab plus chemotherapy for patients with colorectal cancer: a meta-analysis of randomized controlled trials. *Am Health Drug Benefits.* 2016;9(4):221-232.
25. Munoz Martin AJ, Ramirez SP, Moran LO, et al. Pharmacological cancer treatment and venous thromboembolism risk. *Eur Heart J Suppl.* 2020;22(suppl C):C2-C14.
26. Petrelli F, Cabiddu M, Borgonovo K, Barni S. Risk of venous and arterial thromboembolic events associated with anti-EGFR agents: a meta-analysis of randomized clinical trials. *Ann Oncol.* 2012;23(7):1672-1679.
27. Barni S, Labianca R, Agnelli G, et al. Chemotherapy-associated thromboembolic risk in cancer outpatients and effect of nadroparin thromboprophylaxis: results of a retrospective analysis of the PROTECHT study. *J Transl Med.* 2011;9:179.
28. Khorana AA, Kuderer NM, Culakova E, Lyman GH, Francis CW. Development and validation of a predictive model for chemotherapy-associated thrombosis. *Blood.* 2008;111(10):4902-4907.
29. Seng S, Liu Z, Chiu SK, et al. Risk of venous thromboembolism in patients with cancer treated with Cisplatin: a systematic review and meta-analysis. *J Clin Oncol.* 2012;30(35):4416-4426.
30. Key NS, Khorana AA, Kuderer NM, et al. Venous thromboembolism prophylaxis and treatment in patients with cancer: ASCO clinical practice guideline update. *J Clin Oncol.* 2020;38(5):496-520.
31. Merli G, Spiro TE, Olsson CG, et al. Subcutaneous enoxaparin once or twice daily compared with intravenous unfractionated heparin for treatment of venous thromboembolic disease. *Ann Intern Med.* 2001;134(3):191-202.
32. Prandoni P, Lensing AW, Piccioli A, et al. Recurrent venous thromboembolism and bleeding complications during anticoagulant treatment in patients with cancer and venous thrombosis. *Blood.* 2002;100(10):3484-3488.
33. Lee AY, Levine MN, Baker RI, et al. Low-molecular-weight heparin versus a coumarin for the prevention of recurrent venous thromboembolism in patients with cancer. *N Engl J Med.* 2003;349(2):146-153.
34. Raskob GE, van Es N, Verhamme P, et al. Edoxaban for the treatment of cancer-associated venous thromboembolism. *N Engl J Med.* 2018;378(7):615-624.
35. Young AM, Marshall A, Thirlwall J, et al. Comparison of an oral factor Xa inhibitor with low molecular weight heparin in patients with cancer with venous thromboembolism: results of a randomized trial (SELECT-D). *J Clin Oncol.* 2018;36(20):2017-2023.
36. Agnelli G, Becattini C, Meyer G, et al. Apixaban for the treatment of venous thromboembolism associated with cancer. *N Engl J Med.* 2020;382(17):1599-1607.
37. Mulder FI, Bosch FTM, Young AM, et al. Direct oral anticoagulants for cancer-associated venous thromboembolism: a systematic review and meta-analysis. *Blood.* 2020;136(12):1433-1441.
38. Khorana AA, Noble S, Lee AYY, et al. Role of direct oral anticoagulants in the treatment of cancer-associated venous thromboembolism: guidance from the SSC of the ISTH. *J Thromb Haemost.* 2018;16(9):1891-1894.

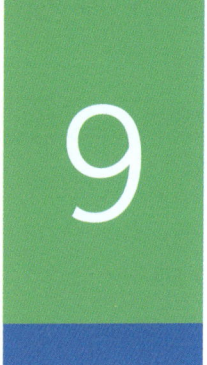

Cardiac Masses

Jonathan D. Wolfe and Daniel J. Lenihan

GENERAL PRINCIPLES

- Cardiac masses, thankfully uncommon, often present significant diagnostic and therapeutic challenges.
- Cardiac masses may be neoplastic or non-neoplastic. Cardiac neoplasms are relatively uncommon compared to non-neoplastic cardiac masses.[1]
- This chapter provides a broad overview of cardiac masses with a more detailed focus on cardiac neoplasms.

CLASSIFICATION OF CARDIAC MASSES

- **Anatomic variants:**
  - Normal or pathologic anatomic variants may be misclassified as cardiac masses, particularly on echocardiography (Table 9-1).
- **Implanted devices:**
  - Pacemaker and defibrillator leads, ventricular assist devices, right heart catheters, occluder devices, prosthetic valves and clips, foreign bodies
- **Thrombus:**
  - Most common intracardiac mass
  - Usually occurs in areas of low flow (eg, alongside an akinetic left ventricular myocardial segment)
- **Vegetations:**
  - Infectious and noninfectious (Libman-Sacks/verrucous)
  - Infectious vegetations typically occur as mobile, oscillating masses on the low-pressure side of valve tissues.
  - Noninfectious vegetations tend to occur as small, nodular, and relatively nonmobile masses on valve leaflet tips.[2]
- **Artifacts:**
  - Most relevant to masses seen on echocardiography[3]
  - Side and grating lobe artifacts, reverberation artifact, beam width artifact, double image artifact, mirror image artifact
- **Neoplasm:**
  - Primary: Originating from the cardiac structures
  - Secondary: Originating in noncardiac structures with metastasis to cardiac structures

TABLE 9-1	Anatomic Variants Mistaken for Cardiac Masses
Location	Findings
Left atrium	Pectinate muscles, Q-tip (warfarin ridge)
Right atrium	Crista terminalis, Eustachian valve, Chiari network
Ventricles	False bands, moderator band, hypertrophy, papillary muscles, noncompaction
Pericardium	Pericardial cysts, epicardial fat
Valves	Lambl excrescences, mitral annular calcification
Other	Lipomatous hypertrophy of interatrial septum, atrial septal aneurysm, hiatal hernia, fat in the atrioventricular groove or transverse sinus, coronary artery aneurysm

CARDIAC NEOPLASMS

Clinical Presentation

- **Cardiac neoplasms are often discovered incidentally on imaging examinations performed for an unrelated indication.**[1]
- Symptoms may vary greatly depending on the underlying neoplasm and location but may include[4]:
  - Cardiovascular: cerebral or peripheral embolism, arrhythmias, heart failure, palpitations, chest pain, dyspnea, syncope
  - Systemic: fever, arthralgias, fatigue, weight loss, paraneoplastic syndromes
  - Obstruction: chamber, valve, venous
  - External cardiac compression
  - Asymptomatic

Diagnostic Testing

- **The clinical context is a critical component in the evaluation of cardiac masses** given their broad differential.[5]
- Example 1: A patient with new-onset heart failure and severe, segmental left ventricular dysfunction after an anterior myocardial infarction presents with echocardiographic evidence of an apical mass. A mass in this context is much more likely to be a thrombus as opposed to a neoplasm.
- Example 2: A patient with a history of metastatic melanoma is found to have a mobile, solid mass on the tricuspid valve on routine cardiac imaging. In the absence of clinical signs and symptoms suggesting infective endocarditis, the mass is concerning for a metastatic lesion to the heart.
- Two-dimensional (2-D) transthoracic echocardiography (TTE) is often the initial imaging modality of choice in the evaluation of cardiac masses as it is noninvasive and widely available.
- Depending on the characteristics of the mass and the known comorbidities of the patient, additional imaging is often undertaken to provide complimentary data regarding tumor extension, metastasis, vascularity, and tissue characterization.[4]
- Additional testing modalities:
  - Electrocardiogram (ECG)

- Three-dimensional (3-D) echocardiography with or without contrast
- Cardiac magnetic resonance imaging (MRI) with gadolinium contrast
- Coronary angiography (to characterize coronary blood flow and identify "tumor blush")
- Positron emission tomography (PET) to provide staging for cancer
- Computed tomography (CT) including CT angiogram, to clarify intrathoracic structures
- Transesophageal echocardiography (TEE) can often provide detailed anatomic information.
- **Evidence of perfusion, often based on contrast enhancement, is a critical imaging characteristic that may distinguish neoplasms from other causes of cardiac masses**.
- Table 9-2 summarizes common imaging characteristics for select cardiac neoplasms.

Classification of Cardiac Neoplasms
- Primary: very rare with an autopsy incidence of 1:2000[1]
  - Benign: 80% to 94% of primary cardiac tumors
  - Malignant: 6% to 20% of primary cardiac tumors and usually pathologically described as sarcomas
  - The location of the tumor is often critical in identifying the type of neoplasm.
- Secondary: 20 to 40 times more common than primary cardiac neoplasms[4,6]
- Table 9-3 summarizes the pathology of cardiac neoplasms.

Benign Primary Cardiac Neoplasms
- Despite their benign nature, **benign cardiac neoplasms often require surgical treatment**.
- **Myxomas** are the most common primary cardiac neoplasm in adults and constitute about 50% of all adult cases.
- Rhabdomyomas are the most common benign primary neoplasms in children and account for 40% to 60% of pediatric cases.
- Benign primary cardiac neoplasms include:
  - Myxoma
  - Rhabdomyoma
  - Papillary fibroelastoma
  - Fibromas
  - Lipomas
  - Hemangiomas
  - Paraganglioma

Myxoma
- The most common benign cardiac tumor in adults (Fig. 9-1)[7]
- Most commonly found in the left atrium (>80%) and found in decreasing frequency in the right atrium, right ventricle, and left ventricle
- Typical location is attached to the fossa ovalis.
- The incidence of cardiac myxoma peaks at 40 to 60 years of age.
- Female to male ratio of 3:1
- Most myxomas are solitary and occur sporadically, but they may rarely be genetically mediated:
  - Carney complex: A genetic syndrome associated with the development of multiple myxomas in atypical locations including the skin, mucosal surfaces, and heart[8,9]

TABLE 9-2 Imaging Characteristics of Cardiac Neoplasms

Cardiac neoplasm	Typical location	Echocardiography	Cardiac CT	Cardiac MRI
Myxoma	LA> RA> ventricle	Mobile mass, **often attached by a stalk to the fossa ovalis**, isoechogenic	Pedunculated, mobile, **heterogeneous**, low attenuation, ~10% are calcified	Isointense to hypointense on T1, hyperintense on T2, heterogeneous enhancement with contrast
Papillary fibroelastoma	Valves (AV> MV> TV)	Small (<10 mm), **highly mobile, "shimmering" edge**, attached by a stalk	Small, pedunculated, mobile, low attenuation	Isointense to hypointense on T1 and T2, **further characterization often not feasible** because of size
Rhabdomyoma	LV> RV	**Bright echogenic mass**, either protruding into the chamber or completely embedded in the wall	**Smooth**, multiple, low attenuation or attenuation similar to myocardium	Isointense on T1, isointense to hyperintense in T2, no/minimal contrast enhancement
Lipoma	Variable	Broad based, **immobile**, homogeneous, hypoechoic in the pericardial space, intracavitary lipomas are hyperechoic	Smooth, encapsulated, **fat attenuation**, no enhancement	Hyperintense bright signal in T1 and T2, **reduced with fat suppression technique**, no contrast enhancement
Paraganglioma	LA	Broad base, echogenic mass	**Heterogeneous**, low attenuation with marked contrast enhancement	Hyperintense on T2

Fibroma	LV > RV	**Homogeneous,** appears brighter than surrounding myocardium, may have hyperintense areas of calcium	Homogeneous, low attenuation, minimal contrast enhancement, **central calcification**	Hypointense in all T1, T2 steady-state free procession, minimal late contrast hyperenhancement
Angiosarcoma	RA > RV, pericardium	**Dense and irregular mass, often nonmobile,** broad based with endocardial to myocardial extension, pericardial effusion	Broad based, irregular, heterogeneous areas of necrosis, low attenuation, infiltrative, pericardial effusion	Heterogeneous in T1 and T2, heterogeneous contrast enhancement **"sunray appearance"**
Primary cardiac lymphoma	RA, RV, may affect the atrioventricular groove or pericardium	Homogeneous, **infiltrating masses associated with restrictive physiology**	Large, focal mass, diffuse soft tissue infiltration, heterogeneous contrast enhancement	Isointense on T1, hyperintense on T2 with scattered areas of hypointense necrosis
Mesothelioma	Pericardium	Pericardial effusion, **tumor encasing the heart**	Multiple contrast-enhancing pericardial masses	Multiple contrast-enhancing pericardial masses

AV, aortic valve; CT, computed tomography; LA, left atrium; LV, left ventricle; MRI, magnetic resonance imaging; MV, mitral valve; RA, right atrium; RV, right ventricle; TV, tricuspid valve.

TABLE 9-3	Pathology of Cardiac Neoplasms
Benign	Myxoma
	Papillary fibroelastoma
	Rhabdomyoma
	Lipoma
	Paraganglioma/pheochromocytoma
	Fibroma
	Other: Hemangioma, neurofibroma, teratoma, leiomyoma, lymphangioma
Malignant	Sarcomas (multiple types)
	Mesothelioma
	Lymphoma
Metastatic	Lung cancer
	Esophageal cancer
	Leukemia
	Lymphoma
	Sarcoma
	Breast cancer
	Renal cell carcinoma
	Cervical cancer
	Melanoma

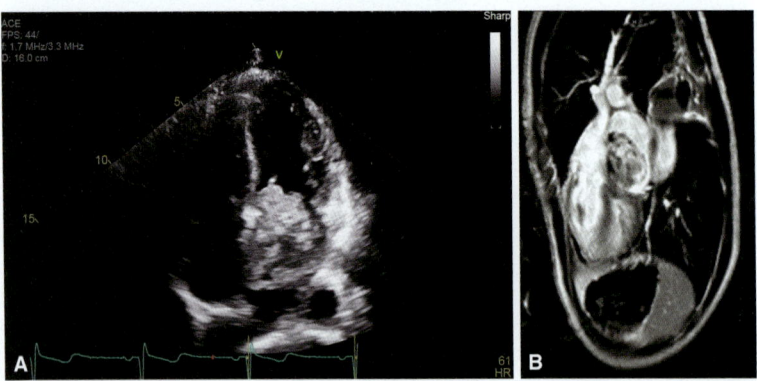

Figure 9-1. Transthoracic echocardiogram: Cardiac myxoma seen within the left atrium on an apical four-chamber view in a 55-year-old woman (A). Cardiac magnetic resonance imaging: Cardiac myxoma seen in the left atrium with heterogeneous contrast enhancement in a 55-year-old woman (B).

- Typically inherited in an autosomal dominant fashion and often associated with the PRKAR1A gene on chromosome 17 (3%-5% of myxoma patients)
- Associated with other systemic features including lentigines, blue nevus, endocrine abnormalities, thyroid cancer or nodules, breast adenomas, and testicular tumors[9]
- Consider Carney complex in younger individuals with myxomas in atypical locations

Etiology and Pathophysiology
- The exact origin of myxoma cells remains uncertain, but they are thought to arise from remnants of subendocardial cells or multipotent mesenchymal cells in the region of the fossa ovalis.[1]
- Histologically, myxomas are composed of spindle- and stellate-shaped cells with myxoid stroma that may also contain endothelial cells, smooth muscle cells, or calcification, all surrounded within an acid mucopolysaccharide coating.
- **Myxomas typically form a pedunculated mass with a short, broad base (85% of myxomas)**, but sessile forms can also occur.
- Grossly, myxomas appear yellowish, white, or brownish with a friable surface.
- Most myxomas are generally smooth, but villous or papillary forms have been reported.
- Myxomas range in size from 1 cm to more than 10 cm.

Clinical Manifestations
- Patients are commonly asymptomatic and the tumor is found incidentally on cardiac imaging.
- When symptoms present, dyspnea (especially positional dyspnea on the left side) is common.
- Clinical presentations may result from valve obstruction (syncope, dyspnea, pulmonary edema) and embolic manifestations (stroke, peripheral embolization, acute coronary syndrome). Nonspecific systemic symptoms and signs such as fatigue, low-grade fever, arthralgia, myalgia, weight loss, and erythematous rash may occur.
- Physical examination may reveal systolic (valve destruction) or diastolic murmurs (valve stenosis) and potentially a tumor plop (a low-pitched diastolic sound heard as the tumor prolapses into the ventricle).

Useful Investigations
- Laboratory tests including complete blood count (CBC), serum electrophoresis, erythrocyte sedimentation rate (ESR), and C-reactive protein (CRP) may reveal anemia, elevated gamma globulin, and elevated inflammatory markers.[1]
- Myxomas do not cause specific ECG findings.
- Chest x-ray findings are nonspecific but may include findings of cardiomegaly, pulmonary edema, or left atrial enlargement. Rarely, the tumor itself is visible because of calcification.
- Echocardiography usually demonstrates a **mass in the atrium (most common location) attached to the interatrial septum by a stalk**. TEE may provide more detail regarding tumor size and origin.
- Cardiac CT and MRI may provide better delineation of the cardiac mass and information on tumor extension in relation to extracardiac structures.

Treatment
- The only definitive treatment is **surgical removal**.
- Generally, myxomas are removed through a right, left, or combined atriotomy and typically require cardiopulmonary bypass and cardioplegic arrest.

- The choice of technique depends on associated conditions requiring intervention including valve repair or replacement and coronary bypass grafting when appropriate.
- Lifelong follow-up is necessary as myxomas may recur. However, limited evidence suggests recurrence rates may be <1%.

Papillary Fibroelastoma

- **Typically attached to valvular structures (>80%),** although may be found anywhere in the endocardium (Fig. 9-2). Left-sided valves are most commonly affected.[10]
- Generally solitary (>90%), although multiple papillary fibroelastomas in the same patient have been reported.
- Grossly appear to be covered in fronds with an appearance resembling a sea anemone.
- Histologically, papillary fibroelastomas are avascular and have a central core of collagen that is surrounded by a layer of acid mucopolysaccharides and covered by endothelial cells.[11]
- Papillary fibroelastomas range in size from 2 to 70 mm with a mean of 9 mm.

Clinical Manifestations

- **Embolism is the most common clinical manifestation** (stroke, peripheral embolization, myocardial infarction) followed by chest pain.
- The source of embolism may be the tumor itself or thrombus that accumulates in the fronds.

Useful Investigations

- A presumptive diagnosis of papillary fibroelastoma can usually be made using echocardiography (often TEE) because of their characteristic appearance.[12]

Treatment

- **Surgery is recommended for patients with symptoms** or those with highly mobile, large (>1 cm), or left-sided tumors.
- For patients that do not require surgery or that are not surgical candidates, antiplatelet agents are often utilized with limited supporting evidence.[13]
- Papillary fibroelastomas may recur after surgical resection though the rates are low (1%-2%).

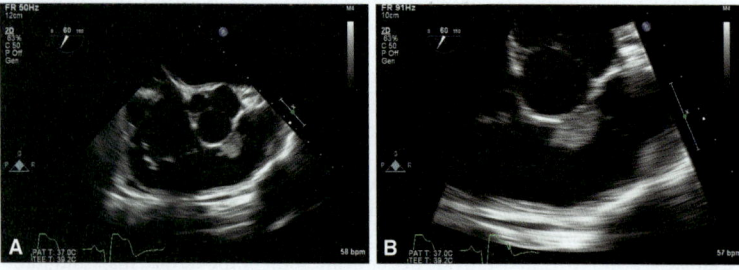

Figure 9-2. Transesophageal echocardiogram: Papillary fibroelastoma seen on the pulmonary valve in a mid-esophageal view of the right ventricular inflow-outflow tract in a 57-year-old female (A). Transesophageal echocardiogram: Zoomed view of a papillary fibroelastoma seen on the pulmonary valve in a mid-esophageal view of the right ventricular inflow-outflow tract in a 57-year-old female (B).

Rhabdomyoma
- The most common benign cardiac tumor in children[14]
- Often occurs in multiples in the ventricles
- Commonly found in patients with signs of or a family history of tuberous sclerosis
- May present clinically with arrhythmias or heart failure
- Tumors may spontaneously regress with age.
- Because of their tendency to regress, surgery can often be avoided unless patients have intractable arrhythmias or heart failure.

Lipoma
- Thought to be the second most common primary cardiac neoplasm (8%-12%)[15]
- Tends to occur in the left ventricle or right atrium but can occur anywhere in the heart including the pericardium
- Classically benign and slow growing
- Frequently asymptomatic. However, if they grow large enough, they may cause obstructive symptoms including of the vena cava (right atrium) or coronary arteries (pericardium) depending on location.
- Treatment is not necessary unless they cause symptoms, in which case surgical removal is indicated.

Paraganglioma
- Exceptionally rare neoplasm composed of chromaffin producing cells **arising from neural crest tissue in the sympathetic and parasympathetic nervous system chains** (Fig. 9-3)[16]
- May be hormonally secretory or nonsecretory
- Histologically, it can be challenging to determine if tumors are benign. Up to 10% will recur after resection with associated metastatic disease.
- **Often located around the roof of the left atrium and aortic root,** but can occur anywhere in the heart including the pericardial space
- **Often associated with large feeding vessels, which may be visualized by CT angiogram or cardiac catheterization**

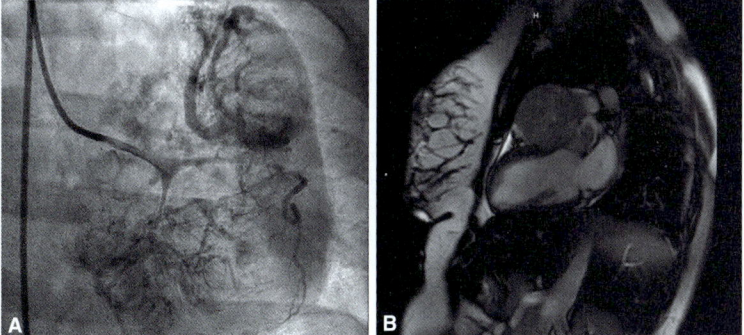

Figure 9-3. Left heart catheterization: A significant "tumor blush" is seen on contrast injection in the left coronary artery in a 26-year-old female with primary cardiac paraganglioma (A). Cardiac magnetic resonance imaging: Large primary cardiac paraganglioma seen in the pericardial space in a 26-year-old female (B).

- Clinical presentation may include hypertension and chest pain.
- **Radical surgical excision is the treatment of choice** but is often difficult because of their hypervascularity. Cardiac autotransplantation (complete removal of the heart with back table resection and reconstruction) has been successfully used in cases with extensive adjacent cardiac involvement.[16-18]

Fibroma
- Histologically composed of fibroblasts or collagen often with central calcification
- Typically occurs in childhood, often in infants
- Often located in the ventricular free wall or interventricular septum and may mimic hypertrophic cardiomyopathy[7]
- Clinical presentation may include chest pain, pericardial effusion, heart failure, arrhythmia
- Cardiomegaly and tumor calcifications may be seen on x-ray.
- Because of their risk of arrhythmia, surgical resection is usually indicated. Fibromas tend not to recur.

Other Rare Benign Cardiac Tumors
- Hemangioma
- Neurofibroma
- Teratoma
- Leiomyoma
- Lymphangioma
- Cystic tumor of the atrioventricular node
- Because of their scarcity, there are limited data to help define expected findings. As a result they are often diagnosed after resection.
- Complete resection is possible with most benign primary cardiac tumors.

Malignant Primary Cardiac Neoplasm
- Sarcomas are the most common histologic type of malignant primary cardiac neoplasm.
- Malignant primary cardiac neoplasms include:
  - Sarcoma
  - Mesothelioma
  - Lymphoma

Sarcomas
- Primary cardiac sarcomas, though extremely rare, account for over 60% to 75% of primary cardiac malignancies with an autopsy incidence of 0.015% (Fig. 9-4).
- The average age of presentation is 40.
- **Approximately 29% of cardiac sarcomas have associated metastatic disease** at the time of presentation, with the lung being the most commonly affected site.
- Unlike sarcomas from other areas, cardiac sarcomas overall have a very poor prognosis with a median survival of 6 to 25 months after diagnosis.
- **The presence of tumor necrosis, metastases, and right-sided sarcomas is associated with particularly poor prognosis.**
- There are numerous histologic subtypes of sarcoma that may occur in the heart:
  - Angiosarcoma: Most common adult cardiac sarcoma, usually originates in the right atrium
  - Leiomyosarcoma: Second most common adult cardiac sarcoma, usually originates in the left atrium

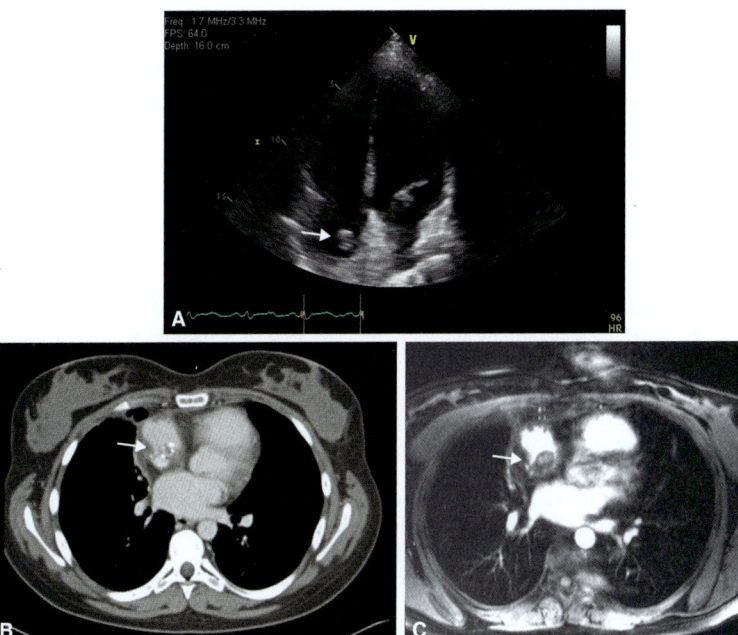

Figure 9-4. Transthoracic echocardiogram: primary cardiac angiosarcoma seen within the right atrium (arrow) in an apical four-chamber view in a 19-year-old female (A). Cardiac computed tomography: primary cardiac angiosarcoma seen within the right atrium (arrow) with heterogeneous areas of necrosis in a 19-year-old female (B). Cardiac magnetic resonance imaging: primary cardiac angiosarcoma seen within the right atrium (arrow) with heterogeneous contrast enhancement ("sunray appearance") in a 19-year-old female (C).

- Rhabdomyosarcoma: Most common pediatric cardiac sarcoma, often affects valves
- Synovial sarcoma
- Osteosarcoma: Usually found in the left atrium
- Fibrosarcoma
- Myxoid sarcoma
- Liposarcoma
- Mesenchymal sarcoma
- Undifferentiated sarcoma

Clinical Manifestations
- Symptoms tend to be caused by three mechanisms: obstruction, embolization, and arrhythmias.
- Pericardial invasion with associated pericardial effusion may be present. Rarely, cardiac tamponade may be the first manifestation of disease.
- Obstructive symptoms include syncope, chest pain, dyspnea, or heart failure.
- Embolism is more commonly associated with left-sided sarcomas.
- **Invasion of tumor across tissue boundaries or planes** may precipitate arrhythmias, and if appreciated on imaging may suggest certain histologic subtypes.

Useful Investigations
- ECG changes are usually nonspecific and may include heart block, ventricular hypertrophy, bundle branch block, and atrial or ventricular arrhythmia.
- Cardiomegaly is a common though nonspecific finding of cardiac sarcomas on chest x-ray.
- TTE is commonly used in the initial diagnosis.
- TEE may provide more specific and detailed imaging than TTE, especially for structures that are more posterior such as the left atrium.
- Cardiac CT and MRI have an important role in the evaluation and assessment of malignant cardiac tumors, especially in the evaluation of myocardial invasion, involvement of mediastinal structures, tissue characterization, and vascularity.
- **Histologic diagnosis of suspected sarcomas should be pursued** when feasible and is often extremely helpful by allowing clinicians to start neoadjuvant chemotherapy.

Treatment
- Complete surgical resection is the optimal goal for surgical treatment.
  - Despite early resection, complete resection is often not possible.
  - For left-sided tumors involving the posteriorly located left atrium, it may be difficult to obtain adequate exposure to achieve complete resection. The technique of cardiac explantation, ex vivo tumor resection, and cardiac reconstruction with reimplantation of the heart altogether termed cardiac autotransplantation was developed to address this challenge and has shown success.[17]
  - Pulmonary artery sarcomas often expand into the pulmonary artery without growing through tissue planes, allowing for removal by endarterectomy.[19]
- Neoadjuvant therapy with adriamycin and ifosfamide has been shown to improve survival with some sarcomas but remains controversial.[20]
- Adjuvant chemotherapy has been shown to improve survival over surgery alone.
- The most commonly used adjuvant chemotherapeutic regimen for cardiac sarcomas is doxorubicin and ifosfamide.[21]
- Other adjuvant chemotherapy options include a combination of docetaxel and gemcitabine, and cyclophosphamide, vincristine, doxorubicin, and dacarbazine (CyVADIC).
- Because of the complexity associated with the care of patients with **cardiac sarcomas, care is often best handled in dedicated centers of excellence with experienced surgical, oncologic, and cardio-oncologic team**.

Lymphoma
- Predominately aggressive B-cell lymphomas with a predilection for the right side of the heart[22]
- **Cardiac metastases from extracardiac forms of lymphoma are much more common than primary cardiac lymphoma**.
- Often seen in immunocompromised individuals
- Symptoms are often nonspecific or systemic (fever, weight loss) but may include arrhythmia and heart failure.
- Treatment may include chemotherapy, immunotherapy, and autologous stem cell transplant.

Mesothelioma
- Very rare neoplasm arising from the pericardial mesothelial cell layer[23]
- There is an assumed association with asbestos exposure. However, because of their rarity, a definitive relationship has not been established.

- Typically found in the pericardium and presents with pericardial effusion
- Highly aggressive neoplasm with a poor prognosis and no standardized treatment strategy. However, treatment may include surgery and chemotherapy.

Secondary (Malignant) Cardiac Tumors

- Significantly more common than primary cardiac tumors with an autopsy incidence of 10% to 12% in cancer patients and 0.7% to 3.5% in the general population[24]
- Cardiac metastases may occur by direct extension, via the blood stream, lymphatics, or by venous spread through the vena cavas.
  - Direct Extension: lung, breast, esophageal, mediastinal
  - Hematogenous: melanoma, breast, lung, genitourinary tract, gastrointestinal tract
  - Lymphatic: leukemia, lymphoma
  - Venous: renal, adrenal, hepatoma, thyroid, leiomyosarcoma, lung
- **The pericardium is the most common location for cardiac metastases (69%)** (Fig. 9-5), followed by epicardial (34%), myocardial (32%), and endocardial (5%) metastases.
- The most common causes of cardiac metastases include lung cancer, esophageal cancer, and hematologic malignancies (Table 9-3).
- Abdominal and pelvic tumors may spread to the right atrium through the inferior vena cava. The most common tumor exhibiting this tendency is renal cell carcinoma (Fig. 9-6).
- Signs and symptoms of cardiac metastases are extremely variable depending on the location of the tumor.
- Paraneoplastic syndromes should be considered.

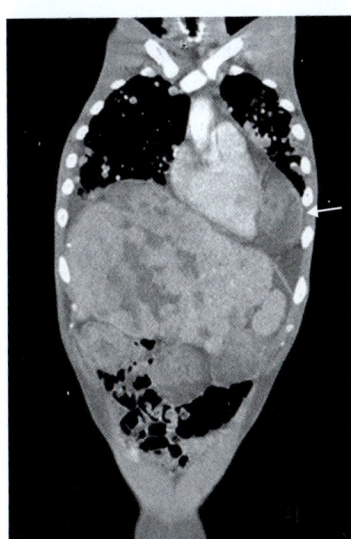

Figure 9-5. Computed tomography chest abdomen pelvis: large pericardial metastasis (arrow) with associated pericardial effusion in a 31-year-old man with metastatic leiomyosarcoma.

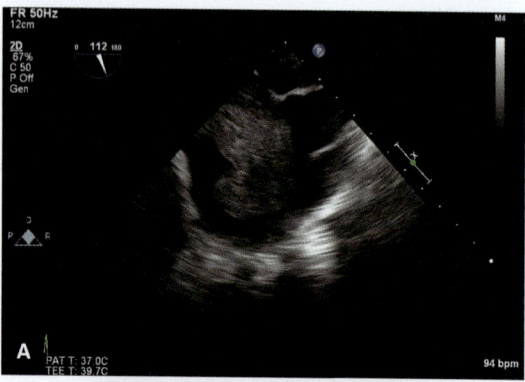

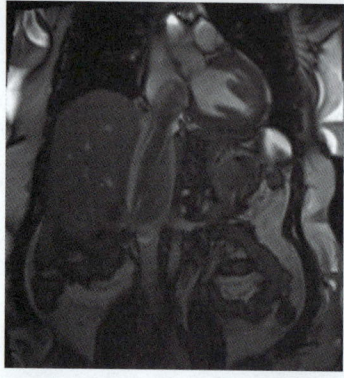

Figure 9-6. Transesophageal echocardiogram: renal cell carcinoma protruding from the inferior vena cava into the right atrium on a mid-esophageal bicaval view in a 48-year-old woman (A). Cardiac magnetic resonance imaging: renal cell carcinoma protruding through the inferior vena cava into the right atrium in a 48-year-old woman (B).

Treatment
- Treatment of metastatic cardiac neoplasms is generally palliative because of their poor prognosis.[25]
- More than 50% of patients with metastatic cardiac neoplasms die within 1 year.
- Palliative radiotherapy and chemotherapy in chemosensitive tumors is recommended.
- Surgical approach can be attempted in highly selected cases, but this is an unusual option.
- The management of a malignant pericardial effusion is typically individualized with close collaboration between oncology and cardiology and may include intrapericardial chemotherapy in select cases.
- End-of-life care should be discussed with patients that have cardiac metastatic disease.

REFERENCES

1. Lenihan DJ, Wusuf SW, Shah A. Tumors affecting the cardiovascular system. In: Zipes DP, Libby P, Bonow RO, Mann DL, Tomaselli GF, Braunwald E, eds. *Braunwald's Heart Disease: A Textbook of Cardiovascular Medicine.* 11th ed. Elsevier; 2019:1866-1878.
2. Basso C, Rizzo S, Valente M, Thiene G. Cardiac masses and tumours. *Heart.* 2016;102(15):1230-1245.
3. Sadhu JS. Cardiac masses. In: Quader N, Makan M, Perez J, eds. *The Washington Manual of Echocardiography.* 2nd ed. Wolters Kluwer; 2017:269-281.
4. Tyebally S, Chen D, Bhattacharyya S, et al. Cardiac tumors. *JACC: CardioOncol.* 2020;2(2):293-311.
5. Mankad R, Herrmann J. Cardiac tumors: echo assessment. *Echo Res Pract.* 2016;3(4):R65-R77.
6. Butany J, Nair V, Naseemuddin A, Nair GM, Catton C, Yau T. Cardiac tumours: diagnosis and management. *Lancet Oncol.* 2005;6(4):219-228.
7. Ekmektzoglou KA, Samelis GF, Xanthos T. Heart and tumors: location, metastasis, clinical manifestations, diagnostic approaches and therapeutic considerations. *J Cardiovasc Med (Hagerstown).* 2008;9(8):769-777.
8. Bussani R, Castrichini M, Restivo L, et al. Cardiac tumors: diagnosis, prognosis, and treatment. *Curr Cardiol Rep.* 2020;22(12):169.
9. Carney JA, Hruska LS, Beauchamp GD, Gordon H. Dominant inheritance of the complex of myxomas, spotty pigmentation, and endocrine overactivity. *Mayo Clin Proc.* 1986;61(3):165-172.
10. Habertheuer A, Laufer G, Wiedemann D, et al. Primary cardiac tumors on the verge of oblivion: a European experience over 15 years. *J Cardiothorac Surg.* 2015;10:56.
11. Sydow K, Willems S, Reichenspurner H, Meinertz T. Papillary fibroelastomas of the heart. *Thorac Cardiovasc Surg.* 2008;56(1):9-13.
12. Cianciulli TF, Soumoulou JB, Lax JA, et al. Papillary fibroelastoma: clinical and echocardiographic features and initial approach in 54 cases. *Echocardiography.* 2016;33(12):1811-1817.
13. Tamin SS, Maleszewski JJ, Scott CG, et al. Prognostic and bioepidemiologic implications of papillary fibroelastomas. *J Am Coll Cardiol.* 2015;65(22):2420-2429.
14. Burke A, Virmani R. Pediatric heart tumors. *Cardiovasc Pathol.* 2008;17(4):193-198.
15. Kassop D, Donovan MS, Cheezum MK, et al. Cardiac masses on cardiac CT: a review. *Curr Cardiovasc Imaging Rep.* 2014;7(8):9281-9281.
16. Ramlawi B, David EA, Kim MP, et al. Contemporary surgical management of cardiac paragangliomas. *Ann Thorac Surg.* 2012;93(6):1972-1976.
17. Reardon MJ, Walkes JC, Defelice CA, Wojciechowski Z. Cardiac autotransplantation for surgical resection of a primary malignant left ventricular tumor. *Tex Heart Inst J.* 2006;33(4):495-497.
18. Chan EY, Ali A, Umana JP, et al. Management of primary cardiac paraganglioma. *J Thorac Cardiovasc Surg.* 2020. doi:10.1016/j.jtcvs.2020.09.100
19. Chan EY, Reardon MJ. Endarterectomy for pulmonary artery sarcoma: too much, too little, or just right? *J Thorac Cardiovasc Surg.* 2018;155(3):1116-1117.
20. McGowan JV, Chung R, Maulik A, Piotrowska I, Walker JM, Yellon DM. Anthracycline chemotherapy and cardiotoxicity. *Cardiovasc Drugs Ther.* 2017;31(1):63-75.
21. Yusuf SW, Bathina JD, Qureshi S, et al. Cardiac tumors in a tertiary care cancer hospital: clinical features, echocardiographic findings, treatment and outcomes. *Heart Int.* 2012;7(1):e4.
22. Gowda RM, Khan IA. Clinical perspectives of primary cardiac lymphoma. *Angiology.* 2003;54(5):599-604.
23. Eren NT, Akar AR. Primary pericardial mesothelioma. *Curr Treat Options Oncol.* 2002;3(5):369-373.
24. Lichtenberger JPI, Dulberger AR, Gonzales PE, Bueno J, Carter BW. MR imaging of cardiac masses. *Top Magn Reson Imaging.* 2018;27(2):103-111.
25. Goldberg AD, Blankstein R, Padera RF. Tumors metastatic to the heart. *Circulation.* 2013;128(16):1790-1794.

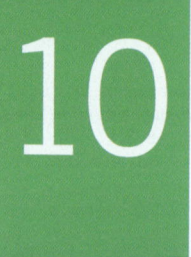

10 Hypertension
Tarun Ramayya and Kathleen W. Zhang

GENERAL PRINCIPLES

- Hypertension is a known adverse effect of multiple cancer therapeutics including vascular endothelial growth factor (VEGF) signaling pathway (VSP) inhibitors, tyrosine kinase inhibitors, proteasome inhibitors, androgen axis inhibitors, and platinum-based chemotherapeutics.
- Uncontrolled blood pressure during cancer treatment may lead to treatment interruption or even treatment discontinuation. Careful blood pressure management is therefore critical to ensure optimal cancer therapy.
- Strategies for management of cancer treatment–related hypertension largely follow established societal guidelines.
- Hypertension is more prevalent among cancer survivors as compared to the general population. Appropriate blood pressure management is therefore an important component of cancer survivorship.[1]

DIAGNOSIS

Definition
- Oncology clinical trials and federal regulatory agencies utilize the Common Terminology Criteria for Adverse Events (CTCAE) as a standardized terminology and grading system for adverse event reporting in cancer patients (Table 10-1).[2]
- In clinical practice, blood pressure management should be guided by standard practice guidelines as issued by the International Society of Hypertension (Table 10-1).[3]

History, Physical Examination, and Diagnostic Testing
History
- **All patients with cancer should be screened for cardiovascular risk factors such as hypertension, diabetes mellitus, chronic kidney disease, smoking, obesity, physical inactivity, and family history of premature cardiovascular disease.**
- Patients should also be screened for history of cardiovascular disease equivalents including coronary artery disease, peripheral vascular disease, cerebrovascular disease, and left ventricular dysfunction.
- A thorough review of the patient's cancer history including cancer type, organs involved, and all prior cancer treatments is necessary.

TABLE 10-1 Comparison of the Common Terminology Criteria for Adverse Events and International Society of Hypertension Grading System for Hypertension

Common Terminology Criteria for Adverse Events

- Grade 1
  - SBP 120-139 mm Hg or DBP 80-89 mm Hg
- Grade 2
  - SBP 140-159 mm Hg or DBP 90-99 mm Hg if previously normal; medical intervention indicated; recurrent or persistent ($\geq$24 hr)
- Grade 3
  - SBP $\geq$160 mm Hg or DBP $\geq$100 mm Hg; medical intervention indicated
- Grade 4
  - Life-threatening consequences (ie, malignant hypertension, transient or permanent neurologic deficit, hypertensive crisis); urgent intervention indicated
- Grade 5
  - Death

International Society of Hypertension

- Normal blood pressure
  - SBP $<$ 130 mm Hg and DBP $<$ 85 mm Hg
- High-normal blood pressure
  - SBP 130-139 mm Hg and/or DBP 85-89 mm Hg
- Grade 1 hypertension
  - SBP 140-159 mm Hg and/or DBP 90-99 mm Hg
- Grade 2 hypertension
  - SBP $\geq$ 160 mm Hg and/or DBP $\geq$ 100 mm Hg

DBP, diastolic blood pressure; SBP, systolic blood pressure.

Derived from Program NCICTE: Common terminology criteria for adverse events. 5.0 ed. 2017. https://ctep.cancer.gov/protocolDevelopment/electronic_applications/ctc.htm#ctc_50; Unger T, Borghi C, Charchar F, et al. 2020 international society of hypertension global hypertension practice guidelines. *Hypertension*. 2020;75(6):1334-1357.

- Secondary causes of hypertension including use of nonsteroidal anti-inflammatory drugs (NSAIDs), corticosteroids, and alcohol as well as presence of obstructive sleep apnea, thyroid disease, and uncontrolled pain should be investigated.
- If the blood pressure is significantly elevated, patients may endorse symptoms of chest pain, dyspnea, peripheral edema, vision changes, or headaches.

Physical Examination
- Careful attention to appropriate in-office blood pressure measurement technique is essential (Table 10-2). Manual confirmation of the blood pressure measurement by the treating clinician is encouraged.[3]
- Cardiovascular findings on physical examination may be normal, especially in patients with new-onset hypertension because of cancer therapy.

TABLE 10-2	Pretreatment Evaluation Prior to Starting on Cancer Therapies Associated With Hypertension
History	
• Cardiovascular risk factors	• Smoking, hypertension, diabetes, chronic kidney disease, obesity, physical inactivity, family history of premature cardiovascular disease (first-degree relative <55 yr [male] or <65 yr [female])
• Cardiovascular disease	• Coronary artery disease, peripheral vascular disease, cerebrovascular disease, left ventricular dysfunction
• Cancer history	• Prior cancer treatment, organs involved
• Secondary causes of hypertension	• Medications (NSAIDs, corticosteroids), alcohol, obstructive sleep apnea, thyroid disease, uncontrolled pain
• Symptoms	• Chest pain, headache, dyspnea, peripheral edema, vision changes
Physical examination	
• Blood pressure measurement	• Patient should remain seated and relaxed for 3-5 min and refrain from talking prior to measurement. • Patient should be seated with mid-arm at heart level, back supported on a chair, legs uncrossed, and feet flat on the floor. • Blood pressure cuff should be sized appropriately for the patient's arm circumference. • For manual devices, the inflatable bladder of the cuff must cover 75%-100% of the arm circumference. • For electronic devices, refer to device instructions. • If the first reading is ≥130/85 mm Hg, up to two additional measurements may be taken 1 min apart and averaged to determine the in-office blood pressure. • Blood pressure of ≥140/90 mm Hg at ≥2 office visits indicates diagnosis of hypertension.
• Cardiovascular examination	• Displaced PMI, S4 gallop suggest long-standing hypertension. • S3 gallop, jugular venous distention, rales, and peripheral edema suggest decompensated heart failure. • Carotid, abdominal, or femoral bruits indicate presence of atherosclerotic disease.
Diagnostic testing	
	• Electrocardiography
	• Basic metabolic panel, hemoglobin A1c, NT-proBNP or BNP
	• If elevated BNP, consider transthoracic echocardiography

BNP, brain natriuretic peptide; NSAIDs, nonsteroidal anti-inflammatory drugs; NT-proBNP, N-terminal pro-brain natriuretic peptide; PMI, point of maximal impulse.
Adapted from Unger T, Borghi C, Charchar F, et al. 2020 international society of hypertension global hypertension practice guidelines. *Hypertension*. 2020;75(6):1334-1357.

Diagnostic Testing
- An electrocardiogram is recommended to screen for underlying cardiac disease.
- Basic metabolic panel, hemoglobin A1c, and brain natriuretic peptide are useful laboratory tests to identify cardiovascular comorbidities that may guide selection of antihypertensive therapy.[3]
- An abnormal brain natriuretic peptide should prompt further evaluation for left ventricular systolic dysfunction with transthoracic echocardiography.

EPIDEMIOLOGY

- Hypertension is common in the general population in the United States, with a lifetime prevalence of >80% for Caucasians and >90% for African Americans and Hispanics.
- Age, tobacco use, and obesity are common risk factors for cancer and hypertension.
- **Standard cardiovascular risk factors increase the risk of adverse consequences of elevated blood pressure (Table 10-3).**
- Hypertension is more prevalent among cancer survivors (40%) as compared to control populations (25%), and prevalence increases significantly with age[4] (see Chapter 17, Section "Cardiovascular Issues in Long-Term Survivors of Cancer Therapy").

TABLE 10-3 Risk Factors for Adverse Cardiovascular Events Because of Cancer Therapy–Associated Hypertension

Risk factors	Definition
Elevated baseline blood pressure	Blood pressure ≥ 140/90
Established cardiovascular disease	Coronary artery disease, peripheral vascular disease, cerebrovascular disease, left ventricular dysfunction
Diabetes mellitus	Hemoglobin A1c ≥6.5
Chronic kidney disease	Proteinuria, glomerular filtration rate <60 mL/min/1.73 m^2
Obesity	Body mass index ≥30 kg/m^2
Multiple (≥3) cardiovascular risk factors	Age (men > 55 yr, women > 65 yr), tobacco use, hyperlipidemia, family history of premature cardiovascular disease (first-degree relative <55 yr [male] or <65 yr [female])

Adapted from Mancia G, De Backer G, Dominiczak A, et al. 2007 Guidelines for the management of arterial hypertension: the Task Force for the Management of Arterial Hypertension of the European Society of Hypertension (ESH) and of the European Society of Cardiology (ESC). *Eur Heart J.* 2007;28(12):1462-1536. doi:10.1093/eurheartj/ehm236

CANCER THERAPIES ASSOCIATED WITH HYPERTENSION

- Several classes of cancer therapy have been associated with increased risk of hypertension. These include the VSP inhibitors, non-VSP tyrosine kinase inhibitors, proteasome inhibitors, androgen axis inhibitors, and platinum-based agents (Table 10-4).
- Several adjunctive therapies commonly used in cancer patients such as corticosteroids, immunosuppressants, erythropoietin, and NSAIDs are also associated with hypertension.

Vascular Endothelial Growth Factor Signaling Pathway Inhibitors

- VSP inhibitors have the strongest association with hypertension.
- The VEGF family of signaling proteins stimulate angiogenesis (growth of blood vessels from preexisting vasculature) and play an important role in maintaining physiologic homeostasis. Angiogenesis is essential for cancer development and growth.
- Inhibition of the VSP is therefore an effective cancer treatment strategy; however, inhibition of angiogenesis is associated with cardiovascular toxicities including hypertension and heart failure.[5-7]

TABLE 10-4 Cancer Therapies Associated With Hypertension

Cancer therapy	Examples	Mechanism for elevated blood pressure	Common indications
VEGF signaling pathway inhibitors	• Bevacizumab • Axitinib • Cabozantinib • Regorafenib • Sorafenib • Sunitinib	• Decreased NO production • Reduced angiogenesis • Impaired natriuresis • Endothelin-1-mediated vasoconstriction	• Renal cell carcinoma • Colonic adenocarcinoma • Hepatocellular carcinoma • Non–small cell lung cancer • Endometrial adenocarcinoma
Tyrosine kinase inhibitors (non-VEGF signaling pathway)	*Bruton tyrosine kinase* • Ibrutinib	• Decreased NO production • Vascular remodeling and fibrosis	• Chronic lymphocytic leukemia • Mantle cell lymphoma • Waldenström macroglobulinemia
	BCR-ABL kinase • Nilotinib • Ponatinib	• Endothelial cell dysfunction • Decreased NO production	• Chronic myelogenous leukemia

TABLE 10-4   Cancer Therapies Associated With Hypertension (continued)

Cancer therapy	Examples	Mechanism for elevated blood pressure	Common indications
	BRAF and MEK • Dabrafenib • Trametinib	• Decreased NO production • RAAS dysregulation • Inhibition of endothelial cell proliferation	• Melanoma • Thyroid carcinomas
Proteasome inhibitors	• Bortezomib • Carfilzomib	• Upregulation of angiotensin II	• Multiple myeloma
Androgen axis inhibitors	• Enzalutamide • Abiraterone	• Mineralocorticoid excess • Metabolic syndrome	• Prostate cancer
Platinum-based agents	• Cisplatin	• Direct toxicity to endothelial cells • Nephrotoxicity	• Sarcomas • Small cell lung cancer • Testicular cancer
Immunosuppressants	• Cyclosporine • Tacrolimus • Mycophenolate mofetil	• Systemic and renal vasoconstriction	• Allogeneic stem cell transplantation

NO, nitric oxide; RAAS, renin-angiotensin-aldosterone system; VEGF, vascular endothelial growth factor.

- VSP inhibitors used in clinical practice include axitinib, bevacizumab, cabozantinib, regorafenib, sorafenib, and sunitinib. Incidence of hypertension on VSP inhibitor therapies ranges from 20% to 40%.[8]

Non–Vascular Endothelial Growth Factor Signaling Pathway Tyrosine Kinase Inhibitors

- Ibrutinib inhibits Bruton tyrosine kinase, an early signaling molecule within the B-cell antigen receptor signaling cascade, and is associated with a three-fold increase in incidence of grade 3 or 4 hypertension.[9] Ibrutinib is used to treat chronic lymphocytic leukemia, mantle cell lymphoma, and Waldenström macroglobulinemia.

- **Nilotinib and ponatinib inhibit the BCR-ABL kinase that is pathologically activated in chronic myelogenous leukemia. Hypertension is the most common adverse cardiovascular event reported on nilotinib and ponatinib.**[10]
- Dabrafenib, vemurafenib (BRAF inhibitors), and trametinib (MEK inhibitor) block signaling pathways that are pathologically activated in BRAF-mutated melanoma. Combination BRAF and MEK inhibitor therapy has a significantly higher relative risk of high-grade hypertension when compared to BRAF monotherapy.[11]

Proteasome Inhibitors

- Bortezomib and carfilzomib are essential components of multiple myeloma treatment that inhibit the essential cellular function of protein degradation.
- **Carfilzomib in particular is associated with hypertension, with an incidence of up to 25% in clinical trials. Risk of cardiotoxicity on carfilzomib is higher in patients with established cardiovascular disease.**[1,12,13]

Platinum-Based Chemotherapeutic Agents

- Cisplatin is a platinum-based agent that interferes with DNA repair and synthesis and is efficacious against various cancers including sarcomas, testicular cancer, and small cell lung cancer.
- Adversely, platinum deposition from cisplatin use is directly toxic to both the kidneys and endothelial cells and is associated with a higher incidence of hypertension as compared to controls in cancer survivors.[1,14]

Androgen Axis Inhibitors

- Enzalutamide and abiraterone both inhibit androgen synthesis and are used to treat castrate-resistant prostate cancer.
- Abiraterone inhibits the cytochrome P450 17A1 enzyme resulting in selective suppression of androgen and cortisol production, which increases adrenocorticotropic hormone (ACTH) levels and results in overproduction of mineralocorticoids. This leads to increased sodium and fluid retention, raising mean arterial pressure.
- **The incidence of hypertension observed in a meta-analysis of several randomized controlled trials was 14% and 21.9% for enzalutamide and abiraterone, respectively.**[15]
- Inhibition of androgen production is also associated with metabolic syndrome, which is a significant risk factor for the development of hypertension and other cardiovascular complications.[15,16]

Immunosuppressants

- Immunosuppressants such as cyclosporine A, tacrolimus, and mycophenolate mofetil are used to prevent acute graft-versus-host disease after allogeneic stem cell transplantation.
- Mechanisms of blood pressure dysregulation on these agents include nephrotoxicity, dysregulation of the renin-aldosterone-angiotensin system, and decreased production of vasodilating prostaglandins.[1,17]
- Randomized studies have demonstrated significantly higher incidence of hypertension in transplant patients treated with cyclosporine (57%) when compared to patients treated with methotrexate (4%).[17]

MANAGEMENT OF CANCER THERAPY–ASSOCIATED HYPERTENSION

- Patients who are expected to start on a cancer therapy associated with hypertension, especially VSP inhibitors, require optimization of blood pressure before and after treatment initiation.
- Although lifestyle modification is an important component of blood pressure management, most patients on cancer therapies associated with hypertension require antihypertensive drug therapy.
- Referral to a cardio-oncologist can facilitate blood pressure surveillance and management.

Pretreatment Evaluation

- A thorough cardiovascular risk assessment should be completed prior to starting on cancer therapy (see Section "History, Physical Examination, and Diagnostic Testing"). This guides the intensity of subsequent blood pressure monitoring and control of blood pressure elevations.
- **In patients with preexisting hypertension, strict blood pressure control (<140/90 in general; <130/80 in patients with specific cardiovascular comorbidities as per standard clinical practice guidelines) should be achieved prior to starting on cancer therapy.**[3,5]

On-Treatment Blood Pressure Surveillance

- Blood pressure should be closely monitored throughout treatment. For patients receiving VSP inhibitors, close monitoring is especially important during the first cycle when the majority of blood pressure elevation is expected to occur.
- Patients are encouraged to monitor blood pressure at home. Instruction in proper blood pressure monitoring technique should be provided (Table 10-2).[5]
- Frequency of in-office blood pressure checks should be individualized based on the patient's cardiovascular comorbidities, severity of blood pressure elevation, and reliability to follow through with home blood pressure monitoring.
- **In general, a blood pressure goal of ≤140/90 should be targeted during cancer therapy. A lower blood pressure goal of ≤130/80 may be appropriate for patients with specific cardiovascular risk factors (ie, diabetes mellitus, chronic kidney disease, or stroke) and in cancer survivors.**[3]

Selection of Antihypertensive Drugs

- **In general, selection of antihypertensive agents should follow standard clinical practice guidelines and is frequently guided by coexisting medical comorbidities (Table 10-5).**[18]
- Commonly used antihypertensive drugs include angiotensin-converting enzyme inhibitors (ACEIs), angiotensin II receptor blockers (ARBs), dihydropyridine calcium channel blockers, beta-blockers, and diuretics.
- Observational data suggest that ACEIs, ARBs, and dihydropyridine calcium channel blockers may be more effective for treatment of hypertension associated with VSP inhibitors. Close monitoring of renal function is necessary on these agents, especially when combined with nephrotoxic chemotherapy and/or underlying renal disease.[8]

TABLE 10-5	Antihypertensive Drugs for Treatment of Cancer Therapy–Associated Hypertension		
Medication class	Examples	Specific indications	Adverse effects
Angiotensin-converting enzyme inhibitor	• Lisinopril • Ramipril • Captopril	• LV dysfunction • Chronic kidney disease • Diabetes mellitus • African Americans	• Hyperkalemia • Angioedema • Cough • Increased serum creatinine
Angiotensin II receptor blocker	• Losartan • Valsartan • Olmesartan • Candesartan	• LV dysfunction • Chronic kidney disease • Diabetes mellitus	• Hyperkalemia • Increased serum creatinine
Dihydropyridine calcium channel blocker	• Amlodipine • Nifedipine	• African Americans	• Peripheral edema
Thiazide diuretic	• Chlorthalidone • Hydrochlorothiazide	• African Americans	• Hyponatremia
Loop diuretic	• Furosemide • Bumetanide • Torsemide	• Hypervolemia	• Hypovolemia • Hypokalemia
Mineralocorticoid receptor antagonist	• Spironolactone • Eplerenone	• LV dysfunction • Hypervolemia	• Hyperkalemia • Gynecomastia • Caution when GFR < 45 mL/min/1.73 m^2 or K > 4.5 mmol/L
β-Blocker	• Carvedilol • Bisoprolol • Propranolol • Metoprolol tartrate, metoprolol succinate	• LV dysfunction • Coronary artery disease • Tachyarrhythmias	• Bradycardia • Fatigue • Bronchospasm (metoprolol, propranolol)

GFR, glomerular filtration rate; LV, left ventricular.

REFERENCES

1. Cohen JB, Geara AS, Hogan JJ, et al. Hypertension in cancer patients and survivors: epidemiology, diagnostics, and management. *JACC: CardioOncology*. 2019;1(2):238-251
2. Program NCICTE. Common terminology criteria for adverse events. 5.0 ed. 2017. https://ctep.cancer.gov/protocolDevelopment/electronic_applications/ctc.htm#ctc_50

3. Unger T, Borghi C, Charchar F, et al. 2020 international society of hypertension global hypertension practice guidelines. *Hypertension.* 2020;75(6):1334-1357. doi:10.1161/HYPERTENSIONAHA.120.15026
4. Armstrong GT, Oeffinger KC, Chen Y, et al. Modifiable risk factors and major cardiac events among adult survivors of childhood cancer. *J Clin Oncol.* 2013;31(29):3673-3680. doi:10.1200/JCO.2013.49.3205
5. Maitland ML, Bakris GL, Black HR, et al. Initial assessment, surveillance, and management of blood pressure in patients receiving vascular endothelial growth factor signaling pathway inhibitors. *J Natl Cancer Inst.* 2010;102(9):596-604. doi:10.1093/jnci/djq091
6. Totzek M, Mincu R, Mrotzek S. Cardiovascular diseases in patients receiving small molecules with anti-vascular endothelial growth factor activity: a meta-analysis of approximately 29,000 cancer patients. *Eur J Prev Cardiol.* 2018;25(5):482-494. doi:10.1177/2047487318755193
7. Eskens F, Verweij J. The clinical toxicity profile of vascular endothelial growth factor (VEGF) and vascular endothelial growth factor receptor (VEGFR) targeting angiogenesis inhibitors: a review. *Eur J Cancer.* 2006;42:3127-3139. doi:10.1016/j.ejca.2006.09.015
8. Brinda BJ, Viganego F, Vo T, et al. Anti-VEGF induced hypertension: a review of pathophysiology and treatment options. *Curr Treat Options Cardiovasc Med.* 2016;18:33. doi:10.1007/s11936-016-0452-z
9. Dickerson T, Wiczer T, Waller A, et al. Hypertension and incident cardiovascular events following ibrutinib initiation. *Blood.* 2019;134(22):1919-1928. doi:10.1182/blood.2019000840
10. Moslehi JJ, Deininger M. Tyrosine kinase inhibitor-associated cardiovascular toxicity in chronic myeloid leukemia. *J Clin Oncol.* 2015;33(35):4210-4218. doi:10.1200/JCO.2015.62.4718
11. Mincu RI, Mahabadi AA, Michel L, et al. Cardiovascular adverse events associated with BRAF and MEK inhibitors: a systematic review and meta-analysis. *JAMA Netw Open.* 2019;2(8):e198890. doi:10.1001/jamanetworkopen.2019.8890
12. Tini G, Sarocchi M, Tocci G, et al. Arterial hypertension in cancer: the elephant in the room. *Int J Cardiol.* 2019;281:133-139. doi:10.1016/j.ijcard.2019.01.082
13. Cornell RF, Ky B, Weiss BM, et al. Prospective study of events during proteasome inhibitor therapy for relapsed multiple myeloma. *J Clin Oncol.* 2019;37(22):1946-1955. doi:10.1200/JCO.19.00231
14. Sagstuen H, Aass N, Fossa SD, et al. Blood pressure and body mass index in long-term survivors of testicular cancer. *J Clin Oncol.* 2005;23(22):4980-4990. doi:10.1200/JCO.2005.06.882
15. Zhu X, Wu S. Risk of hypertension in cancer patients treated with abiraterone: a meta-analysis. *Clin Hypertens.* 2019;25(5):1-9. doi:10.1186/s40885-019-0110-3
16. Bhatia N, Santos, M, Jones LW, et al. Cardiovascular effects of androgen deprivation therapy for the treatment of prostate cancer: ABCDE steps to reduce cardiovascular disease in patients with prostate cancer. *Circulation.* 2016;133(5):537-541. doi:10.1161/CIRCULATIONAHA.115.012519
17. Aad SA, Pierce M, Barmaimon G, et al. Hypertension induced by chemotherapeutic and immunosuppressive agents: a new challenge. *Crit Rev Oncol Hematol.* 2015;93(1):28-35. doi:10.1016/j.critrevonc.2014.08.004
18. Mancia G, De Backer G, Dominiczak A, et al. 2007 Guidelines for the management of arterial hypertension: the Task Force for the Management of Arterial Hypertension of the European Society of Hypertension (ESH) and of the European Society of Cardiology (ESC). *Eur Heart J.* 2007;28(12):1462-1536. doi:10.1093/eurheartj/ehm236

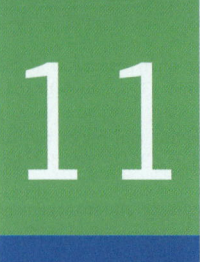

Arrhythmias

Krasimira M. Mikhova and Phillip S. Cuculich

GENERAL PRINCIPLES

- The incidence of **cancer treatment–induced arrhythmias (CTIAs)** is increasing in the context of new cancer therapies and increased survival. This chapter will focus on the diagnosis and treatment of arrhythmias encountered in cardio-oncology, highlighting associations with **conventional chemotherapy agents** and **novel targeted therapies**.
- Though not covered in this chapter, primary and metastatic cardiac malignancies and thoracic irradiation are associated with arrhythmias as well.[1,2]
- The most common rhythm disturbance encountered in cardio-oncology is **atrial fibrillation (AF)**. However, the most directly life-threatening arrhythmia is ventricular fibrillation (VF), which is commonly preceded by **QTc prolongation**.
- Excellent reviews of CTIA exist.[3,4]

Definition

- The **Common Terminology Criteria for Adverse Events (CTCAEs)** developed by the National Cancer Institute lists a number of arrhythmic adverse events as cardiotoxicities that may be reported during oncology trials.
- The clinical and prognostic significance of the rhythm disturbances in this list are highly variable, as it spans sinus tachycardia (not life threatening) to VF (immediately life threatening). Reporting is sometimes incomplete or inaccurate,[5] making the true incidence of specific associated arrhythmias difficult to quantify.

Classification

- CTIA can be classified as **primary** (because of off-target effects of the therapy on molecular pathways that result in arrhythmia) or **secondary** (from therapy-induced cardiotoxicity such as cardiomyopathy or vasculopathy, which subsequently predispose to arrhythmias).[3]
- Most published data on the incidence of arrhythmias with cancer treatments are best described as **associations rather than causative relationships**, because of confounding that cannot be controlled for in oncologic clinical trials. Additionally, although associations listed are attributed to single therapies, cancer therapeutics are often used in combination clinically.

RHYTHM DISTURBANCES

ATRIAL FIBRILLATION

Definition

- AF is characterized by rapid disorganized atrial activation, with variable ventricular conduction.

- The burden of AF is classified as **paroxysmal**, **persistent** (>7 days duration), **long standing** (>12 months), or **permanent** (no longer attempting rhythm control).
- Differentiating AF that is caused by cancer therapy from incidental AF from other risk factors in cancer patients (inflammation, volume depletion, pneumonia, and pulmonary embolism) is difficult.

Associated Drugs/Therapies

- Please refer to Table 11-1 for a comprehensive list of agents associated with elevated risk of AF.
- **Ibrutinib**, a tyrosine kinase inhibitor (TKI) used in hematologic malignancies, is strongly associated with AF.

TABLE 11-1 Therapies Associated With AF and Their Respective Incidence of Severe Thrombocytopenia

Class	Specific agent	AF incidence[3]	Thrombocytopenia expected	Grade 3-4 (<50k)[a]
Alkylating agents	Cyclophosphamide	++	−	
	Melphalan	+++	+++	>50%
Anthracyclines	Doxorubicin	+++	+	<1%
Antimetabolites	Capecitabine	++	+	2%
	Clofarabine	+++	+++	80%
	5-Fluorouracil	++	+++	[b]
	Gemcitabine	++	++	5%
Antimicrotubule agents	Paclitaxel	+	+	<1%
Interleukin-2		++	++	39%
Immunomodulatory drugs	Lenalidomide	++	+++	80%
	Thalidomide	++	−	
Platinum compounds	Cisplatin	+++	+++	25%-30%
Proteasome inhibitors	Carfilzomib	++	+++	45%-64%
Rituximab		++	+	2%
Romidepsin		++	+++	24%-36%
Small molecule TKIs	Ibrutinib	++	++	5%-17%

(*continued*)

TABLE 11-1	Therapies Associated With AF and Their Respective Incidence of Severe Thrombocytopenia (*continued*)			
Class	Specific agent	AF incidence[3]	Thrombocytopenia expected	Grade 3-4 (<50k)[a]
	Ponatinib	++	+++	36%-57%
VEGF pathway inhibitors	Sorafenib	++	+	4%
	Vemurafenib	++	−	

−, rare; +, uncommon (<1%); ++, common (1%-10%); +++, very common (>10%); AF, atrial fibrillation; TKI, tyrosine kinase inhibitor; VEGF, vascular endothelial growth factor.

[a]Incidence of thrombocytopenia obtained from Food and Drug Administration (FDA) package inserts accessed November 29, 2020.

[b]5-Fluorouracil is generally used in combination therapy, and single-agent incidence of thrombocytopenia was not available.

- The mechanism of ibrutinib-induced AF is thought to be off-target inhibition of C-terminal Src kinase.[6]
- Management of AF in the setting of ibrutinib is complicated by **interactions** with commonly used medications for AF, including atrioventricular (AV) nodal blocking agents (calcium channel blockers, digoxin) and anticoagulants (may increase warfarin levels and dabigatran levels; apixaban and rivaroxaban also have potential for interaction).[7]
- AF is also strongly associated with melphalan, a pre–stem cell transplant conditioning regimen.[8] Please refer to Chapter 18 for further discussion of melphalan.
- AF can be a manifestation of cancer treatment–associated cardiomyopathy, such as in the case of doxorubicin, bortezomib, and carfilzomib.[3]

Diagnosis

- **Electrocardiogram** (ECG) shows absence of organized atrial rhythm with P waves replaced by fibrillatory waves, with an irregular ventricular rhythm.
- **Transthoracic echocardiogram** (TTE) is important in assessing left ventricular ejection fraction, presence or absence of mitral valve stenosis, and left atrial size, as these are features that would change prognosis/management.

Management

Acute Management

- AF is generally not a life-threatening rhythm, although rapid ventricular rates can result in hypotension and hemodynamic instability in patients with significant structural heart disease. Hypotension in a patient with AF can be a sign of underlying sepsis or other disease processes (with the arrhythmia being a *symptom* of the underlying disease process rather than a *cause* of hypotension).

- In the case of hemodynamic instability attributed to rapidly conducting AF, **electrical cardioversion** with 120 to 200 J biphasic or 200 J monophasic is appropriate.
- β-**Blockers** or **nondihydropyridine calcium channel blockers** (diltiazem, verapamil) can be used for acute **rate control** with goal heart rate <110 bpm. Calcium channel blockers should be avoided in heart failure with reduced ejection fraction, and in cardiac amyloid.[9] Additionally, nondihydropyridine calcium channel blockers have significant drug-drug interactions that must be considered, often making **beta-blockers the preferred initial agent**.
- **Digoxin** can be useful for rate control in patients whose blood pressure limits the use of first-line agents. Digoxin has often been avoided in cardiac amyloid because of concern for binding with amyloid fibrils and associated toxicity;[10] however, more recent evidence suggests it may be safely used with appropriate patient selection and close monitoring.[11]
- If patients do not like the way that AF makes them feel, a **rhythm-control strategy** can be employed. In patients where the duration of AF is known and is <48 hours, electrical or chemical cardioversion (with agent such as amiodarone) is appropriate. Otherwise, sinus rhythm can be restored if the patient has had **uninterrupted anticoagulation** for 3 weeks prior to cardioversion, or if **transesophageal echocardiogram (TEE)** prior to cardioversion rules out left atrial appendage thrombus.[12]
- In patients without overt symptoms during AF, duration is often not known.
- If an **antiarrhythmic drug** such as amiodarone is employed for a rhythm-control strategy in the setting of a possibly reversible trigger (such as inpatient acute illness, surgery, or chemotherapy initiation), it is reasonable to continue use for 30 days on discharge. Thereafter, decision to continue antiarrhythmic therapy and anticoagulation can be informed by **30-day event monitor** and **patient-centered risk/benefit discussion**, provided suspected trigger has been addressed.
- Electrical or chemical cardioversion of AF **necessitates four subsequent weeks** of **uninterrupted anticoagulation** to minimize the risks of a thromboembolism.[12] Elevated bleeding risk exists in patients with severe thrombocytopenia (platelets <50k) taking oral anticoagulants, so decisions about cardioversion may be affected.

Anticoagulation
- **AF predisposes to embolic stroke**, thus anticoagulation is a key part of AF treatment. In the setting of cancer treatment, anticoagulation is complicated by thrombocytopenias and drug-drug interactions.
- The decision to recommend therapeutic anticoagulation is guided by **CHA2DS2-VASc score** (to estimate ischemic stroke risk; not applicable to AF in the setting of mitral stenosis or hypertrophic cardiomyopathy) and **HAS-BLED score** (to estimate risk of major bleeding and hemorrhagic stroke), while considering anticipated thrombocytopenias and procedures.
- Therapeutic anticoagulation is recommended for a CHA2DS2-VASc of ≥2 in men and ≥3 in women, and may be considered for CHA2DS2-VASc of 1 in men or 2 in women.[12]
- Please refer to Table 11-1 for anticipated thrombocytopenias with cancer therapies.
- Risks (including intracranial hemorrhage) generally outweigh benefits of therapeutic anticoagulation in patients with platelet count <50k.

SUPRAVENTRICULAR TACHYARRHYTHMIAS (SVTS)

Definition
- Rapidly conducted rhythm originating in the atrium
- Sinus tachycardia—rhythm originating in the **sinus node** at a rate >100 bpm that is most often a physiologic response to an underlying process
- AF—see Section "Atrial Fibrillation."
- Atrial tachycardias
  - Focal—Depolarization driven from automatic focus in the atria, outside of the sinus node
  - Multifocal (MAT)—Depolarization driven by numerous foci of automatic activity within the atria
  - Macroreentrant—Depolarization resulting from reentrant circuit within the atria. **Atrial flutter** is the most common macroreentrant SVT.
- AV nodal reentry tachycardia (AVNRT)—Reentrant tachycardia where circuit is within an AV node that has two pathways (**slow pathway and fast pathway**)
- AV reentry tachycardia (AVRT)—Reentrant tachycardia where one limb is through the AV node and the other limb is through an **accessory connection** between the atria and ventricles

Associated Drugs/Therapies
- The most common supraventricular arrhythmia encountered in cardio-oncology is AF, with associations described in the section earlier.
- Clinical trials for chemotherapy agents do not report SVTs with sufficient granularity to classify them by specific type.
- SVT cases have been reported with most classes of conventional and many targeted therapies.[3]

Diagnosis
- ECG during tachycardia can diagnose mechanism.
  - Mechanisms and ECG appearance vary, as represented in Figure 11-1.
  - Sinus tachycardia—Tachycardia (rate >100 bpm) with **P wave that is upright in lead II and biphasic in V1 suggests sinus node origin**.
  - AF—see Section "Atrial Fibrillation."
  - Atrial tachycardias
    - Focal—P-wave morphology during tachycardia that is not consistent with sinus node location
    - Multifocal atrial tachycardia—Three distinct P-wave morphologies during tachycardia
    - Atrial flutter—Recurring regular pattern of atrial activation, described as "sawtooth" in typical atrial flutter
  - AVNRT—Regular narrow complex tachycardia, typically associated with retrograde atrial activation shortly after QRS in typical AVNRT
  - AVRT—Usually narrow complex tachycardia when wave front of activation is going down through the AV node and up the accessory pathway (orthodromic). Wide complex tachycardia if circuit going down the accessory pathway first and up the AV node retrograde (antidromic).
  - When aberrant conduction (wide QRS) is present, it may be difficult to distinguish a supraventricular tachycardia from a ventricular tachycardia (VT). Algorithms exist to help in diagnosis.[13]

SUMMARY ILLUSTRATION

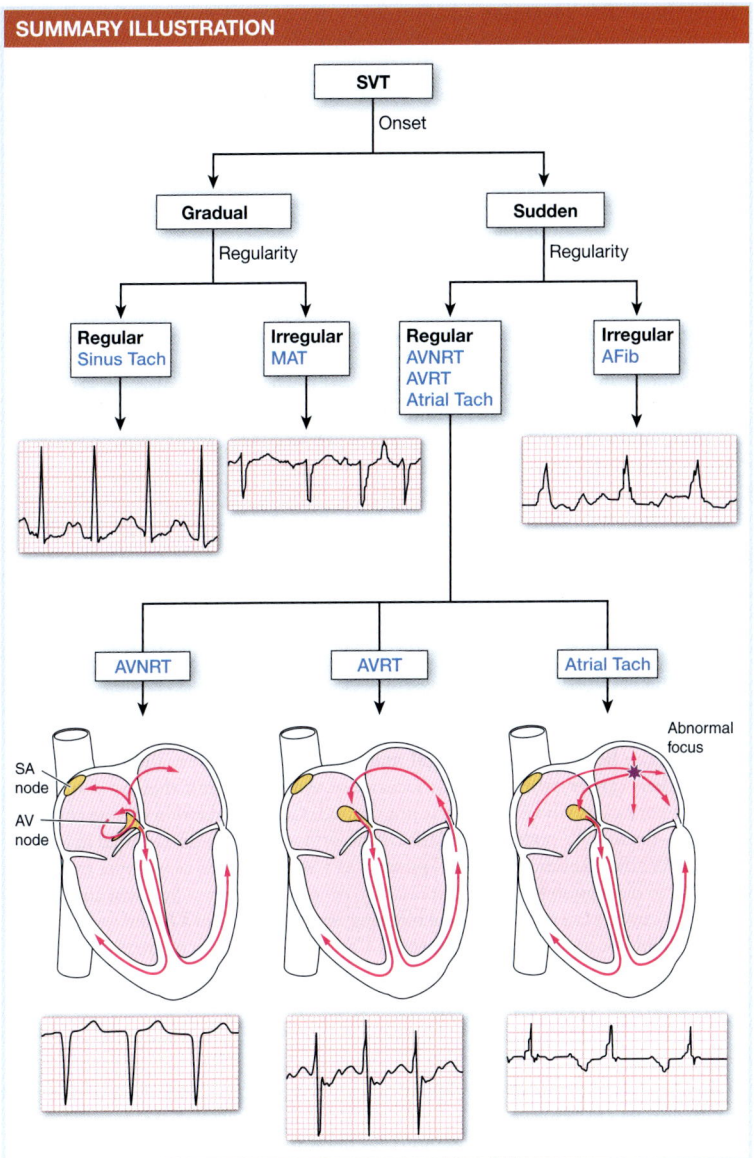

Figure 11-1. Atrial arrhythmias. AV, atrioventricular; AVNRT, AV nodal reentry tachycardia; AVRT, AV reentry tachycardia; MAT, multifocal tachycardia; SA, sinoatrial; SVT, supraventricular tachyarrhythmias. Reprinted with permission from Jackson KP, Daubert JP. Supraventricular tachyarrhythmias. In: Strauss DG, Schocken DD, eds. *Marriott's Practical Electrocardiography.* 13th ed. Wolters Kluwer; 2022:321–344. Summary Illustration 15-1.

- Intravenous (IV) **adenosine** administration can be used to temporarily slow AV conduction and unmask underlying atrial rhythm.
  - Not recommended in patients with significant reactive airway disease, heart transplant recipients, or if there is concern for high-grade conduction system disease.
- ECG in sinus rhythm
  - Sinus rhythm ECG can be compared to tachycardia ECG to identify **retrograde P waves in AVNRT**.
  - **Preexcitation** suggests accessory pathway, making AVRT more likely.

Management

- Sinus tachycardia is most often a secondary response to underlying physiologic cause (such as fever, hypovolemia, anemia, shock, pulmonary embolism, hyperthyroidism, withdrawal from alcohol, and illicit drugs or medications). Management relies on identifying and treating the underlying cause.
  - Inappropriate sinus tachycardia is a diagnosis of exclusion. If heart rate is inappropriately elevated with rest or with minimal exertion despite addressing reversible causes, trial of beta-blockers or ivabradine can be considered.
- AF—see Section "Atrial Fibrillation."
- Atrial tachycardias
  - Focal atrial tachycardia—Nodal blocking agents can slow ventricular rate; antiarrhythmic medication or ablation can also be considered.
  - Multifocal atrial tachycardia—Frequently associated with **chronic obstructive pulmonary disease** and **congestive heart failure**. Treatment of underlying cause is critical, as rate-control agents tend to be ineffective.
  - Atrial flutter is managed like AF (in terms of rate-control or rhythm-control approach, and anticoagulation). In comparison to AF, atrial flutter can be more difficult to rate-control or chemically cardiovert. Atrial flutter is generally sensitive to electrical cardioversion, and ablation can be very effective (as in typical atrial flutter).
- AVNRT can be terminated by **vagal maneuvers**. Beta-blockers and calcium channel blockers can be used to prevent recurrence. Antiarrhythmic therapy is an option in refractory cases where ablation is not desired. Catheter ablation can be curative.
- AVRT—Because AV node is part of the circuit, orthodromic AVRT is treated in a similar way as AVNRT. Antidromic AVRT presents as a wide complex tachycardia and can be difficult to distinguish from VT. Importantly, AF conducting rapidly down an accessory pathway can be exacerbated by nodal blocking agents resulting in **VF**, and expert consultation should be sought if this is suspected. Catheter ablation can be curative in AVRT.

SINUS NODE DYSFUNCTION

Definition

- Sinus bradycardia—Rhythm originating in sinoatrial (SA) node with a rate <60 beats/minute
- Sinus pauses—Periods of time without SA node activity

Associated Drugs/Therapies

- **Crizotinib**, used in non–small cell lung cancer, is associated with sinus bradycardia with an average decrease in heart rate of 26 beats/minute in one study.[14] This was rarely symptomatic and correlated with better clinical response of tumor.

- **Thalidomide** is associated with bradycardia, sometimes necessitating pacemaker placement. In one study of 200 patients (94 of whom were randomized to thalidomide, 106 to placebo), 5 patients required pacemakers for symptomatic bradycardia.[15]
- Anthracyclines, capecitabine, 5-fluorouracil [5-FU], paclitaxel, and TKIs (alectinib, ceritinib, crizotinib) are associated with bradycardia.

Diagnosis
- ECG shows conducted sinus P waves with rate <60 beats/minute.
- Sinus pauses are often identified on telemetry as periods without atrial activity, with or without an escape junctional or ventricular rhythm.
- Single lead examples of arrhythmias of sinus origin can be seen in Figure 11-2.

Management
- Management is guided by **symptoms**. There is no heart rate or pause duration that necessitates intervention.
- Observation alone is sufficient for patients without symptoms or with minimal symptoms.
- Minimize medications that can slow conduction (multiple antihypertensives, antiarrhythmics, and psychoactive medications implicated).[16]
- Screen for **sleep apnea** in patients with sleep-related evidence of sinus node dysfunction.[16]
- After reversible causes have been excluded, patients with symptomatic bradycardia or sinus pauses would benefit from **electrophysiology (EP) consultation** for consideration of EP study or pacemaker therapy.

ATRIOVENTRICULAR BLOCK

Definition
- First-degree AV block is **delay** between atrial and ventricular activation.
- Second-degree AV block
  - Mobitz type 1 (Wenckebach)—Intermittent atrial conduction to the ventricle, with **PR interval prolongation** prior to nonconducted beat
  - Mobitz type 2—Intermittent atrial conduction to the ventricle, without significant PR interval prolongation prior to block
- High-grade AV block—More than two consecutive P waves not conducted, but not meeting criteria for complete heart block
- Third degree (complete) AV block—No atrial conduction to the ventricles, with complete AV dissociation

Associated Drugs/Therapies
- **Immune checkpoint inhibitors (ICIs)** are associated with myocarditis that can result in systolic dysfunction and arrhythmias including heart block, AF, and VT.[17] A case series of 30 patients with suspected ICI-associated cardiotoxicity found that cardiovascular mortality was significantly associated with conduction abnormalities.[18]
- Though **paclitaxel** is most often associated with asymptomatic bradycardia, a study of 47 patients on paclitaxel noted one case of Mobitz type 1 (Wenckebach) that

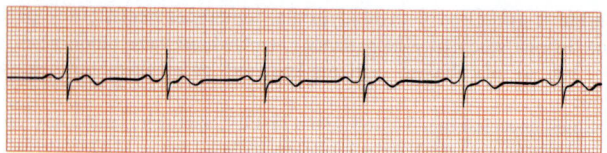

Normal sinus rhythm

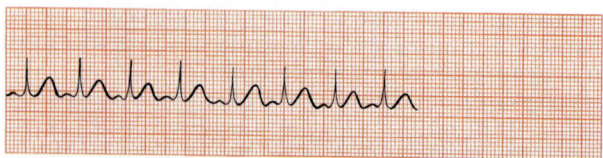

Sinus tachycardia

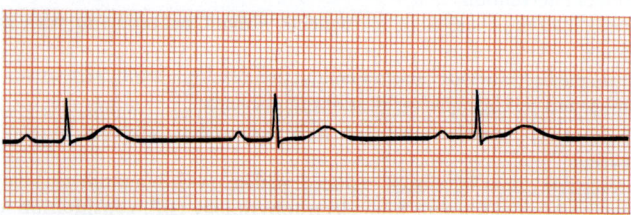

Sinus bradycardia

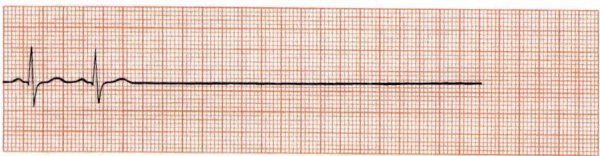

Sinus arrest or exit block

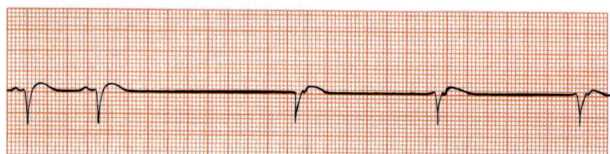

Sinus arrest or exit block with junctional escape

Figure 11-2. Arrhythmias of sinus origin. Reprinted with permission from Thaler M. Arrhythmias. In: *The Only EKG Book You'll Ever Need*. 9th ed. Wolters Kluwer; 2019:103-174. UnFigure 3-15.

resolved 4 hours after infusion each time, and another patient with high-degree AV block that required permanent pacemaker placement.[19]
- There are case reports of complete AV block with cyclophosphamide, busulfan, anthracyclines, capecitabine, 5-FU, arsenic trioxide, all-trans retinoic acid (ATRA),

interleukin (IL)-2, interferons, cisplatin, proteasome inhibitors, nilotinib, ponatinib, cetuximab, rituximab, sorafenib, and a number of vascular endothelial growth factor (VEGF) pathway inhibitors.[3]

Diagnosis
- See "ECG Features in Definition Section."
- Single lead examples of AV block can be seen in Figure 11-3.

Management
- First-degree AV block (AV delay) and second-degree Mobitz type 1 (Wenckebach)
  - Usually reflects conduction delay or block in the AV node, and is generally benign finding, especially in the setting of a narrow QRS. Monitoring for symptoms is appropriate.
- Second-degree Mobitz type 2, complete heart block, high-grade AV block, and complete AV block
  - Mobitz type 2 reflects block below the level of the AV node and is a precursor to high-grade AV block.
  - Pacemaker is recommended regardless of symptoms, provided no reversible cause is identified.[16]
  - In the acute setting:

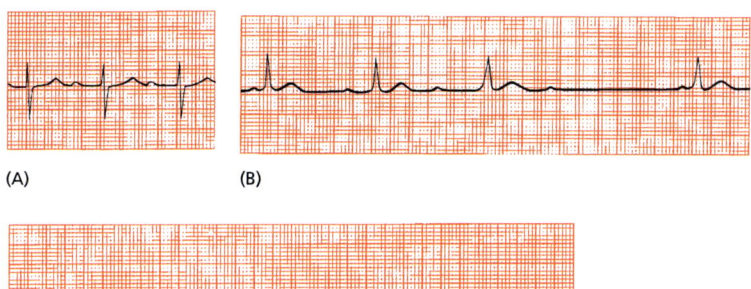

(A)   (B)

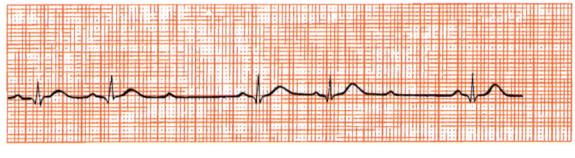

(C)

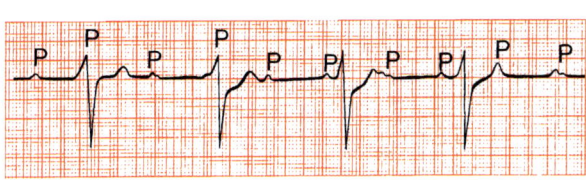

(D)

Figure 11-3. Atrioventricular (AV) block. (A) First-degree AV block. (B) Mobitz type 1 second-degree AV block (Wenckebach block). (C) Mobitz type 2 second-degree AV block. (D) Third-degree AV block. Reprinted with permission from Thaler M. Putting it all together. In: *The Only EKG Book You'll Ever Need.* 9th ed. Wolters Kluwer; 2019:325-350. UnFigure 8-12.

- Emergent temporary pacing may be necessary for hemodynamically unstable or symptomatic patients.
- For hemodynamically stable and asymptomatic patients with high-grade block or complete heart block with a narrow escape rhythm, inpatient telemetry monitoring (with pacer pads physically on the patient and atropine available at bedside) while awaiting definitive device therapy may be sufficient. Stability of **ventricular escape rhythm** is unpredictable—consider temporary transvenous pacemaker or be prepared to place emergently, while awaiting definitive permanent device placement.

QT PROLONGATION

Definition

- The QT interval is measured from the beginning of the Q wave and the end of the T wave on an ECG and reflects ventricular depolarization and repolarization. Prolongation of this interval is usually due to a delay in repolarization.
- **Prolonged repolarization is a risk factor for torsades de pointes (TdP)**, a rare but potentially lethal ventricular arrhythmia (VA) (Fig. 11-4).
- **Sinus bradycardia or sinus pauses** in the setting of QT prolongation further elevate the risk of TdP.

Associated Drugs/Therapies

- **Arsenic trioxide**, an agent that has significantly improved survival in acute promyelocytic leukemia, has a high incidence of QTc prolongation. In one study, 40% of study participants experienced at least one ECG with a QTc >500 ms and 1 out of 40 patients experienced TdP.[20]
- **TKIs** are associated with QT prolongation.[21] In one study, nilotinib, dasatinib, and sunitinib (but not imatinib) increased the action potential duration by inhibition of

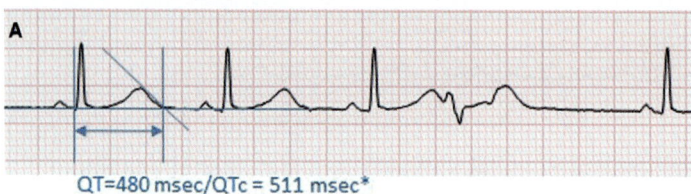

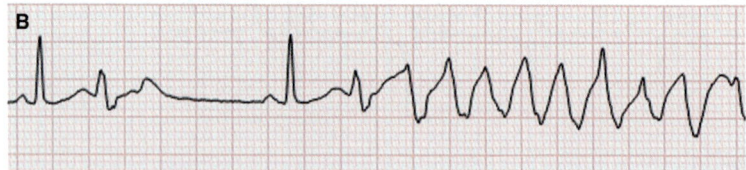

Figure 11-4. Example of QT prolongation (A) with subsequent torsades de pointes (B) in a patient with suspected cardiac metastasis from rhabdomyosarcoma resulting in monomorphic PVCs. Asterisk, QTc calculated by correcting QT via Bazett formula for average heart rate of 68 bpm.

phosphoinositide 3-kinase signaling in canine cardiac myocytes, affecting multiple ion channels.[22]

- Please refer to Table 11-2 for a comprehensive list of agents with elevated risk of QTc prolongation.

TABLE 11-2	Therapies Associated With QTc Prolongation and Their Respective Incidence of Arrhythmia/SCD			
Class	Specific agent	QTc prolongation incidence[a]	Grade 3 QTc prolongation incidence[b]	Arrythmias/SCD (total patients studied)
	Arsenic trioxide	+++	++	24/1 (533)
Antimetabolites	Capecitabine	+++	-	0/0 (52)
	5-Fluorouracil	-	-	0/0 (102)
Antimicrotubule agents	Paclitaxel	++	-	0/0 (290)
Antiangiogenic	Combretastatin	+++	+	0/0 (110)
	Vadimezan	+++	++	0/0 (77)
B-Raf inhibitor	Vemurafenib	++	++	2/0 (3597)
Histone deacetylase inhibitors	Belinostat	++	++	1/0 (195)
	Panobinostat	++	+	0/0 (654)
	Romidepsin	++	−	0/0 (112)
	Vorinostat	+++	++	0/0 (189)
Protease inhibitor	Bortezomib	++	++	0/0 (22)
Protein kinase C inhibitor	Enzastaurin	+++	++	0/0 (135)
Small molecule TKIs	Aflibercept	++	−	0/0 (43)
	Bosutinib	++	−	0/0 (87)
	Ceritinib	+	+	0/0 (130)
	Crizotinib	+	+	0/0 (101)
	Dasatinib	++	+	1/0 (611)
	Dovitinib	++	++	0/0 (49)

(*continued*)

Class	Specific agent	QTc prolongation incidence[a]	Grade 3 QTc prolongation incidence[b]	Arrythmias/SCD (total patients studied)
	Imatinib	++	−	0/0 (897)
	Lapatinib	++	++	0/0 (117)
	Lenvatinib	++	++	0/0 (319)
	Nilotinib	++	+	0/5 (3076)
	Nintedanib	++	++	0/0 (94)
	Pazopanib	+	−	0/1 (99)
	Ponatinib	++	++	0/0 (120)
VEGF pathway inhibitors	Cediranib	+++	++	0/0 (127)
	Sorafenib/ sunitinib	++	++	0/0 (290)
	Vandetanib	++	++	1/0 (2567)

−, ; +, uncommon (<1%); ++, common (1% to 10%); +++, very common (>10%); SCD, sudden cardiac death; TKI, tyrosine kinase inhibitor; VEGF, vascular endothelial growth factor.

[a]QTc prolongation defined in CTCAE by Grade 1 or above (Grade 1 is average QTc 450-480 ms). CTCAE is **Common Terminology Criteria for Adverse Events.**

[b]Grade 3 QTc prolongation is defined in CTCAE as average QTc ≥501 ms or >60 ms change from baseline.

Adapted from Porta-Sánchez A, Gilbert C, Spears D, et al. Incidence, diagnosis, and management of QT prolongation induced by cancer therapies: a systematic review. *J Am Heart Assoc.* 2017;6(12).e007724.

Diagnosis

- The QT interval is manually measured in a single lead from a 12-lead ECG where it is **longest** and in which a prominent U wave is absent; when reported from automated ECG algorithm, it is often the average of the QT complexes.
- The duration of a normal QT interval is dependent on the ventricular rate, denoted as QTc (corrected QT).
  - Many population-derived correction formulas exist:
    ○ Bazett correction: $QTc = QT/RR^{0.5}$
    ○ Widely used clinically but tends to overestimate QT at high heart rates (>90) and underestimate it at lower ones (<60).
    ○ Fridericia correction: $QTc = QT/RR^{0.33}$
    ○ Also reported in drug trials

- Linear regression formulas exist that are more accurate at higher heart rates.
  - Normal QTc is considered **<460 ms in women** and **<450 ms in men. QTc > 500 ms reflects significant QT prolongation**.
- A wide QRS interval reflects prolonged depolarization (as in the setting of bundle branch block) and inherently prolongs the QT interval, though it may not affect repolarization time (and thus risk for TdP).
  - Many correction methods exist to account for this. A suggested method is to normalize the QRS duration to 100 or 110 ms and subtract the difference from the QT interval before correcting for heart rate.[23]

Management

- In patients on a therapy with high incidence of QT prolongation, there is often **Food and Drug Administration (FDA) labeling** for ECG monitoring. For example, the package insert for vandetanib states that ECGs should be obtained at baseline, 2 to 4 weeks, 8 to 12 weeks, and 3 months thereafter.
- If QT prolongation is identified, it is important to correct predisposing **electrolyte abnormalities** (hypokalemia, hypomagnesemia, and hypocalcemia), and to **minimize other QT prolonging medications**. For a comprehensive list of QT prolonging medications, refer to www.crediblemeds.org/.
- Commonly encountered medications in an oncologic population that have a known or possible risk of TdP include ondansetron, tramadol, levofloxacin, and azithromycin.
- Medications that have a risk of TdP in the setting of predisposing risk factors include symptom-relieving drugs such as diphenhydramine, famotidine, hydroxyzine, loperamide, omeprazole and trazodone.
- If QTc remains prolonged despite these interventions, risks and benefits of continuing therapy should be assessed. **Of note, whereas QTc prolongation is associated with many cancer therapies, TdP remains a rare event.**[21]

VENTRICULAR ARRHYTHMIAS

Definition

- VT and VF are life-threatening arrhythmias that require early recognition and intervention.

Associated Drugs/Therapies

- **5-FU** is associated with transient angina and ECG changes attributed to coronary vasospasm.[24] This can rarely result in VT, though routine telemetry with administration, even when selecting for high-risk patients, appears to be low yield.[25]
- **Anthracyclines** are associated with VT, secondary to anthracycline-related cardiomyopathy, at similar rates to those with nonischemic cardiomyopathy.[4]
- **Ibrutinib** is associated with VAs, even for patients without cardiovascular disease. One study showed a relative risk of VAs of 12.4 when compared to the general population (though the study was retrospective, not controlled for presence of hematologic malignancy, and their definition of VAs was more broad than sustained VT and VF).[26]
- **ICIs** are associated with VAs in the setting of myocarditis.[18]
- Therapies associated with QT prolongation can result in TdP, as discussed earlier.

Diagnosis

- ECG, telemetry, or defibrillator (as in the setting of cardiac arrest) can be used for diagnosis.
- Monomorphic VT—Regular wide complex tachycardia with AV dissociation
- Polymorphic VT—VT with an irregular contour. TdP is a specific type of polymorphic VT in the setting of QT prolongation.
- VF—Irregular undulations of varying amplitude.
- Single lead examples of arrhythmias of ventricular origin can be seen in Figure 11-5.

Management

- Follow **advanced cardiovascular life support (ACLS)** guidelines. Emergent external cardioversion is critical for hemodynamically unstable patients
- For monomorphic VT in the absence of hemodynamic instability, IV amiodarone and/or IV lidocaine can be employed to terminate.
- Assess for structural heart disease with echocardiogram. Evaluate for **secondary causes** such as ischemia, electrolyte imbalance, anemia, and drug toxicity.
- Unless reversible cause is identified, defibrillator for **secondary prevention** is recommended, guided by patient preference and life expectancy.

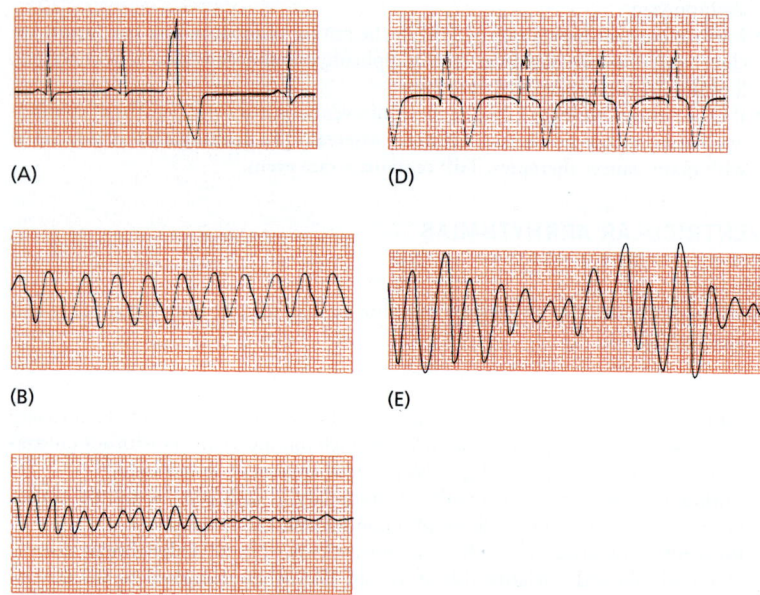

Figure 11-5. Ventricular arrhythmias. (A) Premature ventricular contraction. (B) Ventricular tachycardia. (C) Ventricular fibrillation. (D) Accelerated idioventricular rhythm. (E) Torsades de pointes. Reprinted with permission from Thaler M. Putting it all together. In: *The Only EKG Book You'll Ever Need*. 9th ed. Wolters Kluwer; 2019:325-350. UnFigure 8-11.

Diagnostic Tests
- **ECG**: Key for arrhythmia diagnosis and localization
- **Holter Monitor**: Records continuously for 24 to 48 hours and can quantify arrhythmia burden and help **correlate patient-triggered symptoms** with monitor findings.
- **Event Monitor**: Wearable monitor able to record telemetry for extended periods of time (used when symptoms are not daily). Records automatically triggered events and patient-triggered events.
- **Loop Recorder**: Small monitoring device implanted subcutaneously that can record for over 3 years. Useful to identify rare symptoms. Most often employed in the evaluation of syncope and to look for paroxysmal AF in the setting of stroke.
- **Exercise Stress Test**: Aside from its use in risk stratification for obstructive coronary artery disease, it can be employed to assess for **chronotropic incompetence** and exercise-induced arrhythmias.

REFERENCES

1. Tyebally S, Chen D, Bhattacharyya S, et al. Cardiac tumors: *JACC CardioOncology* state-of-the-art review. *J Am Coll Cardiol CardioOnc*. 2020;2(2):293-311.
2. Gaya AM, Ashford RFU. Cardiac complications of radiation therapy. *Clin Oncol*. 2005;17(3):153-159.
3. Buza V, Rajagopalan B, Curtis AB. Cancer treatment–induced arrhythmias: focus on chemotherapy and targeted therapies. *Circ Arrhythm Electrophysiol*. 2017;10(8):e005443.
4. Rhea I, Burgos PH, Fradley MG. Arrhythmogenic anticancer drugs in cardio-oncology. *Cardiol Clin*. 2019;37(4):459-468.
5. Zhang S, Chen Q, Wang Q. The use of and adherence to CTCAE v3.0 in cancer clinical trial publications. *Oncotarget*. 2016;7(40):65577-65588.
6. Xiao, Ling, Salem, Joe-Elie, Clauss, Sebastian, et al. Ibrutinib-mediated atrial fibrillation due to inhibition of CSK. *Circulation*. 2020;(25):2443-2455.
7. Ganatra S, Sharma A, Shah S, et al. Ibrutinib-associated atrial fibrillation. *JACC Clin Electrophysiol*. 2018;4(12):1491-1500.
8. Feliz V, Saiyad S, Ramarao SM, Khan H, Leonelli F, Guglin M. Melphalan-induced supraventricular tachycardia: incidence and risk factors. *Clin Cardiol*. 2011;34(6):356-359.
9. Pollak A, Falk RH. Left ventricular systolic dysfunction precipitated by verapamil in cardiac amyloidosis. *Chest*. 1993;104(2):618-620.
10. Rubinow A, Skinner M, Cohen AS. Digoxin sensitivity in amyloid cardiomyopathy. *Circulation*. 1981;63(6):1285-1288.
11. Donnelly JP, Sperry BW, Gabrovsek A, et al. Digoxin use in cardiac amyloidosis. *Am J Cardiol*. 2020;133:134-138.
12. January CT, Wann LS, Calkins H, et al. 2019 AHA/ACC/HRS focused update of the 2014 AHA/ACC/HRS guideline for the management of patients with atrial fibrillation: a report of the American College of Cardiology/American Heart Association Task Force on Clinical Practice Guidelines and the Heart Rhythm Society in Collaboration With the Society of Thoracic Surgeons. *Circulation*. 2019;140(2):e125-e151.
13. Vereckei A, Duray G, Szénási G, Altemose GT, Miller JM. New algorithm using only lead aVR for differential diagnosis of wide QRS complex tachycardia. *Heart Rhythm*. 2008;5(1):89-98.
14. Ou S-HI, Tong WP, Azada M, Siwak-Tapp C, Dy J, Stiber JA. Heart rate decrease during crizotinib treatment and potential correlation to clinical response. *Cancer*. 2013;119(11):1969-1975.
15. Fahdi IE, Gaddam V, Saucedo JF, et al. Bradycardia during therapy for multiple myeloma with thalidomide. *Am J Cardiol*. 2004;93(8):1052-1055.

16. Kusumoto FM, Schoenfeld MH, Barrett C, et al. 2018 ACC/AHA/HRS guideline on the evaluation and management of patients with bradycardia and cardiac conduction delay: a report of the American College of Cardiology/American Heart Association Task Force on Clinical Practice Guidelines and the Heart Rhythm Society. *Circulation.* 2019;140(8):e382-e482.
17. Ball S, Ghosh RK, Wongsaengsak S, et al. Cardiovascular toxicities of immune checkpoint inhibitors. *J Am Coll Cardiol.* 2019;74(13):1714-1727.
18. Escudier, Marion, Cautela, Jennifer, Malissen, Nausicaa, et al. Clinical features, management, and outcomes of immune checkpoint inhibitor–related cardiotoxicity. *Circulation.* 2017;136(21):2085-2087.
19. McGuire WP, Rowinsky EK, Rosenshein NB, et al. Taxol: a unique antineoplastic agent with significant activity in advanced ovarian epithelial neoplasms. *Ann Intern Med.* 1989;111(4):273-279.
20. Soignet SL, Frankel SR, Douer D, et al. United States multicenter study of arsenic trioxide in relapsed acute promyelocytic leukemia. *J Clin Oncol.* 2001;19(18):3852-3860.
21. Porta-Sánchez A, Gilbert C, Spears D, et al. Incidence, diagnosis, and management of QT prolongation induced by cancer therapies: a systematic review. *J Am Heart Assoc.* 2017;6(12):e007724.
22. Lu Z, Wu C-YC, Jiang Y-P, et al. Suppression of phosphoinositide 3-kinase signaling and alteration of multiple ion currents in drug-induced long QT syndrome. *Sci Transl Med.* 2012;4(131):131ra50.
23. Zimetbaum P, Buxton A, Josephson M. Practical clinical electrophysiology. In: *Practical Clinical Electrophysiology*. 2nd ed. Wolters Kluwer; 2018:325-333.
24. Jensen SA, Hasbak P, Mortensen J, Sørensen JB. Fluorouracil induces myocardial ischemia with increases of plasma brain natriuretic peptide and lactic acid but without dysfunction of left ventricle. *J Clin Oncol.* 2010;28(36):5280-5286.
25. Pizzolato JF, Baum MS, Steingart RM, Gonan M, Minsky BD, Saltz LB. Cardiac toxicity of 5FU: does prophylactic telemetry monitoring of patients at increased risk for cardiac toxicity improve safety? A 10-year experience. *J Clin Oncol.* 2004;22(14, suppl):8107-8107.
26. Guha A, Derbala MH, Zhao Q, et al. Ventricular arrhythmias following ibrutinib initiation for cancer immunotherapy. *J Am Coll Cardiol.* 2018;72(6):697-698.

12 Intravascular Devices and Thrombotic Complications

Douglas A. Kyrouac, J. Westley Ohman, and Joshua D. Mitchell

PACEMAKER (PM) AND IMPLANTABLE CARDIOVERTER DEFIBRILLATOR (ICD)

GENERAL PRINCIPLES

- Given the significant intersection between patients with cancer and cardiovascular disease, it is not uncommon for patients with cancer to have a previously implanted PM/ICD or to develop an indication for a PM/ICD during or after their therapy.
- PM/ICD in a patient receiving cancer therapy affects **radiation planning** and can be an increased risk of **infection**.
- In patients who develop an indication for a primary prevention ICD, future anticipated **cancer treatments and cancer prognosis are important considerations**. Primary prevention ICDs are generally reserved for patients who have >1 year life expectancy, although some patients who qualify may still opt to forego an ICD depending on their prognosis and goals of care.
- In patients with ICDs having **end-of-life discussions**, it is important to discuss options to have the ICD turned off during shared decision-making.
- Patients with PMs can be classified into categories based on PM use: (a) The patient is **PM dependent**; (b) The patient is bradycardic but asymptomatic without the PM; and (c) The patient is not PM dependent.

Indications

- The **2018 American College of Cardiology/American Heart Association/Heart Rhythm Society (ACC/AHA/HRS) guidelines for PM implantation** provide an outline of which patients may benefit from PM implantation. These guidelines are characterized by strength of indication (ie, class I, II, or III).[1]
- The **2017 AHA/ACC/HRS guidelines for the management of patients with ventricular arrhythmias and prevention of sudden cardiac death** provide an outline of which patients may benefit from ICD therapy.[20]

Radiation Considerations for Patients With PM or ICD

- In patients undergoing radiation therapy, **radiation planning and delivery must take into account the location of the cancer, the location of a preexisting PM or ICD, as well as whether the patient is PM dependent**.
- **Radiation can cause malfunction or failure of a PM** or its parts, either due to ionizing effect or via electromagnetic interference.
  - The complementary metal-oxide-semiconductor has sensitive transistors, such as silicon, which can become irreversibly damaged.

TABLE 12-1 Pacemaker and ICD Indications

Pacemaker		ICD	
Class 1 indications	**Class 2 indications**	**Primary prevention**	**Secondary prevention**
Symptomatic sinus bradycardia or symptomatic chronotropic incompetence	Sinus bradycardia with possible resulting symptoms	Class 1: Ischemic heart disease with LVEF ≤30% despite guideline-directed medical therapy	Class 1: Sudden cardiac arrest due to ventricular tachycardia or ventricular fibrillation
Complete AV block	Sinus node dysfunction with unexplained syncope	LVEF ≤35% with class II or III heart failure despite guideline-directed medical therapy.	Hemodynamically unstable VT not due to a reversible cause
Advanced second-degree type II AV block, with block of 2 or more consecutive p waves	Heart rate <40 bpm with minimal symptoms	Patients with symptomatic long QT syndrome when β-blocker cannot be uptitrated	Stable VT not due to a reversible cause
Second-degree type II AV block with wide QRS or chronic bifascicular block, regardless of symptoms	Asymptomatic second-degree type II AV block with narrow QRS	Patients with arrhythmogenic right ventricular cardiomyopathy at high risk for sudden cardiac death	Unexplained syncope with an inducible sustained monomorphic VT on EP study
Symptomatic second-degree type I AV block	First-degree AV block with hemodynamic compromise related to elongated PR interval	Class 2: Patients with cardiac sarcoid and LVEF >35% who have had syncope or scar noted on CMR or PET. Or if there is an indication for permanent pacing	

Pacemaker		ICD	
Class 1 indications	**Class 2 indications**	**Primary prevention**	**Secondary prevention**
Exercise-induced second- or third-degree AV block not related to ischemia	Bifascicular or trifascicular block associated with syncope	Patients at high risk for ventricular tachycardia/ ventricular fibrillation (HCM w/ risk factors, CHD, etc.)	

AV, atrioventricular; CHD, coronary heart disease; CMR, cardiac magnetic resonance imaging; EP, electrophysiological; HCM, hypertrophic cardiomyopathy; ICD, implantable cardioverter defibrillator; LVEF, left ventricular ejection fraction; PET, positron emission tomography; VT, ventricular tachycardia.

From Kusumoto FM, Schoenfeld MH, Barrett C, et al. 2018 ACC/AHA/HRS guideline on the evaluation and management of patients with bradycardia and cardiac conduction delay: a report of the American College of Cardiology/American Heart Association Task Force on Clinical Practice Guidelines and the Heart Rhythm Society. *J Am Coll Cardiol.* 2019;74(7):932-987. doi:10.1016/j.jacc.2018.10.043; Al-Khatib SM, Stevenson WG, Ackerman MJ, et al. 2017 AHA/ACC/HRS guideline for management of patients with ventricular arrhythmias and the prevention of sudden cardiac death: a report of the American College of Cardiology/American Heart Association Task Force on Clinical Practice Guidelines and the Heart Rhythm Society. *J Am Coll Cardiol.* 2018;72(14):e91-e220. doi:10.1016/j.jacc.2017.10.054. Erratum in: *J Am Coll Cardiol.* 2018;72(14):1760.

- There can be effects on random access memory secondary to scatter radiation or electromagnetic irradiation.
- Aberrant electrical pathways can form within the silicon dioxide insulator and lead to transient or permanent changes in PM function.
- In vitro studies noted a maximum dose rate of only 20 cGy/min was considered "safe." As such, **it is important to avoid direct irradiation to the PM site**.
- Patients who are PM dependent may require movement of the device outside the radiation field before starting radiation therapy.

GUIDELINES/RECOMMENDATIONS FOR PMS AND IRRADIATION

- Patients can be risk stratified based on the necessity of the PM and cumulative radiation dosing to the PM:
  - For PM-independent patients, <2 Gy is low risk, 2 to 5 Gy is medium risk, and >5 Gy or use of neutrons is high risk.
  - **For PM-dependent patients, <2 Gy becomes medium risk, 2 to 5 Gy remains medium risk, and >5 Gy or use of neutrons is high risk.**[3,4]
- If the patient has an ICD, it should be determined whether **antitachycardia pacing** (ATP) can be disabled.[4]
- **Monitoring and follow-up should be based on the abovementioned risk stratification**, as described in Table 12-2.[3,21]

TABLE 12-2 Cardiac Device Follow-Up Monitoring Based on Risk Stratification

<2 Gy (Low Risk)	2–5 Gy (Medium Risk)	>5 Gy or neutrons (High Risk)
• Patient should report any cardiac symptoms during therapy • Have a pacemaker magnet, pulse oximetry, and AED on site • Close audio and visual monitoring of the patient during treatment • Bidirectional communication between radiation physician and cardiology • For ICD patients, turn off antitachycardia pacing or use a magnet when able • Device interrogation before the first radiation treatment and after the last treatment	Low-Risk monitoring PLUS: • Cardiology should have formal involvement in patient care • May consider close monitoring of pacemaker-dependent patients with magnet and pulse oximeter when appropriate • Have cardiac support available for possible complications (ie, crash cart, ECG, magnet, pulse oximeter, AED, transcutaneous pacing with trained staff) • Interrogate the device mid-treatment	Medium-Risk monitoring PLUS: • Weekly ECG interpreted by trained staff • Immediate availability of a cardiologist or pacemaker technologist • Weekly device interrogation once it has received >5 Gy

Of note, a magnet temporarily disables ICDs. The magnet causes pacemakers to fire asynchronously.

AED, automated external defibrillator; ECG, electrocardiogram; ICD, implantable cardioverter defibrillator.

Data from Hurkmans CW, Knegjens JL, Oei BS, et al. Management of radiation oncology patients with a pacemaker or ICD: a new comprehensive practical guideline in The Netherlands. Dutch Society of Radiotherapy and Oncology (NVRO). *Radiat Oncol.* 2012;7:198. doi:10.1186/1748-717X-7-198; Miften M, Mihailidis D, Kry SF, et al. Management of radiotherapy patients with implanted cardiac pacemakers and defibrillators: a report of the AAPM TG-203[†]. *Med Phys.* 2019;46(12):e757-e788.

- Manufacturers also provide specifications and guidelines that are PM specific.
- Importantly, **as low as reasonably achievable (ALARA) radiation should be utilized**.
  - If there is need for direct irradiation because of mediastinal mass, the clinician should first consider PM necessity (ie, PM utilization as discussed earlier).

Chapter 12 Intravascular Devices and Thrombotic Complications | 171

- **If PM is necessary and mediastinal irradiation is required, consideration of switching to a leadless PM may be reasonable.**

ROLE OF LEADLESS PM

- Leadless PMs can circumvent the issue of a bulky implantable pulse generator in the chest wall in the event of infection risk or need for mediastinal radiation (Fig. 12-1).

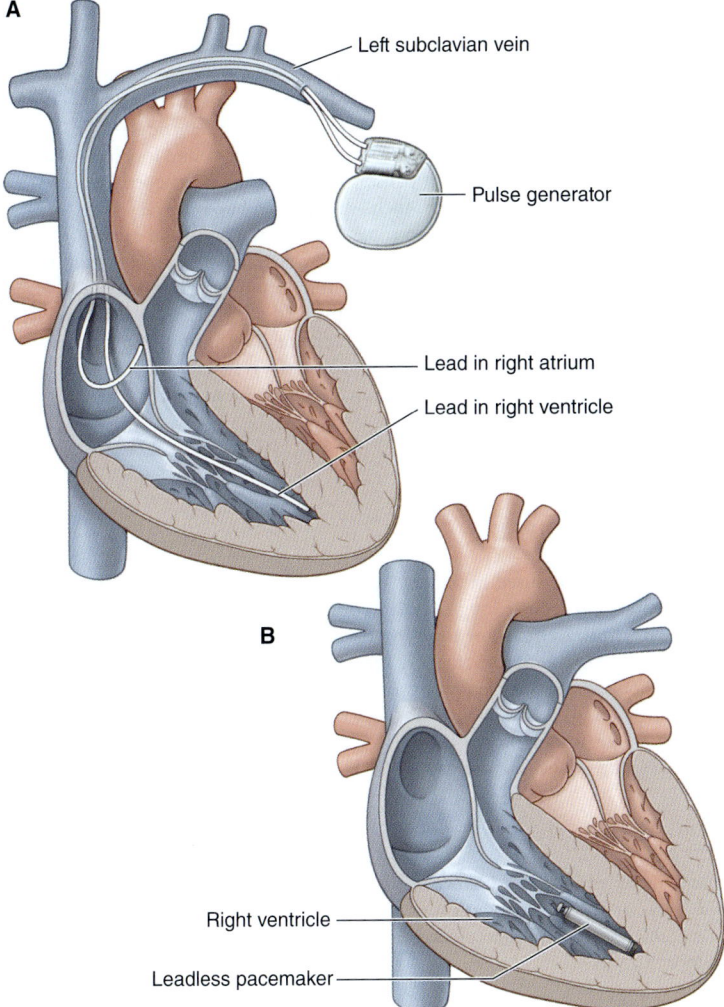

Figure 12-1. (A) Traditional pacemaker with leads in the right atrium and right ventricle. (B) Single chamber leadless pacemaker embedded in the right ventricle.

- Patients with end-stage renal disease (ESRD) are also the prime candidates for leadless PM implantation, because leadless PMs carry less infection risk and do not consume vascular real estate.[5]
- There are **two broad categories of leadless PMs**, with single-component systems currently being predominant with the most data:
  - A **single-component system** contains a battery, electronics, stimulating electrodes, and rate-adaptive sensors within a single device.
  - A **multicomponent system** integrates two or more components, including an energy transducer within the cardiac chamber in addition to a subcutaneous device. The subcutaneous device generates a pacing pulse that it communicates to the intracardiac component via external ultrasound or radio wave energy.
- Single-component leadless PM systems can currently only pace one ventricle. As such, the indications for these leadless PMs are more limited than the general guidelines discussed earlier: chronic atrial fibrillation with atrioventricular (AV) block or significant pauses, sinus rhythm with high-degree AV block and low-level of activity, sinus bradycardia with infrequent pauses, and unexplained syncope with abnormal electrophysiological (EP) findings, such as prolonged HV interval.[5]
- Although it is not recommended to subject a leadless PM to direct radiation, there have been cases where radiation therapy was unavoidable as a result of proximity of the mass to the PM. One patient received maximum proton doses of 30 Gy in 15 sessions to a mediastinal mass. Despite being within the field of radiation, the leadless PM was unaffected. If the PM is within the field of radiation, it is recommended to have close follow-up and interrogation of the device to ensure it is functioning properly.[6]
- A conventional PM outside the radiation field may be more advantageous than a leadless PM within the field.

PORTS

GENERAL PRINCIPLES

- Ports are commonly used in patients receiving cancer treatment. They are suitable for patients who require long-term, intermittent venous access for **chemotherapy administration, frequent or time-intensive infusions, or frequent blood draws**.
- Importantly, common chemotherapy agents are vesicants or irritants that necessitate stable venous access, such as a port, to avoid the potential complication of subcutaneous infiltration, which is much more likely to occur with temporary venous access.[7]
- Ports **may improve quality of life** by providing long-term central venous access while minimizing needlesticks. **Patients may bathe, swim, or exercise after port placement**.

CONSIDERATIONS

- For patients with **breast cancer**, the port should be **placed on the contralateral side** so as to not interfere with surgical management.[8]
- If possible, ports should be **placed 2 weeks before chemotherapy** to allow healing before treatment.[8]

COMPLICATIONS

- Ports have been reported to have an **overall complication rate of up to 27%**.[9] These complications can be divided into early and delayed complications of port placement.

Early Complications
- **Early complications** include malposition, arrhythmia, perforation (which may lead to hemothorax or cardiac tamponade), arterial malpositioning, pneumothorax, thoracic duct injury, or air embolism.

Delayed Complications
- **Delayed complications** include infection, venous thrombosis embolism (VTE)/pulmonary embolism (PE), venous stenosis, catheter pinch-off, fracture and migration, catheter embolization, or air embolism.[9]
- **Symptomatic VTE** may affect patients with cancer with ports, with an incidence of around 5%. However, nearly half of ports may be complicated by some degree of thrombus formation.
  - The majority of these thrombi are subclinical, form gradually, and may be managed conservatively.[8,10]
  - Anticoagulant or antiplatelet use was associated with a lower risk of VTE in retrospective analysis,[7] but prospective studies have not confirmed this finding.[8] Benefits must be weighed against potential risks of therapy.
  - Current guidelines recommend **medical therapy with anticoagulation**, rather than catheter removal, for treatment of **uncomplicated catheter-associated VTE**.
  - A meta-analysis of dialysis **catheter–related atrial thrombi recommended removing the catheter when possible**.[11] Patients with a small thrombus (<6 cm), without major complication, such as PE on anticoagulation or hemodynamic compromise, without contraindications to anticoagulation may receive anticoagulation alone for 6 months.
- **Catheter mechanical complication can be identified during infusion**: prolonged infusion time, inability to inject saline, subcutaneous extravasation of chemotherapy, arm swelling, neck or back pain with infusion, or inability to puncture the port.[9]
- **Blood stream infection is a rare but clinically important complication**.
  - Ports associated with bacteremia should be removed if there are severe complications: severe sepsis, suppurative thrombophlebitis, endocarditis, or persistent bacteremia despite 72 hours of appropriate antimicrobial therapy.
  - Given the proximity to the heart and risk for endocarditis, **high-risk infections due to *Staphylococcus aureus*, *Pseudomonas aeruginosa*, fungi, or mycobacteria necessitate port removal**.[12]
  - Otherwise, bacteremia may be treated with 7 to 14 days of antibiotic therapy and the port may be left in if the microorganism is low risk (coagulase-negative *Staphylococcus*, *Enterococcus*, or non-*Pseudomonas* Gram negative bacilli), susceptible to antibiotics, and there is no evidence of endocarditis.[12]

THROMBOTIC COMPLICATIONS: INFERIOR VENA CAVA FILTER (IVCF), PERCUTANEOUS SUCTION THROMBECTOMY SYSTEMS, STENTING

GENERAL PRINCIPLES

- **Cancer is a major risk factor for VTE, with 4 to 7 times relative risk when compared to the general population**. In fact, thrombotic events are one of the major sources of morbidity and mortality for patients with cancer. In addition to common risk factors, risk for VTE can be related to cancer stage, chemotherapy regimen, and the presence of intravascular devices.[13]

CARDIAC COMPLICATIONS

- Patients may develop **cardiac complications from VTE** by showering pulmonary emboli or by direct clot formation in the cardiac chambers.
- Patients who experience **PE** are at risk of developing **pulmonary hypertension**.
- Pulmonary emboli can be categorized based on their effect on the heart into low risk, intermediate-low risk, intermediate-high risk, or high risk.
  - **Patients with hypotension/shock are high risk.**[14]
  - For patients who are not high risk, a **Pulmonary Embolism Severity Index (PESI) score** can further help risk stratify patients based on their demographics, clinical history, and presentation.
  - **PESI class of I to II signifies low-risk PE** and does not cause hypotension, right ventricle (RV) strain, or myocardial injury.[15]
  - **PESI class of III to IV signifies intermediate-risk PE**. These patients are able to maintain a normal blood pressure but may have evidence of strain on the heart as evidenced by abnormalities on electrocardiogram (ECG), imaging with echocardiogram or computed tomography (CT) scan, or blood work with an elevation in natriuretic peptide or troponin.[15,16]
  - **If RV function is compromised and laboratory testing is positive, then the patient is intermediate-high risk.**[16]
  - If none or one of these is positive, then the patient is intermediate-low risk.[16]
- **Anticoagulation is the gold standard treatment for VTE when feasible**. Anticoagulation prevents further thrombus formation but has no thrombolytic effects. This has led to the development of alternative treatments directed toward high-risk VTE and prevention of post-thrombotic syndrome, as discussed later.[15]

ALTERNATIVE MANAGEMENT

- Often, anticoagulation alone is contraindicated or felt to be insufficient treatment for large VTE, particularly high-risk PE. Additional treatment options include catheter-directed thrombolysis, vena cava filter placement, balloon dilation and venous stenting, and aspiration thrombectomy.[15]

Thrombolytics and Catheter-Directed Thrombolysis

- In contrast to anticoagulation, thrombolytic therapy can restore blood flow by decreasing clot burden. This benefit is not without consequence, as there is a much higher risk of bleeding associated with thrombolytic therapy.
- Based on current evidence, **thrombolysis should be reserved for patients with high-risk PE or patients with large deep vein thrombosis (DVT) with concern for limb loss** due to arterial compromise without intervention.[17]
- **Contraindications to thrombolytic therapy** include ischemic stroke within previous 3 months (>3 months is a relative contraindication), prior intracranial hemorrhage, intracranial mass, vascular malformation, recent major surgery, gastric ulcer, or active bleeding.[14]
- **Catheter-directed thrombolysis** was developed to alleviate the systemic bleeding risk associated with thrombolytic therapy and to ensure that therapy reaches the thrombus location. (1) A 5- to 6-French introducer sheath is placed in a central vein. (2) A pigtail catheter is advanced into the pulmonary artery. (3) Pulmonary artery pressures are measured before therapy as a baseline. (4) Angiography may be performed to identify the thrombus location. (5) A wire-catheter combination is used to pass through the thrombus. (6) The catheter is exchanged for a 5-French multi-side hole infusion catheter, and fibrinolytic therapy is administered.[14]

- **Catheter-based thrombolysis should be considered in patients with intermediate-high risk and high-risk PE who are without contraindications to thrombolytic therapy but still at high risk for bleeding with systemic therapy.**[14]
- Tricuspid or pulmonary valve prosthesis or vegetation, recent myocardial infarction, and left bundle branch block are **contraindications to catheter-directed thrombolytic therapy.**[14]

IVC Filter

- **IVCFs** are small metallic devices that are designed to prevent DVT from progressing to clinically significant PE. They **are not designed to stop all emboli**.
- IVCFs are foreign objects in the vascular system, and there is **a risk of promoting thrombosis**.
- Because IVCF placement is a balance of risks and benefits, multiple societies such as American College of Chest Physicians (ACCP), AHA, American College of Radiology Appropriateness Criteria (ACR), and Society for Interventional Radiology (SIR) have provided, at times conflicting, recommendations on when to offer IVCF to patients. As such, the **ACC published an expert analysis in 2016 outlining the indications for IVCF placement.**[18]

Guidelines

- There is consensus that patients who have had **VTE with contraindication to anticoagulation should have an IVCF placed.**[18]
- Patients who failed anticoagulation should be considered for IVCF placement.[18]
- An IVCF should be considered for patients who are **hemodynamically unstable as an adjunct to anticoagulation** in order to prevent further decompensation. This recommendation is based on retrospective database analysis that demonstrated lower mortality among those patients who underwent IVCF placement. There is not prospective data supporting this recommendation.[18]
- The ACCP, SIR, and ACR recommend patients with high-risk PE treated with thrombolysis or thrombectomy should be considered for filter placement. However, the AHA disagrees with this recommendation.[18]
- Both SIR and ACR recommend IVCF as prophylaxis in high-risk populations. However, ACCP disagrees with this recommendation.[18] We recommend against IVCF in this setting.

Complications of IVCF

- There can be **complications during implantation**, including hematoma or tilting, which may result in lower efficacy.[18]
- While in place, the IVCF is **at risk of promoting thrombus formation**. Newer versions of IVCFs are often **retrievable**; however, retrieval IVCF rates in the United States may be as low as 30% due to follow-up complications.[18] When the filter remains in place, risk of clot perpetuates.
- There is also a risk of **subclinical vessel extrusion of the tines**, with axial imaging identifying involvement of retroperitoneal structures. The clinical importance of these findings must be evaluated on a case-by-case basis.
- **During retrieval, there is risk of IVC perforation.**[18]

Percutaneous Suction Thrombectomy Systems

- **PE with associated right heart thrombi ("clot-in-transit") is associated with high mortality** if untreated.[19] Embolectomy or thrombolysis is possible treatment; however, many patients have either absolute or relative contraindications to thrombolysis as discussed earlier, and many are poor surgical candidates for embolectomy.

- **Mortality with heparin alone has been reported to be nearly 25%. Mortality for patients who undergo thrombolysis is reduced to 11%** and those who undergo embolectomy is 24%.
- The **AngioVac aspiration system** was developed as an alternative to thrombolysis or thrombectomy and is approved for use by the Food and Drug Administration (FDA) in 2009. This system utilizes a **veno-venous extracorporeal bypass circuit with an in-line filter** to remove thrombus, foreign bodies, tumor, or vegetations. The setup utilizes a 22-French suction cannula to aspirate the foreign body; the aspirate is filtered through an extracorporeal circuit and reinfused through a second catheter for blood return. It can avoid the hemodynamic changes associated with surgical thrombectomy or increased risk of bleeding associated with thrombolysis. One study found 12.5% in-hospital mortality for patients who underwent clot removal with AngioVac.[19]
- **In the absence of metastatic disease, AngioVac should be avoided if there is a risk for tumor maceration and venous spread**.
- The same AngioVac system can be used as a last resort method to remove **tricuspid valve endocarditis vegetations** in patients who are at high risk for surgery.[19,20]
- The most common side effect is a decrease in hemoglobin, as blood is circulated through an external circuit. Bleeding, RV free wall perforation, and embolization to pulmonary arteries causing cardiovascular collapse are less common but more serious potential complications.[19]
- See Figure 12-2.

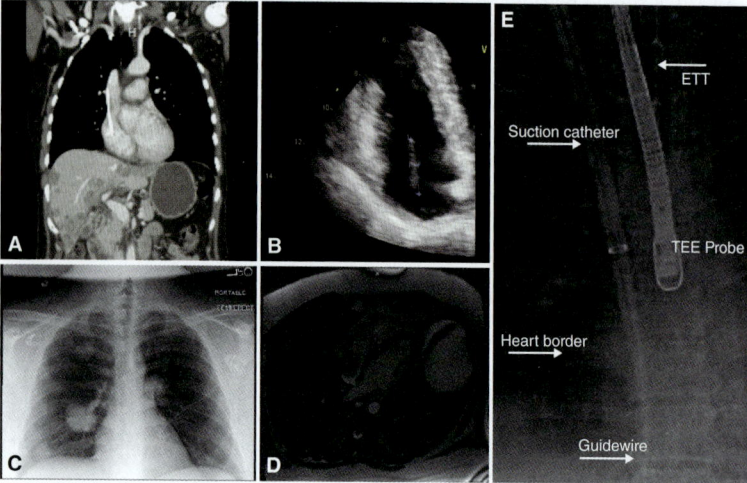

Figure 12-2. Two patients were each found to have a right atrial thrombus. (A) The first patient has a port that terminates in the right atrium as noted on computed tomography. (B) Mobile mass in the right atrium was noted to be 0.4 cm × 2.5 cm. This patient was treated with anticoagulation alone. (C) The second patient had a peripherally inserted central catheter (PICC) that terminated in the right atrium. (D) After PICC removal, he was found to have a right atrial thrombus on magnetic resonance imaging at the site of prior PICC. He was having symptomatic orthostatic hypotension, so the thrombus was removed via suction catheter. (E) Intraprocedural image of AngioVac device removing a right atrial thrombus. The suction catheter is inserted through the right internal jugular vein to remove the thrombus. TEE imaging is used during the procedure to visualize the thrombus removal. ETT, endotracheal tube; TEE, transthoracic echocardiogram.

- Endovascular venous thrombus aspiration systems have been replicated by different companies with similar mechanisms of action.[14]

Stenting

- **Stenting can be done to maintain vessel patency after thrombectomy, but evidence is limited describing its effectiveness.**[15] This is an area of opportunity for future studies.
- Stenting is rarely performed nor needed after thrombectomy for acute thrombus but is **heavily utilized for subacute and chronic thrombi**.
- Patients with **May-Thurner syndrome**, in which the left iliac vein is compressed by an overlapping right iliac artery, may benefit from stent placement when they develop thrombotic complications, as they can form extensive left-sided VTE due to common iliac vein stenosis.[15] However, subclinical compression of the left iliac vein does not require aggressive intervention.
- Likewise, **stenting can be utilized for patients with extrinsic caval compression due to retroperitoneal tumors or metastasis**.

REFERENCES

1. Kusumoto FM, Schoenfeld MH, Barrett C, et al. 2018 ACC/AHA/HRS Guideline on the evaluation and management of patients with bradycardia and cardiac conduction delay: a report of the American College of Cardiology/American Heart Association Task Force on Clinical Practice Guidelines and the Heart Rhythm Society. *J Am Coll Cardiol.* 2019;74(7):932-987. doi:10.1016/j.jacc.2018.10.043
2. Al-Khatib SM, Stevenson WG, Ackerman MJ, et al. 2017 AHA/ACC/HRS guideline for management of patients with ventricular arrhythmias and the prevention of sudden cardiac death: a report of the American College of Cardiology/American Heart Association Task Force on Clinical Practice Guidelines and the Heart Rhythm Society. *J Am Coll Cardiol.* 2018;72(14):e91-e220. doi:10.1016/j.jacc.2017.10.054. Erratum in: *J Am Coll Cardiol.* 2018;72(14):1760.
3. Hurkmans CW, Knegjens JL, Oei BS, et al. Management of radiation oncology patients with a pacemaker or ICD: a new comprehensive practical guideline in the Netherlands. Dutch society of radiotherapy and oncology (NVRO). *Radiat Oncol.* 2012;7:198. doi:10.1186/1748-717X-7-198
4. Miften M, Mihailidis D, Kry SF, et al. Management of radiotherapy patients with implanted cardiac pacemakers and defibrillators: a report of the AAPM TG-203[†]. *Med Phys.* 2019;46(12):e757-e788. doi:10.1002/mp.13838
5. Lee JZ, Mulpuru SK, Shen WK. Leadless pacemaker: performance and complications. *Trends Cardiovasc Med.* 2018;28(2):130-141. doi:10.1016/j.tcm.2017.08.001
6. Martínez-Sande JL, García-Seara J, Rodríguez-Mañero M. Radiotherapy in a leadless pacemaker. *EP Europace.* 2018;20(1):81. doi:10.1093/europace/eux067
7. Skelton WP, 4th, Franke AJ, Welniak S, et al. Investigation of complications following port insertion in a cancer patient population: a retrospective analysis. *Clin Med Insights Oncol.* 2019;13:1179554919844770. doi:10.1177/1179554919844770
8. Walser, E.M. Venous access ports: indications, implantation technique, follow-up, and complications. *Cardiovasc Intervent Radiol.* 2012;35:751-764. doi:10.1007/s00270-011-0271-2
9. Machat S, Eisenhuber E, Pfarl G, et al. Complications of central venous port systems: a pictorial review. *Insights Imaging.* 2019;10(1):86. doi:10.1186/s13244-019-0770-2
10. Shivakumar SP, Anderson DR, Couban S. Catheter-associated thrombosis in patients with malignancy. *J Clin Oncol.* 2009;27(29):4858-4864. doi:10.1200/JCO.2009.22.6126
11. Stavroulopoulos A, Aresti V, Zounis C. Right atrial thrombi complicating haemodialysis catheters. A meta-analysis of reported cases and a proposal of a management algorithm. *Nephrol Dial Transplant.* 2012;27:2936-2944. doi:10.1093/ndt/gfr739

12. Mermel LA, Allon M, Bouza E, et al. Clinical practice guidelines for the diagnosis and management of intravascular catheter-related infection: 2009 update by the Infectious Diseases Society of America. *Clin Infect Dis.* 2009;49(1):1-45. doi:10.1086/599376
13. Kyrouac D, Lenihan DJ, Kates AM, et al. A unique case of orthostasis in a patient with testicular choriocarcinoma. *JACC CardioOncol.* 2019;1(2):326-330. doi:10.1016/j.jaccao.2019.08.015
14. Xue X, Sista AK. Catheter-directed thrombolysis for pulmonary embolism: the state of practice. *Tech Vasc Interv Radiol.* 2018;21(2):78-84. doi:10.1053/j.tvir.2018.03.003
15. Goktay AY, Senturk C. Endovascular treatment of thrombosis and embolism. In: Islam M, ed., *Thrombosis and Embolism: From Research to Clinical Practice. Advances in Experimental Medicine and Biology.* Vol. 906. Springer. 2017:195-213. doi:10.1007/5584_2016_116
16. Konstantinides SV, Torbicki A, Agnelli G, et al. Task force for the diagnosis and management of acute pulmonary embolism of the European Society of Cardiology (ESC). 2014 ESC guidelines on the diagnosis and management of acute pulmonary embolism. *Eur Heart J.* 2014;35(43):3033-3069, 3069a-3069k. doi:10.1093/eurheartj/ehu283. Erratum in: *Eur Heart J.* 2015;36(39):2666. Erratum in: *Eur Heart J.* 2015;36(39):2642.
17. Tritschler T, Kraaijpoel N, Le Gal G, Wells PS. Venous thromboembolism: advances in diagnosis and treatment. *JAMA.* 2018;320(15):1583-1594. doi:10.1001/jama.2018.14346
18. Weinberg I. Appropriate use of inferior vena cava filters. https://www.acc.org/latest-in-cardiology/articles/2016/10/31/09/28/appropriate-use-of-inferior-vena-cava-filters
19. Rajput FA, Du L, Woods M, Jacobson K. Percutaneous vacuum-assisted thrombectomy using angioVac aspiration system. *Cardiovasc Revasc Med.* 2020;21(4):489-493. doi:10.1016/j.carrev.2019.12.020
20. Starck CT, Dreizler T, Falk V. The angioVac system as a bail-out option in infective valve endocarditis. *Ann Cardiothorac Surg.* 2019;8(6):675-677. doi:10.21037/acs.2019.11.04
21. Munshi A, Agarwal JP, Pandey KC. Cancer patients with cardiac pacemakers needing radiation treatment: a systematic review. *J Cancer Res Ther.* 2013;9(2):193-198. doi:10.4103/0973-1482.113348

13 Autonomic Dysfunction
Walter B. Schiffer and Daniel J. Lenihan

GENERAL PRINCIPLES

Definition
- **Autonomic dysfunction (AD)** is characterized by **an imbalance between sympathetic and parasympathetic nervous systems** and may affect multiple organs, including the heart, gastrointestinal tract, urinary tract, skin, and sexual organs.
- Both sympathetic and parasympathetic tone continuously maintain homeostasis in the cardiovascular system by **regulating heart rate, ventricular contractility, and vascular resistance**.
- See Table 13.1.

Classification
- AD may be divided into **neurogenic, non-neurogenic, and iatrogenic** causes.
- Neurogenic causes encompass neurodegenerative diseases, including Parkinson disease, pure autonomic failure, Lewy body dementia, amyotrophic lateral sclerosis, and neuro-infiltrative diseases, including amyloidosis.
- Non-neurogenic causes include heart failure, vasovagal syncope, volume depletion, adrenal insufficiency, and diabetes mellitus.
- Iatrogenic causes include antihypertensive medications and, especially in the cardio-oncology patient population, toxicity from chemotherapy as well as radiation therapy.

Background and Epidemiology
- The prevalence of AD in the cardio-oncology patient population varies widely depending on specific exposures, including the amount and duration of **chemotherapy**, location and amount of **radiation therapy**, or the specific type of amyloid precursor protein in those with **amyloidosis**.
- Older patients are particularly susceptible to AD because of age-related changes in the baroreceptor reflex, stiffening vasculature, and decreased α-1 receptor responsiveness to sympathetic stimuli. In one study of nursing home residents, 18% of those older than 65 had orthostasis.[1]

AntiNeoplastic Chemotherapies
- Peripheral, symmetrical **sensory neuropathy** occurs frequently with both **platinum-based and taxane-based** chemotherapies. The co-occurrence of AD is well described, but its frequency is less well defined.
- **Platinum-based** alkylating chemotherapies, including cisplatin, oxaliplatin, and carboplatin, are associated mainly with peripheral sensory neuropathies that are

TABLE 13-1 Causes of Autonomic Dysfunction and Associated Clinical Findings

Disease or chemotherapy associated with autonomic dysfunction		Cumulative dose threshold	Associated neurologic findings	Associated cardiovascular findings
Antineoplastic chemotherapies	Platinum Based (Cisplatin, Oxaliplatin)	Cisplatin >350 mg/m^2 Oxaliplatin >550 mg/m^2	Progressive distal extremity stocking and glove distribution of sensory neuropathy +/– autonomic involvement	Orthostatic hypotension Arrhythmias Heart failure
	Taxanes (Paclitaxel, Docetaxel)	Paclitaxel 1000 mg/m^2 Docetaxel 400 mg/m^2	Motor symptoms rarely occur at higher doses	
	Thalidomide	>20 g		Hypertension with thalidomide
	Proteasome Inhibitors (Bortezomib)	Bortezomib >16 mg/m^2	Painful distal sensory neuropathy +/– autonomic involvement	Orthostatic hypotension Myocardial ischemia (rare)
Systemic amyloidosis	AL ATTR	N/A N/A	Distal sensory and motor neuropathies Autonomic dysfunction	Orthostatic hypotension Heart failure and arrhythmias (common)
Radiation therapy		>60 Gy to cranial nerves or carotid sinus	Cranial nerve dysfunction	Labile blood pressure Arrhythmias Valvular and vascular calcification
Head and neck surgery		N/A	Cranial nerve and carotid sinus dysfunction	Labile blood pressure Tachycardia
Paraneoplastic syndromes (Anti-Hu)		N/A	Encephalomyelitis Sensory neuropathy	Orthostatic hypotension

AL, light chain amyloidosis; ATTR, transthyretin amyloidosis.

dose-dependent. For patients undergoing chemotherapy with cisplatin, for example, over 90% experience neuropathic symptoms at a cumulative dose of 500 to 600 mg per m^2.[2] AD may occur, especially in those with more severe sensory involvement.
- **Taxanes**, including paclitaxel and docetaxel, are similarly associated with peripheral sensory neuropathy, which may be accompanied by AD.[3] Neuropathic symptoms are usually dose-related and occur more frequently in patients receiving cumulative doses of 1000 mg per m^2 of paclitaxel and 400 mg per m^2 of docetaxel. The reported prevalence of neuropathic symptoms in those receiving taxanes varies widely from 21% to 83%,[4] although paclitaxel consistently carries a higher risk for neuropathic side effects than docetaxel. AD is considered to be an uncommon side effect and almost always co-occurs with sensory neuropathy.
- **Proteasome inhibitors, especially intravenous bortezomib**, may cause sensory and autonomic disturbances. Between 60% and 75% of patients receiving bortezomib report neuropathy of any kind, and AD occurs in about 10% to 15% of patients.[5] Specific autonomic side effects include gastrointestinal symptoms and orthostatic hypotension.[5,6] Other proteasome inhibitors, including carfilzomib and ixazomib, are less frequently implicated in causing neuropathic symptoms and AD, and with less severity.
- **Thalidomide** causes neuropathy in roughly half of patients receiving it as a first-line therapy, which may manifest as a sensory, motor, or autonomic neuropathy. Autonomic symptoms include orthostasis, erectile dysfunction, and gastrointestinal dysmotility.[7] Other thalidomide analogues, including **lenalidomide and pomalidomide**, are associated with much lower rates of **neuropathy and AD**, although it may occur or exacerbate existing neuropathic symptoms.

Amyloidosis

- Both **light chain (AL) amyloidosis and transthyretin (ATTR) amyloidosis frequently cause autonomic and sensory neuropathies**. AD occurs more frequently in ATTR amyloid, especially in certain hereditary forms, such as V3OM mutation, where between 50% and 75% of patients have been reported to experience orthostasis.[8] Neuropathy also tends to occur earlier in the disease process in ATTR. By comparison, between 17% and 35% of patients with AL experience neuropathy. In contrast to neuropathies because of antineoplastic therapies, the severity of sensory involvement is not always correlated with AD in amyloidosis, and **orthostasis may be the presenting symptom**.[9] Other autonomic symptoms are also common, particularly in hereditary TTR amyloid, including gastrointestinal dysmotility, erectile dysfunction, and bladder dysfunction. Hereditary variants of TTR amyloid may present with different phenotypes with respect to cardiac and neuropathic symptoms. The most common mutation in the United States is V122L, which is cardiomyopathic predominant and is seen commonly in patients with African American or Caribbean heritage.[8,10]

Radiation Therapy and Surgery

- **Radiation therapy to the mediastinum and neck** is associated with AD, which may be delayed in onset for many years. In one study of patients with Hodgkin lymphoma, those receiving thoracic radiation were more likely to have abnormal heart rate recovery and blood pressure response to exercise as compared to controls.[11] About 4% of patients receiving head and neck radiotherapy experience cranial nerve (CN) deficits,[12] which may lead to AD, though the frequency of patients experiencing symptoms was not defined.

- **Surgical treatment of head and neck cancer** may also cause direct damage to CNs IX and X, which impairs afferent coordination of the carotid baroreceptor reflex. The frequency of AD after surgery is not well described, though one study of 889 patients with oropharyngeal cancer found evidence of lower CN palsy (including CN IX and X) in 5% of those treated with either radiation therapy or surgery.[13]

Paraneoplastic Autonomic Dysfunction
- Anti-Hu antibodies are a rare cause of AD that has been described in case series of patients with small cell lung cancer.

ANATOMY AND PATHOPHYSIOLOGY

Autonomic Nervous System
- A broad understanding of the organization of the Autonomic Nervous System (ANS) is essential to interpreting clinical symptoms of AD and identifying potential causes.
- The ANS controls blood flow in every organ of the body through afferent (sensory) and efferent (output) limbs.
- Afferent sensory neurons include glossopharyngeal and vagus nerves, which monitor hemodynamic changes in the carotid sinus and aortic arch baroreceptors, respectively. This information is then communicated to the solitary nucleus of the medulla, which coordinates sympathetic and parasympathetic output to the heart, vascular smooth muscle, and kidneys (Fig. 13-1).
- Parasympathetic innervation predominates in the resting state and helps to restore homeostasis after exercise by reducing heart rate and heart contractility.
- Sympathetic activity allows for increased systemic vascular resistance and cardiac output in response to positional changes and exercise.
- Upon standing, approximately 500 to 800 mL of intravascular volume pools in the lower extremities, requiring a compensatory response that is coordinated by the ANS.[14] Increased sympathetic output and parasympathetic inhibition allow blood pressure drop and heart rate increase to be minimized to within 5 to 10 mm Hg and 10 to 25 beats per minute, respectively.

Mechanisms of Neurotoxicity
- The pathogenesis and resulting manifestations of AD differ depending on the underlying toxin or disease process.

Antineoplastic Agents
- Multiple mechanisms have been proposed for neuropathy resulting from antineoplastic chemotherapies.
- **Platinum-based chemotherapies are thought to directly cause neuropathic damage through mitochondrial dysfunction** and oxidative stress and may also induce cellular apoptosis by altering nuclear and mitochondrial DNA structure. They may also indirectly damage neurons through **capillary dysfunction and impaired blood supply**. These adverse changes primarily affect peripheral neurons and those in the dorsal root ganglion.[15]
- Taxanes disrupt microtubule formation and are thought to cause neuropathy by interfering with axon transport in both the dorsal root ganglion and peripheral nerve cells, as well as provoking immune-mediated **neuronal inflammation**.[16,17]
- Proteasome inhibitors exert their antiproliferative effects through **proteasomal degradation of ubiquitinated proteins**. The mechanism by which they induce

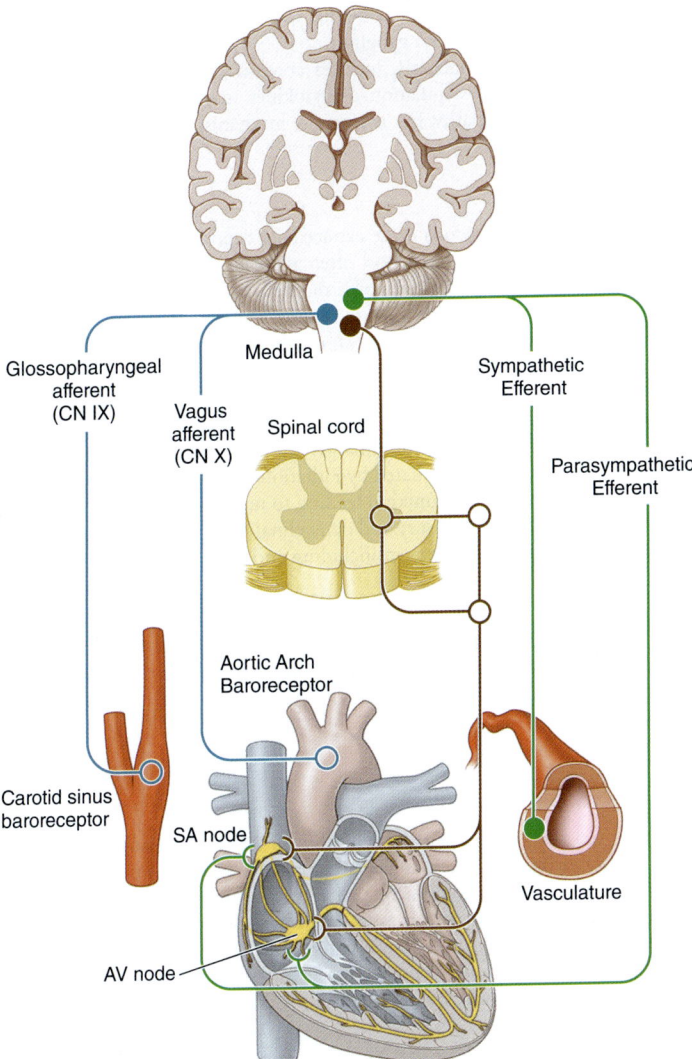

Figure 13.1. Anatomy of the Autonomic Nervous System. The autonomic nervous system relies on both afferent (blue lines) and efferent (black and green lines) to sustain homeostatic balance of blood pressure and heart rate. The glossopharyngeal nerve communicates information from the carotid baroreceptor to the solitary nucleus of the medulla. Likewise, the aortic arch baroreceptor conveys blood pressure information to the medulla, which then coordinates efferent output through parasympathetic (green lines) and sympathetic (black lines) signaling. The sympathetic efferent pathway runs through the paraspinal sympathetic chain, which starts at T1. The parasympathetic efferent runs through the vagus nerve and innervates the heart, including the sinoatrial and atrioventricular nodes, and the smooth muscle of the vasculature. Sympathetic neurons also affect renin excretion from the kidney (not shown), which further aids in increasing systemic vascular tone.

neuropathy remains unclear, but may be due to accumulation of ubiquitinated aggregates in cells of the dorsal root ganglion.
- Thalidomide inhibits angiogenesis, induces apoptosis, and upregulates T-cell response to cancer cells. Dysregulation of cytokines may cause **demyelination of neurons** leading to neuropathy, but the precise mechanism remains unknown.[18]

AMYLOIDOSIS

- Both AL and ATTR amyloidosis cause extracellular deposits of insoluble protein aggregates in peripheral nerve fibers, most often affecting efferent sympathetic output. These protein deposits are thought to cause mechanical compression of the nerve and induce an inflammatory reaction leading to fibrosis. There is also evidence that amyloid deposits promote glycosylation of basement membranes, similar to diabetes mellitus.

Radiation and Surgery

- External beam radiation uses photon beams that create double-stranded DNA breaks causing cell cycle arrest, predominantly affecting rapidly dividing cancer cells. Neuropathy is thought to be mediated by radiation-induced **fibrosis causing nerve compression**, perivascular dysfunction leading to nerve ischemia, **and direct damage to nerves** through axonal injury and demyelination.[19] Direct damage to afferent nerves may also be caused by surgery, including endarterectomy and angioplasty.[12]

PARANEOPLASTIC SYNDROMES

- Anti-Hu antibody targets RNA-associated proteins in neurons and may cause encephalitis, sensory neuropathy, and AD.

DIAGNOSIS

Differential Diagnosis for Orthostasis

- Orthostasis is a common presenting symptom of AD but is nonspecific. A broad differential for orthostasis, including neurogenic, non-neurogenic, and iatrogenic etiologies, should be considered in any patient presenting **with postural symptoms of orthostatic hypotension, dizziness, and/or presyncope** (Fig. 13-2).
- Another important consideration in the cardio-oncology population is that antineoplastic therapies and amyloidosis may independently cause heart failure, which may also contribute to orthostatic symptoms.

History

- A thorough history of the patient's symptoms should be obtained with an emphasis on onset, time course, and associated cardiac or neurologic symptoms.
- Patients should be asked specifically about postural symptoms, including **syncope and presyncope, visual blurring, cognitive impairment, neck and shoulder pain, chest pain, and dyspnea**.
- History should also clarify potential sources of volume depletion, such as vomiting, recent bleeding, or diarrhea.
- For amyloidosis, the natural time course for neuropathy and AD is indolent and progressive.

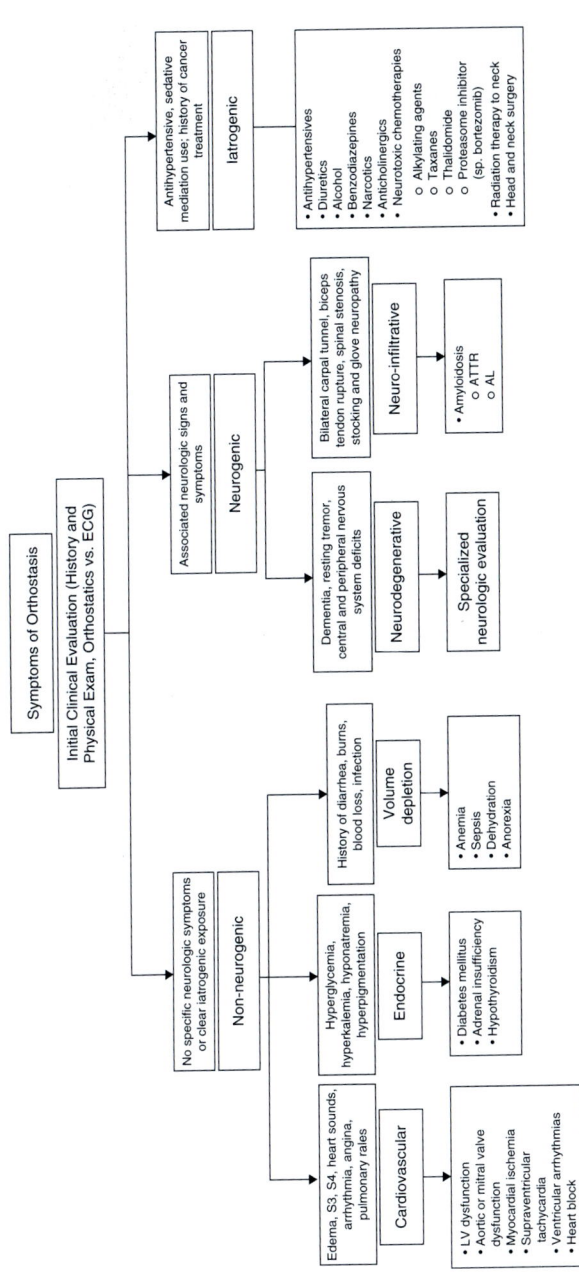

Figure 13.2. Differential diagnosis for orthostasis in the cardio-oncology patient. AL, light chain amyloidosis; ATTR, transthyretin amyloidosis; ECG, electrocardiogram; LV, left ventricular.

- Antineoplastic chemotherapies often cause slowly progressive neuropathic symptoms that correlate with cumulative treatment dose.
  - One exception is paclitaxel, which may cause an acute demyelinating polyneuropathy during or immediately after infusion.[15]
- Neuropathy caused by radiation therapy may not occur until months or years after the last radiation treatment.
- A detailed cancer history and treatment course should be obtained in those patients with a cancer diagnosis. This should include type and amounts of chemotherapies, as well as doses and treatment fields of any radiation therapy.
- Family history should also be scrutinized to evaluate for any familial cardiomyopathies or neuropathies, as may be present with hereditary ATTR.
- Detailed medication review should also be undertaken, with a particular focus on antihypertensives including **alpha blockers, diuretics, atrioventricular nodal blocking agents**, antihyperglycemic, and sedating medications.
- Social history and nutritional history should be obtained with consideration of alcohol use and appropriate vitamin intake.

Physical Examination and Bedside Maneuvers

- For patients with symptoms of AD, thorough bedside cardiovascular and neurologic examinations should be performed.
- Heart and lung examination should focus on heart rate, rhythm, presence of extra heart sounds, carotid bruits, pulmonary crackles or rales, jugular venous pressure, and lower extremity edema.
- Neurologic examination should test sensory function, including fine touch, pain, and vibration, as well as cerebellar and motor pathways.
  - Amyloidosis usually causes ascending, bilateral, and symmetric sensory neuropathy similar to that found in diabetes mellitus.
  - Antineoplastic chemotherapies also typically cause neuropathy that involves the distal extremities in a symmetric "stocking and glove" pattern.
- **Orthostatic vital signs** should also be obtained as follows: record blood pressure after lying down for 5 minutes, then repeat blood pressure measurement after standing for 3 minutes. A fall in systolic blood pressure of at least 20 mm Hg or a fall in diastolic blood pressure of at least 10 mm Hg qualifies as orthostatic hypotension.
  - Patients with neurogenic AD will have an impaired blood pressure response as well as a blunted heart rate response to standing, which can be quantified by the ratio of heart rate increase to the decrease in systolic blood pressure. A ratio below 0.5 is sensitive and specific for neurogenic baroreflex dysfunction.[20]
- Evaluating blood pressure changes after Valsalva maneuver may also help to identify AD. In one study, the median decrease in systolic blood pressure after a 15-second Valsalva (phase two) was 37 mm Hg in those with AD as compared to 5 mm Hg in controls.[21]

Diagnostic Testing

Cardiovascular Diagnostic Testing

- Electrocardiography is important to evaluate for potential arrhythmias that may cause episodes of presyncope and dizziness similar to orthostasis. It may also help to screen for underlying structural heart disease. Ambulatory monitoring should also

be considered depending on the frequency of symptoms and if orthostatic symptoms are not clearly correlated with positional movements.
- Ambulatory blood pressure monitoring for 24 hours can help define blood pressure and heart rate variability, which may elucidate underlying AD, as well as clinical predictors of future AD, such as postprandial hypotension. Moreover, blood pressure variability is informative as a prognostic marker, as it identifies those at increased risk for cardiovascular events.[11,22]
- Transthoracic echocardiogram will help differentiate AD from primary cardiac dysfunction, especially low-output heart failure and aortic stenosis.

Neurologic Diagnostic Testing
- Tilt table testing provides another way of measuring positional blood pressure change in patients who cannot safely stand or whose symptoms do not manifest soon after standing. Head-up tilt table testing typically places the patient 60 to 70 degrees from supine position for 10 minutes or longer while serially measuring blood pressure and heart rate.
- The quantitative sudomotor axon reflex test (QSART) provides a measure of sympathetic function by measuring sweat volumes after acetylcholine application but is rarely used in clinical practice.
- **Nerve conduction studies** are used to define the extent and type of nerve fiber involvement.

Lab Evaluation
- Basic metabolic panel may reveal evidence of intravascular volume depletion through elevations in blood urea nitrogen (BUN) to creatinine ration. It may also indicate electrolyte imbalance as a result of diarrhea or emesis and can identify potassium derangement in the case of adrenal insufficiency.
- **Complete blood count** should be obtained to rule out anemia.
- **Serum** N-terminal pro-brain natriuretic peptide (**NT-proBNP**) may be drawn to screen for evidence of heart failure.
- **Troponin** should be obtained if there is concern for cardiac ischemia.
- Blood glucose and hemoglobin A1c should be obtained to screen for diabetes mellitus.
- When amyloidosis is suspected, laboratory testing should be performed to evaluate for **light chains**, including serum free light chain ratio, serum and urine protein electrophoresis, and immunofixation.
- Serum vitamin B_{12} may be obtained in patients with clinical history consistent with subacute combined degeneration.
- **AM cortisol level** can evaluate potential underlying adrenal insufficiency.

TREATMENT

- A primary goal in the management of AD is to maintain arterial blood pressure and prevent ischemic end organ damage. To this end, oral sympathomimetic medications are often used to elevate mean arterial pressure and prevent hypotensive episodes (Table 13-2). However, these drugs may also result in supine hypertension and resting tachycardia, and long-term use of some agents can result in adverse cardiovascular effects.

TABLE 13-2 Pharmacologic Manipulation

Drug	Dose	Mechanism	Side effects
Midodrine	2.5–15 mg PO 2–3 times daily	α-1 receptor agonist; increases systemic vascular resistance	Supine hypertension
Droxidopa	100–600 mg PO 2–3 times daily	Enzymatically converted to norepinephrine	Headache, supine hypertension
Fludrocortisone (in nonadrenally insufficient patients)	0.05–0.2 mg PO once daily	Mineralocorticoid receptor agonist; pressor response after 3–5 days	Hypokalemia, supine hypertension; long term may cause heart and renal failure, sudden death during sleep
Yohimbine	5.4 mg PO 2–3 times daily	α-2 antagonist	Supine hypertension, headache
Atomoxetine	10–18 mg, PO 2 times daily	Norepinephrine reuptake inhibitor	Insomnia, reduced appetite
Pyridostigmine	30–60 mg, PO 2–3 times daily	Reversible acetylcholinesterase inhibitor	Diarrhea, urinary frequency, bradycardia
Recombinant erythropoietin	50 mg/kg SQ, 2–3 times weekly	Increases red blood cell production and intravascular volume	Hypertension
Octreotide	100 μg SQ, 2–3 times daily	Somatostatin analogue, increases splanchnic vascular tone	Nausea, hyperglycemia
Desmopressin	0.05 mg intranasal spray, nightly	Vasopressin agonist	Hyponatremia
Ivabradine	2.5–7.5 mg PO 2 times daily	Sinoatrial node f-channel antagonist	Bradycardia, hypertension, atrial fibrillation

CI, confidence interval; SBP, systolic blood pressure. (From Kaufmann H, Norcliffe-Kaufmann L, Palma JA. Baroreflex dysfunction. *New England Journal of Medicine.* 2020;382(2):163-178.)

- **Nonpharmacologic strategies** center on intravascular volume expansion and elimination of aggravating factors, including warm ambient temperatures, hot baths, large meals, and prolonged standing.[14] **Rapid intake of 500 mL of water** may alleviate orthostatic symptoms, as may use of abdominal binders, compression stockings, and physical counter-maneuvers, including leg crossing and isotonic muscle contraction (Table 13-3).[23] Careful medication review should also be employed to discontinue antihypertensive medications and sedating medications, including benzodiazepines.
- In the case of AD related to neurotoxic chemotherapies, collaboration with the patient's oncologist is important to determine if an alternative chemotherapy may be used or if the current therapy may be administered less frequently.
- The treatment of AD associated with amyloidosis relies in part on treatment of the underlying light chain paraproteinemia or ATTR fibril deposition. Here the goal is to reduce the burden of amyloid infiltration of the peripheral nerves and halt symptom progression (see chapters on "treatment of amyloidosis").
- Gastrointestinal dysmotility and urinary symptoms of AD are also treated symptomatically with medications that mitigate diarrhea or constipation, as well as urinary retention or overflow incontinence. Of note, sildenafil and other phosphodiesterase inhibitors should be avoided in patients with AD-related erectile dysfunction, as these medications may exacerbate **orthostatic hypotension**.

TABLE 13-3 Nonpharmacologic Interventions for Treatment of Orthostatic Hypotension

Nonpharmacologic strategies for improving orthostatic hypotension are presented. All patients should avoid triggers that may exacerbate orthostasis, including hot baths, large meals, and prolonged standing. Water bolus was defined as ingestion of 480 mL of tap water within 5 minutes. Physical counter-maneuver consisted of isometric contraction of lower limbs, including leg crossing. Abdominal compression includes use of an elastic belt or abdominal binder.

Intervention	Increase in standing SBP	Efficacy (SBP drop attenuated by ≥10mm Hg)
Water bolus	12 mm Hg (CI: 4–12)	56%
Lower extremity support hose	7.5 mm Hg (CI: −1–13)	32%
Abdominal compression	10 mm Hg (CI: 2–18)	52%
Physical counter-maneuver	7 mm Hg (CI: −1–16)	44%

SBP, systolic blood pressure. (Derived from Newton JL, Frith J. The efficacy of nonpharmacologic inter-vention for orthostatic hypotension associated with aging. *Neurology*. 2018;91(7): e652–e656.)

PROGNOSIS

- AD is an independent risk factor for cardiovascular events and mortality, regardless of the underlying cause.[24]
- Neuropathies associated with antineoplastic chemotherapies may improve after cessation or less frequent dosing of the offending agent, but many patients are left with permanent symptoms.
- Autonomic symptoms because of amyloidosis may improve with treatment of the underlying disease process. In a trial that examined patients with ATTR amyloid who were treated with patisiran (RNA silencer), patients reported improvement in autonomic symptoms.[25]
- Despite improvements in the administration of antineoplastic agents, as well as increased awareness and earlier recognition of amyloidosis, neuropathic sequelae and AD remain highly morbid and challenging to treat. The complex assessment and management of these patients highlight the need for interdisciplinary collaboration to advance diagnosis and treatment strategies.

REFERENCES

1. Rutan GH, Hermanson B, Bild DE, Kittner SJ, Labaw F, Tell GS. *Orthostatic Hypotension in Older Adults. The Cardiovascular Health Study*. Hypertension. 1992;19:508-519.
2. Park SB, Goldstein D, Krishnan AV, et al. Chemotherapy-induced peripheral neurotoxicity: a critical analysis. *CA: A Cancer Journal for Clinicians*. 2013;63(6):419-437. Doi: 10.3322/caac.21204.
3. Dermitzakis EV, Kimiskidis VK, Lazaridis G, et al. The impact of paclitaxel and carboplatin chemotherapy on the autonomous nervous system of patients with ovarian cancer. *BMC Neurology*. 2016;16(1):190. Doi: 10.1186/s12883-016-0710-4.
4. Rivera E, Cianfrocca M. Overview of neuropathy associated with taxanes for the treatment of metastatic breast cancer. *Cancer Chemotherapy and Pharmacology*. 2015;75(4):659-670. Doi: 10.1007/s00280-014-2607-5.
5. Stratogianni A, Tosch M, Schlemmer H, et al. Bortezomib-Induced severe autonomic neuropathy. *Clinical Autonomic Research*. 2012;22(4):199-202. Doi: 10.1007/s10286-012-0164-8.
6. Meregalli C. An overview of bortezomib-induced neurotoxicity. *Toxics*. 2015;3(3):294-303. Doi: 10.3390/toxics3030294.
7. Waage A, Gimsing P, Fayers P, et al. Melphalan and prednisone plus thalidomide or placebo in elderly patients with multiple myeloma. *Blood*. 2010;116(9):1405-1412. Doi: 10.1182/blood-2009-08-237974.
8. Maurer MS, Hanna M, Grogan M, et al. Genotype and phenotype of transthyretin cardiac amyloidosis. *Journal of the American College of Cardiology*. 2016;68(2):161-172. Doi: 10.1016/j.jacc.2016.03.596.
9. Gertz MA, Dispenzieri A. Systemic amyloidosis recognition, prognosis, and therapy: a systematic review. *JAMA—Journal of the American Medical Association*. 2020;324(1):79-89. Doi: 10.1001/jama.2020.5493.
10. Loavenbruck AJ, Singer W, Mauermann ML, et al. Transthyretin amyloid neuropathy has earlier neural involvement but better prognosis than primary amyloid counterpart: an answer to the paradox? *Annals of Neurology*. 2016;80(3):401-411. Doi: 10.1002/ana.24725.
11. Groarke JD, Tanguturi VK, Hainer J, et al. Abnormal exercise response in long-term survivors of Hodgkin lymphoma treated with thoracic irradiation: evidence of cardiac autonomic dysfunction and impact on outcomes. *Journal of the American College of Cardiology*. 2015;65(6):573-583. Doi: 10.1016/j.jacc.2014.11.035.
12. Norcliffe-Kaufmann L., Palma JA. Blood pressure instability in head and neck cancer survivors. *Clinical Autonomic Research*. 2020;30(4):291-293. Doi: 10.1007/s10286-020-00711-3.

13. Aggarwal P, Zaveri JS, Goepfert RP, et al. Symptom burden associated with late lower cranial neuropathy in long-term oropharyngeal cancer survivors. *JAMA Otolaryngology—Head and Neck Surgery.* 2018;144(11):1066-1076.
14. Freeman R, Abuzinadah AR, Gibbons C, Jones P, Miglis MG, Sinn DI. Orthostatic Hypotension: JACC State-of-the-Art review. *Journal of the American College of Cardiology.* 2018;72(11):1294-1309. Doi: 10.1016/j.jacc.2018.05.079.
15. Zajaczkowską R, Kocot-Kępska M, Leppert W, Wrzosek A, Mika J, Wordliczek J. Mechanisms of chemotherapy-induced peripheral neuropathy. *International Journal of Molecular Sciences.* 2019;20(6):1451. Doi: 10.3390/ijms20061451.
16. LaPointe NE, Morfini G, Brady ST, Feinstein SC, Wilson L, Jordan MA. Effects of eribulin, vincristine, paclitaxel and ixabepilone on fast axonal transport and kinesin-1 driven microtubule gliding: implications for chemotherapy-induced peripheral neuropathy. *NeuroToxicology.* 2013;37:231-239. Doi: 10.1016/j.neuro.2013.05.008.
17. Peters CM, Jimenez-Andrade JM, Kuskowski MA, Ghilardi JR, Mantyh PW. An evolving cellular pathology occurs in dorsal root ganglia, peripheral nerve and spinal cord following intravenous administration of paclitaxel in the rat. *Brain Research.* 2007;1168(1):46-59. Doi: 10.1016/j.brainres.2007.06.066.
18. Richardson PG, Delforge M, Beksac M, et al. Management of treatment-emergent peripheral neuropathy in multiple myeloma. *Leukemia.* 2012;26(4):595-608. Doi: 10.1038/leu.2011.346.
19. Delanian S, Lefaix J-L, Pradat P-F. Radiation-induced neuropathy in cancer survivors. *Radiotherapy and Oncology.* 2012;105(3):273-282. Doi: 10.1016/j.radonc.2012.10.012.
20. Kaufmann H, Norcliffe-Kaufmann L, Palma JA. Baroreflex Dysfunction. *New England Journal of Medicine.* 2020;382(2):163-178. Doi: 10.1056/nejmra1509723.
21. Novak P. Assessment of sympathetic index from the Valsalva maneuver. *Neurology.* 2011;76(23):2010-2016. Doi: 10.1212/WNL.0b013e31821e5563.
22. Lakoski SG, Jones LW, Krone RJ, Stein PK, Scott JM. Autonomic dysfunction in early breast cancer: incidence, clinical importance, and underlying mechanisms. *American Heart Journal.* 2015;170(2):231-241. Doi: 10.1016/j.ahj.2015.05.014.
23. Newton JL, Frith J. The efficacy of nonpharmacologic intervention for orthostatic hypotension associated with aging. *Neurology.* 2018;91(7):e652-e656. Doi: 10.1212/WNL.0000000000005994.
24. Curtis BM, O'Keefe J. Autonomic tone as a cardiovascular risk factor: the dangers of chronic fight or flight. *Mayo Clinic Proceedings.* 2002;77(1):45-54. Doi: 10.4065/77.1.45.
25. Palma JA, Gonzalez-Duarte A, Kaufmann H. Orthostatic hypotension in hereditary transthyretin amyloidosis: epidemiology, diagnosis and management. *Clinical Autonomic Research.* 2019;29(1):33-44. Doi: 10.1007/s10286-019-00623-x.

14 Echo Techniques for Cardiac Safety During and After Cancer Treatment

Christopher Fine and Joshua D. Mitchell

- With significant improvements in cancer treatment and cancer-related survival, the potential long-term cardiovascular (CV) toxicity of cancer therapy, and its significant impact on the morbidity and mortality of cancer survivors, has become more apparent.
- Ongoing CV evaluations and screening in patients with cancer at increased CV risk—before, during and following cancer treatment—have proven importance in **assessing for subclinical adverse CV effects, helping direct early therapy, and mitigating further toxicity**.
- **Echocardiography has remained the cornerstone** of pretreatment and surveillance monitoring in the cancer patient owing to its wide availability, reproducibility, unmatched safety profile, lack of radiation exposure, and the comprehensive nature of evaluation for cardiac manifestations of toxicity.[1-3]

GENERAL PRINCIPLES

The Role of Echocardiography in Surveillance

- Cancer survivors are at significantly increased risk for CV disease. It is the leading competing cause of morbidity and mortality in patients with cancer.
- The **goal of screening is to identify any cardiotoxicity early in its course to help direct management and mitigate more severe progression.** Ultimately, the objective is to **maximize delivery of cancer therapy** while limiting associated toxicity (Fig. 14-1).
- Studies have shown that initiating **cardioprotective medications**, such as angiotensin converting enzyme inhibitors (ACE-I), angiotensin receptor blockers, or β-blockers, after early signs of cardiotoxicity (troponin elevation, drop in global longitudinal strain [GLS]), can reduce risk of future left ventricular (LV) dysfunction (see Chapter 20, Table 20-1).[4,5]
- In 2014, the American Society of Echocardiography (ASE) and the European Association of Cardiovascular Imaging (EACVI) produced the first expert consensus statement detailing recommendations for CV imaging of patients during and after cancer therapy.[6]
- Since then, other guidelines committees of various clinical foci have also reinforced the importance of routine surveillance in this patient population. Identifying high-risk patients and those who develop signs of subclinical cardiotoxicity for early clinical intervention is the unified goal. (Table 14-1).[3,7]
- Recommended **screening intervals** are based on **expert opinion** derived from available cohort studies and factoring in the expected incidence of cardiac dysfunction given the **patient's risk factors and cancer treatment**.

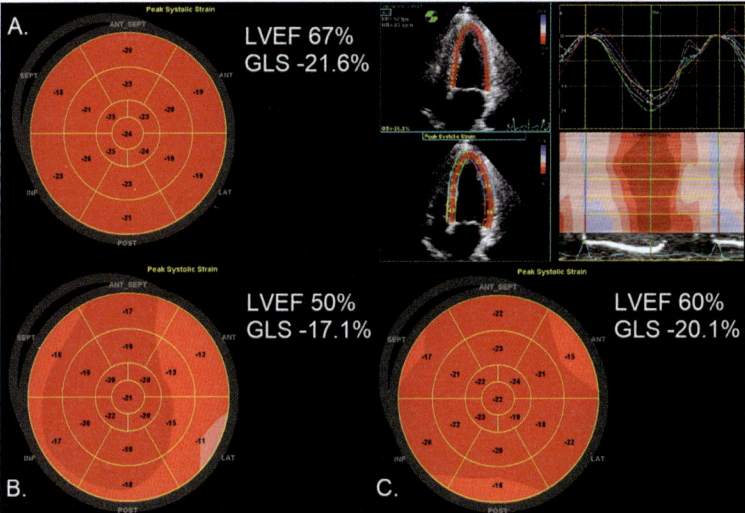

Figure 14-1. A 41-year-old undergoing treatment for breast cancer Stage IIB invasive ductal carcinoma. A. Baseline TTE shows normal LV systolic function (LVEF 67%, GLS −21.6%). B. On screening echocardiogram after five cycles of paclitaxel, carboplatin, and trastuzumab, the patient has an asymptomatic drop in her LVEF to 50% with a GLS reduction to −17.1%. Trastuzumab is held, and she is referred to cardio-oncology. She is started on carvedilol and lisinopril, and her cancer therapy with trastuzumab is resumed. C. Three months later, her LVEF has normalized to 60% with GLS of −20.1%. GLS, global longitudinal strain; LVEF, left ventricular ejection fraction; TTE, transthoracic echocardiogram.

- While screening protocols have generally been derived primarily to detect early signs of LV systolic dysfunction, echocardiogram provides comprehensive information for other forms of cardiotoxicity as well (pulmonary hypertension, right ventricular [RV] dysfunction, valvular dysfunction, etc.).
- Although the diagnosis of cardiotoxicity should prompt a timely multidisciplinary review of the patient's care, it should not automatically trigger discontinuation or modification of cancer therapy (see Chapter 20).

DEFINITIONS

Cardiotoxicity

- There has been some **heterogeneity in the specific definition of "cardiotoxicity,"** both in clinical studies, as well as guidelines and consensus statements.
- Classically, the term "cardiotoxicity" has referred primarily to **reduction in the left ventricular (LV) ejection fraction** (LVEF) and has most commonly been defined as a **drop in LVEF of ≥5% in symptomatic patients or a drop in ≥10% to an LVEF of <53% in asymptomatic patients** (Table 14-2).[2,8,9]
- Certain large registries of cardio-oncology patients have adopted similar definitions but expanded them to include severity of LVEF reduction and added other

TABLE 14-1 Transthoracic Echocardiographic Surveillance Strategies in the Cancer Patient

Cancer therapy	Baseline evaluation[a]	During treatment[a]	Following treatment[a]
Anthracyclines	Recommended	• After >240 mg/m^2 doxorubicin equivalent • Every additional 100-150 mg/m^2 doxorubicin equivalent or every 2 cycles	6-12 mo after final cycle Consider annually for 2-3 yrs in high-risk patients, otherwise 5-yearly review
HER2 receptor antagonists	Recommended	Every 3 mo until treatment conclusion	6-12 mo after treatment in patients who received anthracyclines or are at otherwise high CV risk
Alkylating agents	Consider	If change in clinical status	[b]
Antimetabolites	Consider	If change in clinical status	[b]
Proteasome inhibitors	Consider, especially with carfilzomib and to evaluate for AL in patients with MM	If change in clinical status	[b]
ICIs	Consider	Consider in patients at high risk (combination ICI, other cardiotoxic treatments, high baseline CV risk)	[b]
Anti-VEGF TKIs	Recommended	• Consider every 4 mo during first year of treatment • Consider 6-12 monthly TTE thereafter	[b]

BCR-ABL TKIs (second and third generation)		• Consider 6-12 monthly TTE	b
Dasatinib	Recommended to assess for baseline pulmonary HTN	• Low threshold if cardiac symptoms develop	b
XRT	Consider, especially if high CV risk or in combination with other cardiotoxic treatments	Monitoring during XRT itself generally not required owing to brief treatment times	In patients with AC chemotherapy, 6-12 mo after treatment Further TTE based on CV risk: High: every 5 yr Moderate/low: 10 yr after treatment conclusion, then every 5 yr

Suggested transthoracic echocardiographic surveillance strategies derived from expert consensus statements and from known incidence of cardiovascular events associated with treatment.

AL, light-chain amyloidosis; CV, cardiovascular; HER2, human epithelial growth factor; HTN, hypertension; ICIs, immune checkpoint inhibitors; MM, multiple myeloma; TKIs, tyrosine kinase inhibitors; XRT, radiation.

[a] Consider the summative patient risk based on existing CV disease and cancer therapy, both planned and delivered.

[b] Not required if asymptomatic and normal LV function during treatment.

Adapted from Onishi T, Fukuda Y, Miyazaki S, et al. Practical guidance for echocardiography for cancer therapeutics–related cardiac dysfunction. *J Echocardiogr.* 2021;19(1):1-20. doi:10.1007/s12574-020-00502-9

TABLE 14-2 Cardiotoxicity Classification Criteria for Screening in Cancer Patients

	Severity		
	Mild	**Moderate**	**Severe**
Cardiac Review and Evaluation Committee; Definition of Chemotherapy-Induced Cardiotoxicity[32]	Any one of the following: 1. reduction of LVEF, either global or specific, in the interventricular septum; 2. symptoms of congestive HF; 3. signs associated with HF, such as S3 gallop, tachycardia, or both; 4. reduction in LVEF from baseline ≥5% to <55% in the presence of signs or symptoms of HF or a reduction in LVEF ≥10% to <55% without signs or symptoms of HF		
CTCAE v5.0 Ejection Fraction Decreased	**Grade 2** Resting ejection fraction (EF) 50%-40%; 10%-19% drop from baseline	**Grade 3** Resting ejection fraction (EF) 39%-20%; ≥20% drop from baseline	**Grade 4** Resting ejection fraction (EF) <20%
Package Insert Guidelines to Hold Cancer Therapy Due to LV Dysfunction	**Trastuzumab** ≥16% absolute decrease in LVEF or ≥10% drop to below institutional limits of normal	**Pertuzumab** ≥10% drop in LVEF to <50% for early breast cancer, ≥10% drop in LVEF to 40%-45% for metastatic breast cancer, or drop to <40%	
2014 ASE/EACI Echo Guidelines for Subclinical LV Dysfunction[6]	**Subclinical LV Dysfunction** >15% relative drop in GLS from baseline	**CTRCD** Drop in LVEF of >10 percentage points to a level <53%. Should be confirmed by repeat testing.	
2016 ESC Position Statement	**Mild (Asymptomatic)** LVEF <50% or LVEF reduction >10% from baseline, should be repeated within 3-4 wk	**Moderate (Symptomatic From HF)** LVEF <50%	

	Mild (Asymptomatic)	All Cancer Therapy	Anthracycline or Trastuzumab Related	Moderate	Severe
2020 ESMO Guideline[3]	LVEF >15% from baseline if LVEF >50%			Symptomatic HF regardless of LVEF	LVEF <40%
				LVEF ≥10% from baseline, or Any drop of LVEF to <50% but ≥40%	
2021 ICOS Universal Definition for Asymptomatic CTRCD (with or without additional biomarkers)	**Mild** New LVEF reduction with fall in GLS by >15% ±new rise in cardiac biomarkers[a]			**Moderate** New LVEF reduction to >10% and to 40%-49%	**Severe** New LVEF <40%
				New LVEF reduction by <10% and to 40%-49% AND new fall in GLS by >15% ±new rise in cardiac biomarkers[a]	

Various definitions of cardiotoxicity for asymptomatic patients undergoing screening, with some select definitions in symptomatic patients included when important for clarity. See Table 1-1 for more complete definitions in symptomatic patients.

ASE, American Society of Echocardiography; CTCAE, Common Terminology Criteria for Adverse Events; CTRCD, cancer therapeutics–related cardiac dysfunction; EACI, European Association of Cardiovascular Imaging; GLS, global longitudinal strain; HF, heart failure; LVEF, left ventricular ejection fraction; NYHA, New York Heart Association.

[a]Cardiac troponin I/T >99th percentile, BNP ≥35 pg/mL, NT-proBNP ≥125 pg/mL.

parameters such as global longitudinal strain (GLS), diastolic dysfunction, and serum cardiac biomarkers.[9]
- While definitions of cardiotoxicity have notably focused on LV dysfunction, **cardiotoxicity from cancer therapy can take many forms, including diastolic dysfunction, valvular damage, pericardial disease, pulmonary hypertension, arterial thromboembolism, and RV dysfunction**. Echocardiography can be useful in all of these disease processes.

HISTORY OF SAFETY MONITORING

- It was not long after the initial discovery of anthracyclines in the early 1960s that there was also a recognition of their potential for LV dysfunction and the development of clinical heart failure (HF).[10]

Early Modalities for Cardiac Evaluation

- Early use of radionuclides in the form of equilibrium radionuclide angiography (ERNA), multiple gated acquisition (MUGA), and single-photon emission computed tomography (SPECT)-ERNA were widely used to assess LV function (both systolic and diastolic) owing to availability, accuracy, and reproducibility.[1]
- MUGA using technetium-99m labeled red blood cells, especially before echo technology became more sophisticated, was noted to lower inter- and intraobserver variability compared to early two-dimensional (2D) echocardiography.

The Evolution of Echocardiography

- As echo capabilities have advanced over the last 70 years (Fig. 14-2), reliability has significantly improved and echocardiography has become the screening test of choice owing to its wide availability, safety profile, lack of additional radiation doses and its comprehensive capabilities in evaluating diastology, RV function, cardiac valves, the aorta, and the pericardium.[2]
- Edler and Hertz are credited with the development of early M-mode (motion-mode) technology in the mid-1950s as a means of diagnosing mitral stenosis in

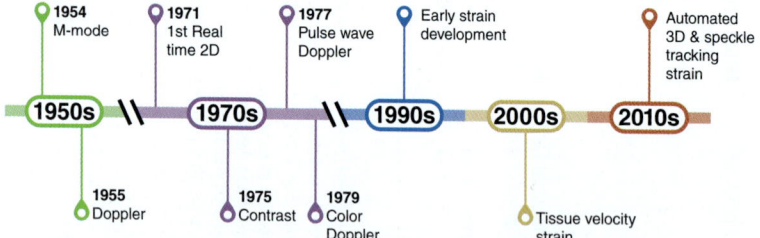

Figure 14-2. A historical timeline of echocardiography techniques. An abbreviated timeline highlighting echocardiographic landmarks in technology advancement that provides the foundation for a comprehensive cardiac evaluation. Although Edler and Hertz are credited with the original echo machine with clinical applicability, there have been countless contributors over the last 70 years that have made this imaging modality what it is today.

patients often at the end of their lives.[11] Roughly at the same time, investigators in Japan were developing the first Doppler applications in ultrasound.
- The 1970s saw significant advancements with the development of the first real-time 2D imaging, echo contrast agents (initially described in intracardial shunt identification), pulse wave Doppler for hemodynamic assessment of valvular stenosis severity, and color Doppler developments.
- The 1990s brought the first attempts at myocardial strain assessment, later becoming more refined and reproducible with incorporation of myocardial tissue velocities in the 2000s and then speckle tracking in the 2010s.
- Automated 3D and full volume acquisitions became more widely available across different vendors around the same time as various strain packages.

ECHOCARDIOGRAPHIC TECHNIQUES FOR MONITORING

Two-Dimensional Imaging
- The workhorse and most widely utilized method of cardiac assessment in echocardiography is that of the 2D image, although consideration of its limitations is important to maximize its usefulness.
- When calculating LVEF, the method chosen needs to limit geometric assumptions as much as possible, which is done most readily (though not perfectly) with the Simpson biplane method of disks from the apical 4- and 2-chamber views.
- Despite this significantly improved method of 2D assessment compared to more complex calculations of the past, the **Simpson method has still been noted to have approximately 10% inter- and intraobserver variability.**[7]
- 2D LVEF assessment can be negatively impacted by **foreshortening** and poor **endocardial definition**; **contrast enhancement** can help mitigate these limitations (see further on).
- The 10% inter- and intraobserver variability in LVEF measurements can potentially have a significant impact given the 10% cutoff for many definitions of cardiotoxicity. **When assessing for cardiotoxicity**, especially when considering changes in cancer therapy, it is vital to **compare prior images side by side** and consider other available information, such as myocardial strain, when available (Fig. 14-3).
- Other applications of 2D echo include chamber size, pericardial thickening, valvular calcification, increased myocardial thickening, and presence of a pericardial effusion with or without chamber collapse in the setting of clinical cardiac tamponade (Table 14-3).[3,12]

Doppler
- Doppler in all its forms (pulse wave, continuous wave, color, and tissue velocity) is an integral part of the comprehensive echo exam.
- Diastolic function assessment, particularly in survivors of childhood cancer and breast cancer survivors who have received anthracycline-based regimens, has been correlated with prognostication and is done by collecting peak mitral flow velocity (E), mitral septal and lateral early diastolic velocity (e′), E/e′, and tricuspid valve regurgitation velocity (along with LA volume).[13,14]
- Notably, **survivors of chest RT** are also at **17 times the risk of diastolic heart failure** within the first 6 years of follow-up owing to radiation-induced myocyte damage and fibrosis.[15]

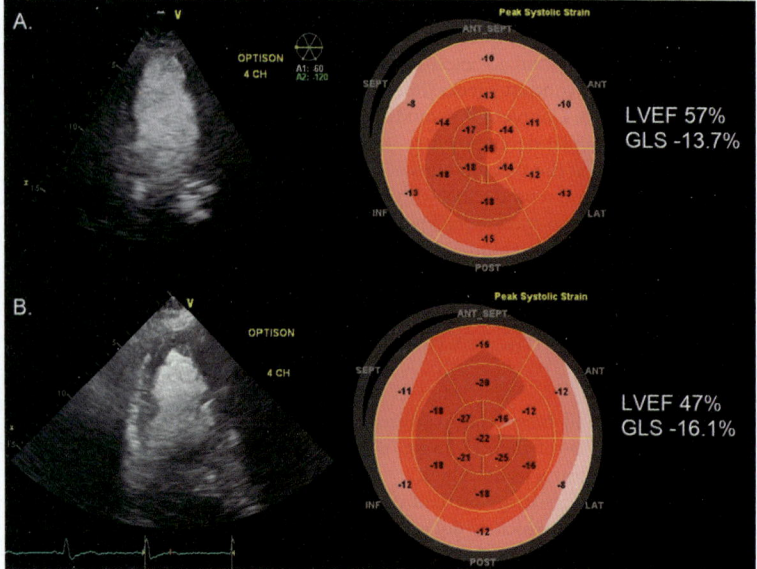

Figure 14-3. A 71-year-old female with metastatic leiomyosarcoma receiving doxorubicin with concurrent dexrazoxane on trial is on the 16th cycle of anthracycline-based therapy (cumulative doxorubicin dose 1200 mg/m^2). A. Her most recent TTE 6 weeks ago showed LVEF of 57% with GLS of −13.7%. B. Her TTE performed today is read in a standard clinical fashion with an LVEF of 47%, and she is subsequently removed from study on concerns of cardiotoxicity. However, her LV strain, a measure with reduced variability, is stable, if not improved, compared to previous measures (GLS −16.1%). Subsequent blinded analysis of her echocardiograms from the research central core lab showed that her LVEF had actually remained unchanged (prior LVEF 60.7% with current LVEF 57.4%). Thus, the patient was erroneously removed from the clinical trial, and her cancer therapy was altered as a result of an incomplete interpretation of her LV function. GLS, global longitudinal strain; LVEF, left ventricular ejection fraction; TTE, transthoracic echocardiogram.

TABLE 14-3	Echocardiographic Techniques for Cardiac Evaluation in the Cancer Patient	
	Clinical application	**Normal reference range**
2D[33]	• Chamber sizes • LV function (Simpson biplane method of disks) • Myocardial thickness • Valvular assessment • Presence of pericardial effusion	**LVEF (biplane)** • 52%-72% (M), 54%-74% (F) **LVEDV** • 62-150 mL (M), 46-106 mL (F) **LVESV** • 21-61 mL (M), 14-42 mL (F) **Indexed LA volume** • 16-34 mL/m^2 (M/F) **LV mass** • 96-200 g (M), 66-150 g (F) **RWT** • 0.22-0.42 (M/F)

TABLE 14-3	Echocardiographic Techniques for Cardiac Evaluation in the Cancer Patient (*continued*)	
	Clinical application	**Normal reference range**
Doppler (Color, PW, CW, TDI)[34]	• Diastolic function • RV function • Pulmonary pressures • Valvular assessment	• E/A ratio (0.8-2.0) • E/e' ratio (<14) • lateral e' (>10 cm/s) • septal e' (>7 cm/s) • TR jet velocity (<2.8 m/s)
3D[33]	• Chamber size/function • Valvular assessment • Cardiac mass evaluation	*No current consensus on 3D-specific chamber quantification guidelines*
Myocardial strain[3]	• Subclinical ventricular dysfunction	• 18%-22% (vendor specific)
Contrast-enhancing agents	• Technically difficult 2D images with poor myocardial border definition • LV apex evaluation for thrombi	N/A

2D, 2-dimensional; 3D, 3-dimensional; A, late diastolic filling velocity; CW, continuous wave; E, early diastolic filling velocity; e', early relaxation tissue velocity; F, females; g, grams; LA, left atrium; LV, left ventricle; LVEDV, left ventricular end diastolic volume; LVESV, left ventricular end systolic volume; M, males; mL, milliliters; PW, pulse wave; RWT, relative wall thickness; STE, speckle-tracking echo; TDI, tissue Doppler imaging.

Three-Dimensional Imaging

- LV geometric assumptions, foreshortening of the LV apex, and operator skill have been noted to be limiting factors for accurate evaluation by echo, and these are mitigated with 3D imaging.
- **3D utilization** has been shown to **reduce temporal variability** of serial imaging in patients (especially when taking into account images obtained by multiple sonographers, which are then interpreted by multiple echo readers) from the typical 10% quoted on 2D assessment to that of **only 5%**.[16]
- Other potential advantages of 3D echo include **less variability in chamber size quantification** compared to 2D assessment alone.[17]
- The use of 3D can also allow for more refined assessment of **valvular calcification** and **vegetations**, as well as valvular or chamber **thrombi**.
- There is also a growing body of literature accumulating for the clinical use of **3D-derived speckle-tracking echocardiography** (STE), particularly in breast cancer patients having previously received anthracycline-based treatment regimens, that suggests feasibility in the assessment of myocardial subclinical dysfunction compared to 2D-derived data, as well as MUGA and magnetic resonance imaging (MRI).[18,19]
- Despite the promise of 3D echo, it is important to note that 2D echo with contrast-enhancing agents has been found to be more reliable than 3D assessment without contrast in at least one series.[20] Some variation in 3D reliability would be expected among nonresearch echo labs based on software packages used as well as sonographer experience and training. Quality control at each center is vital for any technique.

Myocardial Strain and Early Detection of Left Ventricular Dysfunction

- Since a drop in LVEF can be a late finding, after significant cardiotoxicity has already occurred, other measures of subclinical myocardial dysfunction can be important early signs of cardiotoxicity.
- **GLS has emerged as the primary measure of subclinical myocardial dysfunction** and has proven utility across multiple cancer patient populations and cancer treatments for predicting subsequent LVEF reductions and adverse outcomes.[10,21,22]
- **Strain** is **defined as** a change in the length of the myocardium divided by its original length (yielding a negative value) and is a closer measure of **myocardial contractility** then LVEF.
- Originally measured by assessing the myocardial tissue velocities of each individual myocardial segment (a very labor-intensive process prone to error), myocardial strain analysis is now done by automated or semiautomated **speckle tracking.**
- In an analysis of the **survivors of childhood cancer database** (SJLIFE), among survivors with a preserved LVEF by 3D assessment, a **GLS reduction** was seen in 28% of patients (particularly those who had received prior chest radiation exposure), which translated into **worse cardiovascular outcomes** long term compared to those with normal GLS values.[13]
- In the **SUCCOUR trial**, cardioprotective medicines (ACE inhibitors or angiotensin receptor blockers, followed by β-blocker) initiated after a **relative drop in** GLS **of 12%** prevented subsequent decline in LVEF in patients treated with anthracyclines at increased risk for HF.[5]
- Meta-analyses and systematic reviews have consistently found GLS performs well in identifying high-risk patients compared to 2D-derived echo data alone in patients receiving anthracyclines and/or human epithelial growth factor 2 (HER2)–targeted therapy.[23,24]
- In addition to ability to detect subclinical myocardial dysfunction, GLS is also a **more reproducible measure** of LV function with **reduced interobserver variability**.[25] There is known **variability across different vendor packages**, however, which should be recognized when comparing different examinations.

Contrast-Enhancing Agents

- Suboptimal echo images are commonly encountered for a number of reasons (body habitus, advanced pulmonary disease, prior mediastinal or breast radiation, mastectomy, etc.). In such cases, **endomyocardial border definition can be significantly improved by the administration of a contrast-enhancing agent** at the time of echo image acquisition.
- Contrast-enhancing agents can also **improve detection of the blood-flow Doppler** signal across valves but at times can also overestimate velocities depending on the agent dose and the bolus injection timing.

ECHOCARDIOGRAPHY SCREENING FOR CARDIOVASCULAR TOXICITY OF CANCER THERAPY

- There are numerous classes of cancer treatments that pose potential harm to the CV system before, during, and long after the treatments are completed, which are covered in more detail in their respective chapters.

- It is, however, noteworthy to consider specific applications of echocardiography in the monitoring of patients on select cancer treatments known to have the highest incidence of adverse cardiac events.
- Echocardiography **screening protocols** are optimally **individualized** to the patient based on the **incidence of cardiotoxicity** of the patient's cancer therapy, the patient's **known and estimated cardiovascular risk**, and collaboration between the oncologist and cardiologist (Table 14-1).[7]

Cancer Treatment–Related Cardiac Dysfunction (CTRCD)

- The most widely appreciated CTRCD is **LV dysfunction** and cardiomyopathy from **anthracyclines** and **HER2** receptor inhibitors.
- However, many other agents have been associated with either clinical or subclinical LV dysfunction throughout treatment, such as **alkylating agents** (cyclophosphamide, ifosfamide), **proteasome inhibitors** (carfilzomib), **vascular endothelial growth factor inhibitors** (bevacizumab, pazopanib, sunitinib, sorafenib, axitinib), and other select **tyrosine kinase inhibitors** (ponatinib, trametinib).
- **Myocarditis** is also a potential acute manifestation of CTRCD during treatment with **immune checkpoint inhibitors** (e.g., ipilimumab, nivolumab, pembrolizumab).
- Echo plays a critical role in pretreatment cardiac evaluation and monitoring during and after treatment with these agents.

Valvular Heart Disease

- Valvular heart disease most commonly occurs in survivors of mediastinal or left chest **radiation**, often occurring **years after treatment**.
- Progression is usually gradual with fibrosis and calcification resulting in valvular dysfunction with stenosis and/or regurgitation.[26]
- The **incidence of radiation-induced valve disease** has been observed in those with prior mediastinal radiation to be **7% to 39% at 10 years and 12% to 60% at 20 years** in asymptomatic patients, most often affecting the mitral and aortic valves.[27]
- Surveillance strategies in radiation survivors should take into account clinical risk factors, other cancer treatments (such as anthracyclines), and the dose and location of radiation exposure. A recent expert consensus statement from the International Cardio-Oncology Society recommends consideration of echocardiography as early as 6 to 12 months after completion of therapy and as often as every 5 years to screen for cardiomyopathy, valvular dysfunction, and pericardial disease.[28]

Pericardial Disease

- Pericardial disease can be found commonly in radiation survivors as well, but can also occur in patients with a wide range of cancer types regardless of cancer treatment (see Chapter 7).
- Most guidelines use >30Gy of cumulative prior radiation exposure as the qualifier of lower versus higher risk, comparatively, but there can still be significant cardiac exposure with mean heart doses >10 Gy.[29]
- With significant cardiac radiation exposure, the **incidences of pericarditis and pericardial effusion can be as high as 20% and 36%**, respectively.[22,26]
- In this regard, **echo is a first-line imaging modality** for the assessment of diastolic function, ventricular interdependence, and evidence of elevated intracardiac pressures in the setting of a pericardial effusion.

Vascular Toxicity

- **5-FU and capecitabine** (antimetabolites) has been shown to cause **coronary vasospasm**, especially during continuous infusion, resulting in acute coronary syndrome, which can be observed on echo as wall motion abnormalities in a coronary distribution.[2]
- Similarly, **nilotinib** (tyrosine kinase inhibitor), **immune checkpoint inhibitors**, and **radiation** therapy have been associated with **accelerated coronary atherosclerosis**, which can prompt consideration of additional screening for ischemia.
- **Systemic hypertension** can also be found both during therapy and long after therapy has been completed in certain alkylating agents (cisplatin), proteasome inhibitors (bortezomib), tyrosine kinase inhibitors (ibrutinib, nilotinib, trametinib), and vascular endothelial growth factor inhibitors, which can manifest as **left ventricular hypertrophy and diastolic dysfunction on echo assessment**.
- **Dasatinib** (tyrosine kinase inhibitor) has been associated with the development of **pulmonary hypertension** and can be evaluated noninvasively with Doppler-derived hemodynamic assessments.

LIMITATIONS OF ECHOCARDIOGRAPHY

- No imaging modality is without limitations, and echo is no exception.
- Despite multiple studies from robust core labs indicating adequate reproducibility, repeatability, and reliability, there can still be **temporal variability** in LVEF measurement that can be as high as 8% to 10% for 2D echo.[1,30,31]
- The utilization of more complex, though now automated, methods of cardiac assessment such as **3D has been shown to improve accuracy and reproducibility but may not be widely available** in all laboratories. Additionally, **use of contrast** may provide more reliability than 3D for clinical evaluations outside of core labs.
- The interpretability and usefulness of a comprehensive echo evaluation rely on **adequate image acquisition,** which can be negatively impacted by body habitus or comorbidities such as pulmonary disease.
- In this situation, it would be appropriate to consider other imaging modalities, such as cardiac MRI, to assess for signs of cardiotoxicity (Table 14-4).

TABLE 14-4 Comparison of Imaging Modalities for the Initial Evaluation and Surveillance in the Cancer Patient

Modality	Strengths	Weaknesses
Echo	• Lack of radiation, no adverse side effects • Availability • Versatility • Comprehensive cardiac evaluation • Primary study for valvular assessment • Primary study for diastolic assessment • Assessment for subclinical LV dysfunction with strain analysis	• Inter- and intraobserver variability • Imaging quality variability based on body habitus

TABLE 14-4	Comparison of Imaging Modalities for the Initial Evaluation and Surveillance in the Cancer Patient (*continued*)

Modality	Strengths	Weaknesses
CT	• Assessment for coronary calcification • Pericardial disease • Cardiac masses (best spatial resolution)	• Radiation dose • Nephrotoxicity of contrast when needed • Limited ability to evaluate for subclinical cardiac disease
MRI	• Gold standard for LVEF • Gold standard for chamber sizes • Lack of radiation • Cardiac masses (best tissue characterization) • Assessment for subclinical LV dysfunction with strain analysis and other parameters	• Cost, limited availability • Inability to use in certain patients with metallic cardiac devices • Risk of nephrogenic fibrosis with contrast in patients with severe renal disease • Patient tolerance (length of exam, claustrophobia)
MUGA	• Limited variability between studies and interpreters • Highly reproducible	• Radiation dose • Limited diastolic function and subclinical dysfunction assessment • No valvular information • Variability in LVEF assessment relative to MRI
PET	• Assessment of myocardial perfusion and metabolism • Ability to visualize avid metastatic lesions	• Radiation dose • Cost • Availability • Limited subclinical dysfunction assessment currently

CT, computed tomography; LVEF, left ventricular ejection fraction; MRI, magnetic resonance imaging; MUGA, multiple gated acquisition; PET, positron emission tomography.

REFERENCES

1. Awadalla M, Hassan MZO, Alvi RM, Neilan TG. Advanced imaging modalities to detect cardiotoxicity. *Curr Probl Cancer.* 2018;42(4):386-396.
2. Plana JC, Thavendiranathan P, Bucciarelli-Ducci C, Lancellotti P. Multi-modality imaging in the assessment of cardiovascular toxicity in the cancer patient. *JACC Cardiovasc Imaging.* 2018;11(8):1173-1186.
3. Curigliano G, Lenihan D, Fradley M, et al. Management of cardiac disease in cancer patients throughout oncological treatment: ESMO consensus recommendations. *Ann Oncol.* 2020;31(2):171-190.
4. Cardinale D, Colombo A, Sandri MT, et al. Prevention of high-dose chemotherapy-induced cardiotoxicity in high-risk patients by angiotensin-converting enzyme inhibition. *Circulation.* 2006;114(23):2474-2481.

5. Thavendiranathan P, Negishi T, Somerset E, et al. Strain-guided management of potentially cardiotoxic cancer therapy. *J Am Coll Cardiol*. 2021;77(4):392-401.
6. Plana JC, Galderisi M, Barac A, et al. Expert consensus for multimodality imaging evaluation of adult patients during and after cancer therapy: a report from the American Society of Echocardiography and the European Association of Cardiovascular Imaging. *J Am Soc Echocardiogr*. 2014;27(9):911-939.
7. Celutkiene J, Pudil R, Lopez-Fernandez T, et al. Role of cardiovascular imaging in cancer patients receiving cardiotoxic therapies: a position statement on behalf of the Heart Failure Association (HFA), the European Association of Cardiovascular Imaging (EACVI) and the Cardio-Oncology Council of the European Society of Cardiology (ESC). *Eur J Heart Fail*. 2020;22(9):1504-1524.
8. Larsen CM, Mulvagh SL. Cardio-oncology: what you need to know now for clinical practice and echocardiography. *Echo Res Pract*. 2017;4(1):R33-R41.
9. Lopez-Sendon J, Alvarez-Ortega C, Zamora P, et al. Classification, prevalence, and outcomes of anticancer therapy-induced cardiotoxicity: the CARDIOTOX registry. *Eur Heart J*. 2020;41(18):1720-1729.
10. Tanaka H. Echocardiography and cancer therapeutics-related cardiac dysfunction. *J Med Ultrason (2001)*. 2019;46(3):309-316.
11. Feigenbaum H. Evolution of echocardiography. *Circulation*. 1996;93(7):1321-1327.
12. Liu J, Banchs J, Mousavi N, et al. Contemporary role of echocardiography for clinical decision making in patients during and after cancer therapy. *JACC Cardiovasc Imaging*. 2018;11(8):1122-1131.
13. Armstrong GT, Joshi VM, Ness KK, et al. Comprehensive echocardiographic detection of treatment-related cardiac dysfunction in adult survivors of childhood cancer: results from the St. Jude Lifetime Cohort Study. *J Am Coll Cardiol*. 2015;65(23):2511-2522.
14. Nagiub M, Nixon JV, Kontos MC. Ability of nonstrain diastolic parameters to predict doxorubicin-induced cardiomyopathy: a systematic review with meta-analysis. *Cardiol Rev*. 2018;26(1):29-34.
15. Saiki H, Petersen IA, Scott CG, et al. Risk of heart failure with preserved ejection fraction in older women after contemporary radiotherapy for breast cancer. *Circulation*. 2017;135(15):1388-1396.
16. Bottinor WJ, Migliore CK, Lenneman CA, Stoddard MF. Echocardiographic assessment of cardiotoxic effects of cancer therapy. *Curr Cardiol Rep*. 2016;18(10):99.
17. Coutinho Cruz M, Moura Branco L, Portugal G, et al. Three-dimensional speckle-tracking echocardiography for the global and regional assessments of left ventricle myocardial deformation in breast cancer patients treated with anthracyclines. *Clin Res Cardiol*. 2020;109(6):673-684.
18. Walker J, Bhullar N, Fallah-Rad N, et al. Role of three-dimensional echocardiography in breast cancer: comparison with two-dimensional echocardiography, multiple-gated acquisition scans, and cardiac magnetic resonance imaging. *J Clin Oncol*. 2010;28(21):3429-3436.
19. Zhang KW, Finkelman BS, Gulati G, et al. Abnormalities in 3-dimensional left ventricular mechanics with anthracycline chemotherapy are associated with systolic and diastolic dysfunction. *JACC Cardiovasc Imaging*. 2018;11(8):1059-1068.
20. Hoffmann R, Barletta G, von Bardeleben S, et al. Analysis of left ventricular volumes and function: a multicenter comparison of cardiac magnetic resonance imaging, cine ventriculography, and unenhanced and contrast-enhanced two-dimensional and three-dimensional echocardiography. *J Am Soc Echocardiogr*. 2014;27(3):292-301.
21. Clasen SC, Scherrer-Crosbie M. Applications of left ventricular strain measurements to patients undergoing chemotherapy. *Curr Opin Cardiol*. 2018;33(5):493-497.
22. Quintana RA, Bui LP, Moudgil R, et al. Speckle-tracking echocardiography in cardio-oncology and beyond. *Tex Heart Inst J*. 2020;47(2):96-107.
23. Bergamini C, Dolci G, Truong S, et al. Role of speckle tracking echocardiography in the evaluation of breast cancer patients undergoing chemotherapy: review and meta-analysis of the literature. *Cardiovasc Toxicol*. 2019;19(6):485-492.

24. Oikonomou EK, Kokkinidis DG, Kampaktsis PN, et al. Assessment of prognostic value of left ventricular global longitudinal strain for early prediction of chemotherapy-induced cardiotoxicity: a systematic review and meta-analysis. *JAMA Cardiol.* 2019;*4*(10):1007-1018.
25. Karlsen S, Dahlslett T, Grenne B, et al. Global longitudinal strain is a more reproducible measure of left ventricular function than ejection fraction regardless of echocardiographic training. *Cardiovasc Ultrasound.* 2019;*17*(1):18.
26. Desai MY, Windecker S, Lancellotti P, et al. Prevention, diagnosis, and management of radiation-associated cardiac disease: JACC Scientific Expert Panel. *J Am Coll Cardiol.* 2019;*74*(7):905-927.
27. Negishi T, Miyazaki S, Negishi K. Echocardiography and cardio-oncology. *Heart Lung Circ.* 2019;*28*(9):1331-1338.
28. Mitchell JD, Cehic DA, Morgia M, et al. Cardiovascular manifestations resulting from therapeutic radiation: a multidisciplinary statement from the International Cardio-Oncology Society. *JACC CardioOncol.* 2021;*3*(3):360-380.
29. Lancellotti P, Nkomo VT, Badano LP, et al. Expert consensus for multi-modality imaging evaluation of cardiovascular complications of radiotherapy in adults: a report from the European Association of Cardiovascular Imaging and the American Society of Echocardiography. *Eur Heart J Cardiovasc Imaging.* 2013;*14*(8):721-740.
30. Khouri MG, Ky B, Dunn G, et al. Echocardiography core laboratory reproducibility of cardiac safety assessments in cardio-oncology. *J Am Soc Echocardiogr.* 2018;*31*(3):361-371.e3.
31. Bunting KV, Steeds RP, Slater LT, Rogers JK, Gkoutos GV, Kotecha D. A practical guide to assess the reproducibility of echocardiographic measurements. *J Am Soc Echocardiogr.* 2019;*32*(12):1505-1515.
32. Seidman A, Hudis C, Pierri MK, et al. Cardiac dysfunction in the trastuzumab clinical trials experience. *J Clin Oncol.* 2002;*20*(5):1215-1221.
33. Lang RM, Badano LP, Mor-Avi V, et al. Recommendations for cardiac chamber quantification by echocardiography in adults: an update from the American Society of Echocardiography and the European Association of Cardiovascular Imaging. *J Am Soc Echocardiogr.* 2015;*28*(1):1-39.e14.
34. Nagueh SF, Smiseth OA, Appleton CP, et al. Recommendations for the evaluation of left ventricular diastolic function by echocardiography: an update from the American Society of Echocardiography and the European Association of Cardiovascular Imaging. *J Am Soc Echocardiogr.* 2016;*29*(4):277-314.

15 Biomarkers as a Tool for Cardiac Safety

Courtney M. Campbell and Daniel J. Lenihan

GENERAL PRINCIPLES

Definitions
- A biomarker is any substance, structure, or process that can be measured in the body (or its products) that influences or predicts the incidence or outcome of a disease.
- Useful biomarkers are **accurate**, **easy to measure**, and **provide important information** relative to treatment outcome. Biomarkers can include physiologic tests, clinical images, genetic variants, tissue biopsies, and blood sample–derived values.
- Traditional cardiovascular (CV) imaging tests, such as electrocardiography and transthoracic echocardiogram, have limited sensitivity and specificity for early detection of myocardial injury.
- This chapter focuses on **blood-based biomarkers** that have shown the most promise in predicting and monitoring for **cancer therapy–related cardiovascular dysfunction (CTRCD)**. Importantly, the sensitivity, specificity, and negative predictive value of these biomarkers vary depending on the clinical scenario.

Cardio-Oncology Biomarkers

Troponin
- Troponins are a group of proteins found in skeletal and heart muscle fibers that regulate muscular contraction via myosin. Troponin is part of a complex with tropomyosin and actin.
- There are three types of troponin: **troponin I (TnI), troponin T (TnT),** and troponin C (TnC). TnI and TnT are cardiac specific.
- Troponin is released rapidly after myocardial injury (3-6 hours) and remains elevated for 7 to 10 days.
- **Troponin is established as a biomarker for myocardial injury** in other cardiac disease processes such as acute coronary syndrome.
- **Elevated TnI has been associated with left ventricular ejection fraction (LVEF) depression and adverse cardiac events** after cancer therapy, particularly with **anthracycline therapy**.

Natriuretic Peptides
- **Natriuretic peptides (NPs)** are produced by cardiomyocytes and **released in response to wall stress** caused by increased pressure or volume overload.
- Pro–brain natriuretic peptide (proBNP) is a polypeptide prohormone stored in secretory granules. It is cleaved to form the inactive amino-terminal proBNP (NT-proBNP) and biologically active hormone BNP. Both **NT-proBNP and BNP** are secreted into the blood in equimolar amounts.

- BNP has broad physiologic effects, including reduced renal sodium reabsorption to decrease blood volume, reduced aldosterone secretion, vascular smooth muscle relaxation, and increased lipolysis.
- **BNP and NT-proBNP are useful diagnostic tools in predicting or detecting heart failure** and left ventricular systolic dysfunction.
- In the cardio-oncology (C-O) setting, BNP and NT-proBNP have been associated with predicting cancer therapy–related cardiotoxicity and detecting heart failure.

C-reactive Protein
- C-reactive protein (CRP) is an annular, pentameric protein produced by the liver that increases after macrophage and T-cell secretion of interleukin-6.
- CRP is considered an acute-phase reactant and marker of inflammation.
- In the Justification for the Use of Statins in Primary Prevention: An Intervention Trial Evaluating Rosuvastatin (JUPITER) trial, patients with an elevated high-sensitivity (hs) CRP >2 mg/L and low-density lipoprotein (LDL) cholesterol <130 mg/dL benefited from statin therapy with a lower rate of CV events.
- Initial CRP increase and then decline are associated with cancer response to immune checkpoint inhibitors (ICI). Persistent elevation is associated with poor prognosis. **Monitoring CRP can be considered for ICI myocarditis surveillance** and monitoring resolution.
- Elevated high-sensitivity hs-CRP demonstrated good sensitivity in predicting LVEF decrease in a single study of breast cancer patients.

Investigational Biomarkers
- Additional blood-derived biomarkers have been evaluated in cardio-oncology (C-O), but validation studies are needed.[1,2] Examples include the following:
  - *Inflammatory marker:* growth-differentiation factor-15 (GDF-15)
  - *Vascular remodeling markers:* placental growth factor (PGF) and soluble fms-like tyrosine kinase receptor-1 (sFlt-1)
  - *Fibrosis marker:* galectin-3
  - *Amyloidosis markers:* **plasma hepatocyte growth factor (HGF),**[3] neurofilament light chain (NfL).[4]
- Myeloperoxidase (MPO) is an enzyme secreted by polymorphonuclear leukocytes that scavenges nitric oxide, inhibits nitric oxide synthase, and promotes lipid peroxidation. MPO has atherogenic and prooxidant effects.
  - Anthracycline toxicity may be caused by topoisomerase II-beta inhibition, leading to oxidative stress, resulting in elevated MPO levels. In a 2014 study of 78 patients with breast cancer undergoing doxorubicin and trastuzumab therapy, early increases in TnI and MPO were associated with increased risk of cardiotoxicity.[1]
- **MicroRNAs (miRs) are small, highly conserved non–protein-coding RNA molecules involved in regulating gene expression.** Although human clinical trials are needed, animal models of cancer therapy–related cardiotoxicity support miRs as potential cardio-oncology biomarkers.[5]
  - miR-34a upregulation, associated with heart failure, preceded doxorubicin-induced cardiac injury in a mouse model.
  - miR-150 downregulation preceded doxorubicin-induced cardiac injury in a dose-dependent manner in a mouse model.

- miR-208b upregulation, associated with myosin expression and impaired contractility, was elevated in a dose-dependent relationship in a mouse model of doxorubicin-induced cardiac injury.

BIOMARKERS IN PRACTICE

- Although biomarkers are widely used in C-O practice, prospective, systematic studies have been conducted only in a few practice scenarios discussed in this section.
- The exact role and timing of biomarker measurement in patients undergoing potentially cardiotoxic cancer therapy is yet to be determined.

Anthracyclines

- Anthracyclines are topoisomerase II inhibitors that inhibit DNA and RNA synthesis resulting in cell death.
- Anthracyclines are used to treat multiple malignancies, including breast cancer, urothelial cancers, gynecologic cancer, gastric esophageal cancer, acute lymphoblastic/myeloid leukemia, lymphoma, and sarcoma.
- Drugs in this class include doxorubicin, daunorubicin, epirubicin, and idarubicin.
- Cumulative anthracycline exposure is associated with permanent myocardial damage in a dose-response relationship. Cardiomyopathy risk increases with doses >250 mg/m^2, but cardiotoxicity can occur at lower doses.
- **Both NPs and troponins have been studied as biomarkers for LV dysfunction related to anthracycline therapy.**[6]
- **Troponin elevations are best associated with monitoring for anthracycline-induced cardiomyopathy**, as established in early studies.[7]
  - In a 2002 study of 211 high-risk breast cancer patients receiving high-dose chemotherapy, LVEF progressively decreased in the TnI positive group, but not the TnI negative group over the 1-year follow-up.
  - In a 2004 study of 703 patients undergoing high-dose chemotherapy for aggressive malignancies, elevated TnI soon after therapy and 1 month later was associated with 84% positive predictive value for future cardiac events. No TnI elevation was associated with a 99% negative predictive value for future cardiac events.
- However, not all studies firmly supported troponin as a stand-alone biomarker for early detection of anthracycline cardiotoxicity.[8]
  - In a 2011 study of 53 patients with breast cancer treated with adjuvant anthracycline therapy, elevated BNP, but not TnI, was associated with LVEF depression of ≥10%.
  - In a 2012 study of 81 patients with human epidermal growth factor receptor 2 (HER2)–positive breast cancer treated with anthracyclines followed by taxanes and trastuzumab, both ultrasensitive TnI and peak systolic longitudinal strain predicted subsequent development cardiotoxicity. Together, the sensitivity of cardiotoxicity detection was 87%, with a negative predictive value of 91%.
- Although initial studies of BNP elevation preceding anthracycline toxicity were mixed, more recent studies show that **persistent NP elevations can precede LVEF decline and other adverse CV events.**
  - In a 2014 study of 333 cancer patients, both BNP (>100 pg/mL) and LVEF <50% predicted heart failure development, but only BNP was predictive of overall mortality.

- In a 2016 study of 111 patients receiving anthracycline chemotherapy, BNP was more effective than LVEF evaluation in predicting the occurrence of adverse cardiac events.[9]
- Recommendation: Consider using **troponins and NPs at baseline, during, and after anthracycline treatment to identify high-risk individuals** for cardiotoxicity and adverse CV events.

Trastuzumab

- Trastuzumab is a humanized monoclonal antibody that blocks the activation of human epidermal growth factor receptor (HER)-2/neu receptor, resulting in impaired cell growth and survival. Not all HER-2 targeted therapies are associated with cardiotoxicity.
- Trastuzumab is used primarily to treat breast cancer.
- Cardiotoxicity typically presents as an asymptomatic decrease in LVEF, is not related to cumulative dose, and is often reversible.
- Prospective studies have identified biomarkers linked to trastuzumab cardiotoxicity.
  - In a 2010 study of 251 patients undergoing trastuzumab therapy for breast cancer, elevated TnI was an independent predictor of cardiotoxicity and lack of LVEF recovery.[10] Patients previously treated with anthracycline were more likely to have elevated TnI.
  - In a 2017 study of 452 patients with HER2-positive breast cancer, elevated TnI or TnT was associated with increased risk of cardiac dysfunction.[11] Higher NT-proBNP increases from baseline were seen in patients with significant LVEF drop.
  - In a 2012 study of 54 patients with HER-2-positive breast cancer treated with trastuzumab, abnormal hs-CRP, not TnI or BNP, was associated with clinically significant LVEF decrease.[12] Elevated hs-CRP predicted LVEF decreased with 92% sensitivity and 46% specificity; the negative predictive value was 94%.
- Recommendation: Consider incorporating **troponin, NT-proBNP, and hs-CRP biomarkers during trastuzumab therapy.**

Vascular Endothelial Growth Factor Inhibitors

- Vascular endothelial growth factor (VEGF) inhibitors are a subset of tyrosine kinase inhibitors (TKIs). Tyrosine kinases are enzymes that catalyze protein phosphorylation and are important in cell growth, proliferation, and angiogenesis.
- VEGF inhibitors are small molecules used to treat a range of cancers, including renal cell carcinoma, hepatocellular carcinoma, thyroid cancers, endometrial cancers, and sarcomas.
- Drugs in this class include axitinib, cabozantinib, lenvatinib, pazopanib, regorafenib, sorafenib, sunitinib, and vandetanib.
- Hypertension is the most common adverse CV event related to VEGF inhibitor use (21%-80%). However, LV dysfunction (1%-2.5%) and ischemia (1.4%-3%) are also observed.[13]
  - In a 2013 study of 159 patients with renal cell carcinoma treated with VEGF inhibitors, **NT-pro-BNP was associated with LV dysfunction.**[14]
  - Treating blood pressure decreases the risk of LV dysfunction and lowers the risk of vascular events.[14,15]
- Recommendation: **Consider monitoring for VEGF inhibitor CV toxicity with NPs.**

Proteasome Inhibitors

- Proteasome inhibitors (PIs) are peptides that block the function of proteasomes, complexes that break down proteins and result in cancer cell apoptosis.
- PIs are used commonly in the treatment of multiple myeloma, mantle cell lymphoma, and light chain amyloidosis.
- Drugs in this class include bortezomib, carfilzomib, and ixazomib.
- Adverse cardiac events related to PIs include hypertension, arrhythmia, heart failure, ischemic heart disease, cardiomyopathy, thromboembolic events, pulmonary hypertension, and sudden cardiac death.
- In a 2019 study of 95 patients receiving PIs, patients underwent serial NPs, troponins, electrocardiograms, and transthoracic echocardiogram.[16] Adverse CV events occurred in 51% of patients, with 86% occurring in the first 3 months.
  - Elevated NPs at baseline and mid–first cycle were associated with a significantly higher risk of subsequent CV adverse events (odds ratio, 10.8 and 36.0, respectively).
  - PI therapy was resumed in 89% of patients, but 41% of patients required chemotherapy modifications such as dose delay or reduction.
- Recommendation: Consider using **NPs at baseline and mid–chemotherapy cycle to monitor for adverse CV events related to PI use, especially with carfilzomib**.

Immune Checkpoint Inhibitors

- Immunotherapy drugs called **immune checkpoint inhibitors (ICIs) are monoclonal antibodies directed at checkpoint proteins**. ICIs remove the natural brakes placed on T-cell-mediated response and increase the immune system's ability to scavenge for and identify foreign cells.
- ICIs are eligible for use in almost 50% of cancer patients, including patients with breast, colon, lung, and skin cancer.
- Drugs in this class include:
  - Programmed cell death 1 (PD-1) inhibitors: cemiplimab, nivolumab, pembrolizumab
  - Programmed death-ligand 1 (PD-L1) inhibitors: atezolizumab, avelumab, durvalumab
  - Cytotoxic T-lymphocyte-associated protein 3 (CTLA-4) inhibitor: Ipilimumab
- CRP kinetics, with an initial increase and then a decline, are associated with beneficial cancer response to ICI.[17]
- Myocarditis is a potentially fatal adverse cardiac event related to ICI use. Other adverse CV events include pericarditis, LV dysfunction, Takotsubo-like syndrome, coronary vasospasm, arrhythmias, and myocardial infarction.
- In a registry of patients who received ICIs, most patients who developed myocarditis had an elevated troponin (94%), and many (46%) developed a major adverse cardiac event (MACE). **Elevated TnT was associated with a fourfold increased risk of MACE**.[18]
- Other biomarkers such as CRP and NPs can also be used to monitor for myocarditis, but baseline levels should be established.[19]
- Recommendation: **Consider using TnT, hs-CRP, and NPs** at baseline and **to monitor for ICI myocarditis**.

Amyloidosis

- Amyloid cardiomyopathy occurs when misfolded proteins aggregate into fibrils and deposit into the myocardium, leading to organ dysfunction.
- Patients with amyloid cardiomyopathy often have a stable, mildly elevated troponin. Recognition of this finding in clinical practice should prompt further diagnostic evaluation.

- **Cardiac biomarkers, NPs and troponins, are often used for prognosis, disease progression, and treatment response.**
  - Decreases in troponin or NPs can indicate treatment response or heart failure management optimization.
  - Increases in troponin or NPs indicate disease progression or reflect acute decompensation of heart failure.
- For light chain amyloidosis, the 2012 Mayo Staging system uses three criteria[20]:
  - TnT (>0.025 ng/mL)
  - NT-proBNP (>1800 pg/mL)
  - Free light chain difference >18 mg/dL
  - Patients are staged from 1 to 4 depending on the number of criteria met.
  - Recent median survival by stage was 118, 76, 64, and 27 months, for stages 1 to 4, respectively.[21]
- For wild-type transthyretin amyloidosis, the 2016 Boston University staging system uses two criteria[22]:
  - TnT (>0.05 ng/mL)
  - NT-proBNP (>3000 pg/mL)
  - The median overall survival was 55, 42, and 20 months for individuals who met none, one, or both criteria, respectively.
- For both wild-type and hereditary variant transthyretin amyloidosis, another staging system uses NT-proBNP and estimated glomerular filtration rate (eGFR)[23]:
  - NT-proBNP (>3000 ng/L)
  - eGFR (<45 mL/min)
  - The median survival was 69, 47, and 24 months for individuals who met none, one, or both criteria, respectively.
- Recommendation: **Consider routine monitoring for disease progression with troponins and NPs in the care of patients with amyloid cardiomyopathy.**

Integration of Biomarkers into Cardio-Oncology Care

- Cardiotoxicity is frequently a treatment-limiting side effect of many cancer therapies. Biomarkers can assist in early identification of patients at increased risk of cardiotoxicity or detection of cardiac injury at the earliest, subclinical, timepoint.
- Early initiation of cardioprotective strategies may prevent or reduce the need to modify life-saving cancer therapies. Biomarkers can have a role before initiation of cancer therapy, throughout cancer therapy, and during cancer survivorship.
- Before cancer therapy and during cancer survivorship, assessment of biomarkers may:
  - Identify subclinical CV issues such as heart failure
  - Recognize patients at high risk of CV adverse events
  - Prompt medication optimization
  - Provide prognostic information
  - Encourage referral for C-O evaluation
- During cancer therapy, biomarkers can be used:
  - To detect congestion or myocardial injury, independent of detectable changes in LVEF, and prompt further evaluation
  - For identifying patients that may benefit from initiation of cardioprotective strategies, CV medications, and increased monitoring
  - To monitor the resolution of acute cardiac adverse events
- Biomarker monitoring strategies can be personalized on the basis of the patient's CV risk and the planned cancer treatment regimen (Figure 15.1).

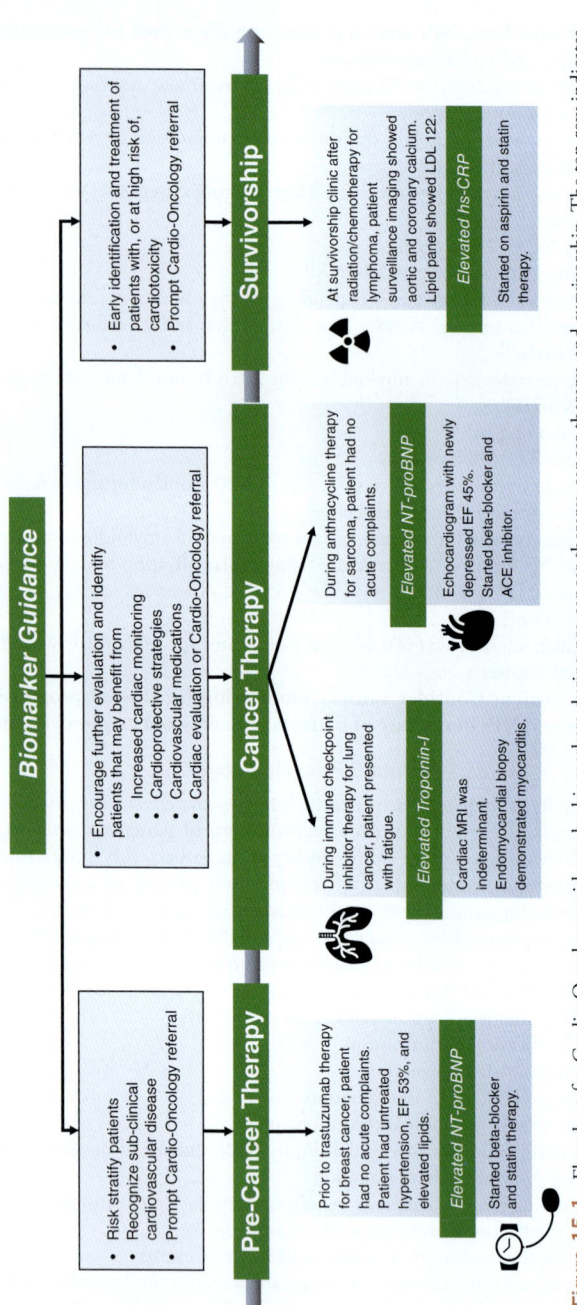

Figure 15-1. Flowchart for Cardio-Oncology guidance by biomarkers during pre-cancer therapy, cancer therapy, and survivorship. The top row indicates clinical uses of biomarkers during clinical cancer care. The bottom row provides example scenarios of clinical decisions guided by biomarkers.

Cardiac Biomarker Profiles

- NPs and troponin are the most commonly used biomarkers. Elevated NP indicates congestion or left ventricular stress, and elevated troponin indicates myocardial injury.
- **Different profiles of cardiac biomarkers should prompt evaluation, and a broad differential diagnosis should be considered.**[24]
  - **Profile I: (-) NP, (-) Troponin**
  - **Profile II: (+) NP, (-) Troponin**
  - **Profile III: (-) NP, (+) Troponin**
  - **Profile IV: (+) NP, (+) Troponin**

Initial Cardiac Biomarker–Based Workup

- Abnormalities in a biomarker alone should not prompt treatment modification but should elicit further investigation with clinical symptom evaluation, CV imaging, electrocardiogram, or more frequent monitoring.
- Workup based on biomarkers can include:
  - Routine CV surveillance (I)
  - CV risk factor modification (I, II, III, IV)
  - Blood pressure and heart rate (II, III, IV)
  - Weight (II, IV)
  - 12-lead electrocardiogram (III, IV)
  - Assessment of left ventricular function (+/− strain) (II, III, IV)
  - Chest imaging (IV)
  - Consider referral to C-O (II, III, IV)

Diagnosis and Intervention

- Differential diagnosis related to CV toxicity can include acute coronary syndrome, myocarditis, heart failure, cardiomyopathy, amyloidosis, arrhythmia, arterial/venous/pulmonary thromboembolism, or hypertension.

Acute Setting

- Acute presentations, such as acute coronary syndrome, myocarditis, or pulmonary embolism, should be treated promptly.[25] Additional workup may include left heart catheterization, coronary angiogram, endomyocardial biopsy, or cardiac magnetic resonance imaging (MRI).
  - For serious adverse events, cancer therapy may need to be held or discontinued and treatment started.
  - Resolution of elevated biomarkers can signal effectiveness of treatment.

Outpatient Setting

- If there is evidence of hypertension, consider initiation or optimization of antihypertensives. Hypertension induced by TKIs responds best to calcium channel blockers and potassium-sparing diuretics.[13]
- If there is evidence of heart failure or cardiomyopathy, consider:
  - Increased imaging surveillance frequency
  - Optimization or initiation of guideline-directed therapy, including beta-adrenergic antagonists (ie, carvedilol or metoprolol succinate) and angiotensin-converting enzyme inhibitor (ie, lisinopril) or angiotensin II receptor blocker (ie, losartan)
  - Initiation of diuretic for volume overload

- Reduction in intravenous fluid volume during chemotherapy infusions or as part of standard imaging order sets
- Using protocols that minimize fluid shifts, such as extending an autologous stem cell transplant from 1 to 2 days
- If there is evidence of myocardial injury, consider:
  - Increased frequency of imaging surveillance
  - Alternative chemotherapeutic options or prolongation of chemotherapy infusion time
  - Initiation of cardioprotective medications, such as beta-adrenergic antagonists, angiotensin-converting enzyme inhibitors or angiotensin II receptor blockers, and mineralocorticoid antagonists. The regimen will vary depending on the patient and cancer treatment type.

CLINICAL VIGNETTES

Case 1: Breast Cancer

- *A 54-year-old female with HER2+ breast cancer was initiated on docetaxel, carboplatin, trastuzumab, and pertuzumab. After four cycles, she had an echocardiogram as part of her preoperative risk assessment for a mastectomy. Her LVEF had dropped from 55% to 44%. She is referred to a cardio-oncology clinic for further assessment.*
- She reported fatigue during her chemotherapy and weight loss of 10 lbs attributable to anorexia. At the time of her clinic visit, she walked 3 miles/day without dyspnea and had no limitations on her daily activities.
  - Blood pressure: 150/82; heart rate 84 bpm
  - Biomarkers: TnI <0.03; NT-proBNP 768; hs-CRP 6
  - No coronary or aortic calcification on imaging studies
  - *Biomarker guidance:*
    - With elevated blood pressure, elevated NT-proBNP, and drop in LVEF, cardioprotective therapy with lisinopril was started.
    - No further cardiac testing was recommended before surgery, given her excellent exercise capacity and no clinical evidence of decompensated heart failure.
- The patient underwent a mastectomy with no acute complications. The patient was continued on trastuzumab by her oncologist.
- One year later, her LVEF recovered to 55%, and her blood pressure was stable at 128/78.
- *Learning point:*
  - **Abnormalities in biomarkers can prompt the initiation of cardioprotective medications, especially in the setting of concomitant hypertension.**

Case 2: Immune Checkpoint Inhibitors

- *A 67-year-old male with advanced non–small cell lung cancer presents 1 week after a witnessed cardiac arrest with rapid CPR initiation and return of spontaneous circulation after one shock by emergency medical services (EMS). The rhythm was ventricular fibrillation. At an outside facility, the patient underwent a coronary angiogram with no evidence of obstructive disease. He is referred to a C-O clinic for further evaluation. He started pembrolizumab 3 weeks ago.*
  - EKG: normal sinus rhythm with nonspecific ST changes
  - Biomarkers: TnI 10, BNP 98, hs-CRP 22
  - *Biomarker guidance:*

- Elevated TnI and hs-CRP with recent cardiac arrest resulting from ventricular fibrillation are concerning for ICI myocarditis and workup initiated.
- Cardiac MRI showed a normal LVEF of 58% with minimal diagnostic evidence of myocarditis.
- An endomyocardial biopsy revealed cellular infiltration consistent with myocarditis.
- The patient was treated with corticosteroids, and pembrolizumab was held.
- *Learning point:*
  - **Even without convincing evidence of myocarditis by imaging, elevated biomarkers should prompt definitive diagnosis with endomyocardial biopsy in the setting of recent ICI initiation.**

CASE 3: ANTHRACYCLINE THERAPY

- *A 70-year-old female with uterine leiomyosarcoma treated with surgical resection followed by gemcitabine and taxotere 3 years ago was found to have metastatic disease during routine surveillance imaging. She was referred to a C-O clinic before the initiation of possible cardiotoxic therapy with doxorubicin.*
  - TnI: <0.03, NT-proBNP: 131
  - Echocardiogram: Normal left and right systolic function with impaired diastolic function
  - *Biomarker guidance:*
    - Given normal baseline biomarkers and echocardiogram with only diastolic dysfunction, recommended biomarker assessment before each chemotherapy cycle, and echocardiogram every 6 months during therapy. No initiation of CV therapy was recommended.
    - Recommended consideration of coadministration with dexrazoxane if planned dose exceeded 300 mg/m^2
- The patient's first three cycles proceeded uneventfully with only mild fatigue. Biomarkers before the patient's fourth cycle of doxorubicin with dexrazoxane were increased from baseline.
  - Biomarkers: TnI: 0.07; NT-proBNP 530
  - *Biomarker guidance:*
    - Given the new elevation of biomarkers, an echocardiogram was ordered, which revealed a reduced LVEF of 45%. The patient was started on carvedilol 6.25 mg twice daily and lisinopril 5 mg.
- The patient completed her chemotherapy course as planned. At the end of therapy, her LVEF was 55%.
- *Learning point:*
  - **Baseline biomarkers can help guide the C-O surveillance strategy**. Even in the absence of symptoms, **alterations in biomarkers** can prompt changes to the C-O monitoring plan, such as **earlier cardiac imaging and cardioprotective medications**.

CASE 4: AMYLOIDOSIS

- *A 76-year-old male with a history of poorly controlled hypertension presents to the hospital with persistent dyspnea after his first set of tennis that did not resolve with rest. Six months ago, he could complete a full game.*
  - Blood pressure 165/90; heart rate 92 bpm

- Electrocardiogram without evidence of acute ischemic changes
- Biomarkers: Serial TnT 0.142, 0.136, 0.140; BNP 450 pg/mL
- The physical exam is notable for bilateral lower extremity edema to his ankles and mildly elevated jugular venous distention. He was treated as a non–ST-elevation myocardial infarction.
  - Coronary angiogram: Mild luminal irregularities and no obstructive disease
  - Echocardiogram: LV hypertrophy, intraventricular septum diameter of 1.6 cm, LVEF 50%, normal global longitudinal strain pattern
- The patient was treated with intravenous diuretics with the resolution of his swelling and improvement of his dyspnea.
  - *Biomarker guidance:*
    - Given left ventricular hypertrophy, elevated BNP, and a stable troponin elevation, a diagnostic workup for amyloidosis was completed with quantitative free light chains, serum/urine electrophoresis and immunofixation, and nuclear technetium-99 pyrophosphate (PYP) scan was completed.
    - PYP scan revealed heart–contralateral lung ratio of 1.8, visual score grade 3, and myocardial uptake of single photon emission computed tomography (SPECT). Genetic testing was negative for transthyretin mutation.
- The patient was diagnosed with wild-type transthyretin amyloidosis and started on tafamidis.
- He then presented to an amyloidosis clinic as an outpatient 1 month later. He had no swelling of his ankles, and his dyspnea had significantly improved. He was euvolemic on exam.
  - Biomarkers: TnT 0.086, BNP 154, NT-proBNP 1852, eGFR 61
  - *Biomarker guidance:*
    - With his volume status optimized, his biomarkers can be used for prognostication. His elevated troponin places him in the stage II category of the Boston 2016 system, with a prognosis of 42 months. However, his NT-proBNP <3000 and eGFR >45 place him at stage I in the 2018 staging system with a prognosis of 69 months.
- *Learning point:*
  - **In amyloidosis, cardiac biomarkers should be used in diagnosis and in prognostication**.

CASE 5: CANCER SURVIVORSHIP

- *A 46-year-old female with a history of lymphoma treated with an anthracycline-based therapy (total dose 250 mg/m^2 doxorubicin) and thoracic radiation 5 years ago presented to survivorship clinic with new-onset hypertension.*
  - Blood pressure: 142/85
  - Lipid panel: Total cholesterol 180, HDL 65, LDL 115
  - Biomarkers: BNP 98 pg/mL, hs-CRP 7 mg/L
- Her 10-year atherosclerotic cardiovascular disease (ASCVD) risk score was 1.3% (low risk).
- A review of her most recent thoracic imaging demonstrated evidence of mild coronary artery calcification.
- An antihypertensive agent is started.
  - *Biomarker guidance:*

- Given her elevated CRP and **evidence of atherosclerotic disease on imaging**, aspirin 81 mg and rosuvastatin 10 mg are started—despite having a low ASCVD risk score.
- *Learning point:*
  - CRP can help risk-stratify patients with a higher risk of CVD attributable to cancer therapy (ie, chest wall radiation and certain chemotherapies). These patients may not have many traditional ASCVD risk factors, such as older age, male sex, elevated cholesterol, diabetes, tobacco use, or hypertension.

ADDITIONAL RESOURCES

For additional resources, see Tables 15-1 and 15-2.

TABLE 15-1 Biomarkers in Cancer Care

Context	Biomarkers	Frequency	Utility in clinical decisions	Strength of association
Cancer Clinical Context				
Prior to cancer treatment initiation	Tn, NPs	Once	Establish baselines, prompt medical optimization, recognize high-risk patients, help identify patients for cardio-oncology referral.	Moderate
During cancer treatment	Tn, hs-CRP, NPs	Varies by cardiotoxic potential of therapies	Detect congestion or myocardial injury prior to changes in imaging or symptoms, prompt further evaluation, identify patients that may benefit from cardioprotective strategies, monitor resolution of acute cardiac events.	Moderate
After cancer treatment	NPs	At least once, depending on prior treatment regimen, or change in clinical status	Prompt medical optimization, detect long-term cardiotoxic effects prior to symptoms or imaging changes.	Moderate

(continued)

TABLE 15-1	Biomarkers in Cancer Care (*continued*)			
Context	Biomarkers	Frequency	Utility in clinical decisions	Strength of association
Specific Cancer Treatments				
Anthracyclines	NPs, Tn	Baseline and during therapy. Consider prior to each cycle.	Elevated biomarkers should prompt cardiac evaluation and initiation of cardioprotective strategies.	Moderate/High
Trastuzumab	NPs, hs-CRP, Tn	Baseline and during therapy. Consider prior to each cycle.	Elevated biomarkers should prompt evaluation of LVEF and consideration of cardioprotective medication initiation.	Moderate
Vascular Endothelial Growth Factor Inhibitors	NPs	Baseline and during therapy: Consider at 1 mo and then every 3 mos.	Elevated NP should prompt evaluation of LVEF and assessment for possible HF symptoms.	Fair
Immune Checkpoint Inhibitors	Tn, hs-CRP, NPs	Baseline and during therapy. Consider every 1-2 wk for first 6 wks and/or once per cycle	Elevated biomarkers in the context of vague symptoms can prompt workup for myocarditis and allow for early intervention.	Moderate
Proteasome Inhibitors	NPs	Baseline and mid-chemotherapy cycle.	Elevations associated with adverse cardiac events. After full cardiac evaluation, consider dose reduction or dose delay, especially with carfilzomib.	Moderate/High

hs-CRP, high-sensitivity-C-reactive protein; LVEF, left ventricular ejection fraction; NP, natriuretic peptides; Tn, troponin.

TABLE 15-2 Biomarkers in Amyloidosis

Context	Biomarkers	Frequency	Utility in clinical decisions	Strength of association
Diagnosis	TnT, NPs	Once	In the context of HFpEF due to amyloidosis, NPs will be elevated. Stable elevated serial troponin should raise clinical suspicion of amyloidosis.	High
Prognosis	TnT, NT-proBNP	Once, when clinically optimized	Multiple staging systems for light chain and transthyretin amyloidosis rely on biomarkers	High
Disease progression	TnT, NPs	3-6 mos	Slow steady rise may indicate disease progression. Stabilization or improvement can indicate treatment efficacy. In clinical trials, patients started to see decreases in NPs after 9 mos of tafamidis treatment.	High
HF management	NPs	3-6 mos or clinical change	Abrupt relative increase may indicate acute heart failure exacerbation.	Moderate

NP, natriuretic peptides; NT-proBNP, amino-terminal pro–brain natriuretic peptide; TnT, troponin T.

REFERENCES

1. Ky B, Putt M, Sawaya H, et al. Early increases in multiple biomarkers predict subsequent cardiotoxicity in patients with breast cancer treated with doxorubicin, taxanes, and trastuzumab. *J Am Coll Cardiol*. 2014;63(8):809-816. doi:10.1016/j.jacc.2013.10.061
2. Arslan D, Cihan T, Kose D, et al. Growth-differentiation factor-15 and tissue doppler imaging in detection of asymptomatic anthracycline cardiomyopathy in childhood cancer survivors. *Clin Biochem*. 2013;46(13-14):1239-1243. doi:10.1016/j.clinbiochem.2013.06.029
3. Zhang KW, Miao J, Mitchell JD, et al. Plasma hepatocyte growth factor for diagnosis and prognosis in light chain and transthyretin cardiac amyloidosis. *JACC CardioOncol*. 2020;2(1):56-66. doi:10.1016/j.jaccao.2020.01.006
4. Ticau S, Sridharan GV, Tsour S, et al. Neurofilament light chain (NfL) as a biomarker of hereditary transthyretin-mediated amyloidosis. *Neurology*. 2021;96(3):e412-e422. doi:10.1212/wnl.0000000000011090
5. Desai VG, J CK, Vijay V, et al. Early biomarkers of doxorubicin-induced heart injury in a mouse model. *Toxicol Appl Pharmacol*. 2014;281(2):221-229. doi:10.1016/j.taap.2014.10.006
6. Curigliano G, Lenihan D, Fradley M, et al. Management of cardiac disease in cancer patients throughout oncological treatment: ESMO consensus recommendations. *Ann Oncol*. 2020;31(2):171-190. doi:10.1016/j.annonc.2019.10.023

7. Cardinale D, Sandri MT, Colombo A, et al. Prognostic value of troponin I in cardiac risk stratification of cancer patients undergoing high-dose chemotherapy. *Circulation*. 2004;109(22):2749-2754. doi:10.1161/01.cir.0000130926.51766.cc
8. Sawaya H, Sebag IA, Plana JC, et al. Assessment of echocardiography and biomarkers for the extended prediction of cardiotoxicity in patients treated with anthracyclines, taxanes, and trastuzumab. *Circ Cardiovasc Imaging*. 2012;5(5):596-603. doi:10.1161/circimaging.112.973321
9. Lenihan DJ, Stevens PL, Massey M, et al. The utility of point-of-care biomarkers to detect cardiotoxicity during anthracycline chemotherapy: a feasibility study. *J Card Fail*. 2016;22(6):433-438. doi:10.1016/j.cardfail.2016.04.003
10. Cardinale D, Colombo A, Torrisi R, et al. Trastuzumab-induced cardiotoxicity: clinical and prognostic implications of troponin I evaluation. *J Clin Oncol*. 2010;28(25):3910-3916. doi:10.1200/jco.2009.27.3615
11. Zardavas D, Suter TM, Van Veldhuisen DJ, et al. Role of troponins I and T and N-terminal prohormone of brain natriuretic peptide in monitoring cardiac safety of patients with early-Stage human epidermal growth factor receptor 2-Positive breast cancer receiving trastuzumab: a herceptin adjuvant study cardiac marker substudy. *J Clin Oncol*. 2017;35(8):878-884. doi:10.1200/jco.2015.65.7916
12. Onitilo AA, Engel JM, Stankowski RV, Liang H, Berg RL, Doi SA. High-sensitivity C-reactive protein (hs-CRP) as a biomarker for trastuzumab-induced cardiotoxicity in HER2-positive early-stage breast cancer: a pilot study. *Breast Cancer Res Treat*. 2012;134(1):291-298. doi:10.1007/s10549-012-2039-z
13. Waliany S, Sainani KL, Park LS, Zhang CA, Srinivas S, Witteles RM. Increase in blood pressure associated with tyrosine kinase inhibitors targeting vascular endothelial growth factor. *JACC CardioOncol*. 2019;1(1):24-36. doi:10.1016/j.jaccao.2019.08.012
14. Hall PS, Harshman LC, Srinivas S, Witteles RM. The frequency and severity of cardiovascular toxicity from targeted therapy in advanced renal cell carcinoma patients. *JACC Heart Fail*. 2013;1(1):72-78. doi:10.1016/j.jchf.2012.09.001
15. McKay RR, Rodriguez GE, Lin X, et al. Angiotensin system inhibitors and survival outcomes in patients with metastatic renal cell carcinoma. *Clin Cancer Res*. 2015;21(11):2471-2479. doi:10.1158/1078-0432.ccr-14-2332
16. Cornell RF, Ky B, Weiss BM, et al. Prospective study of cardiac events during proteasome inhibitor therapy for relapsed multiple myeloma. *J Clin Oncol*. 2019;37(22):1946-1955. doi:10.1200/jco.19.00231
17. Riedl JM, Barth DA, Brueckl WM, et al. C-reactive protein (CRP) levels in immune checkpoint inhibitor response and progression in advanced non-small cell lung cancer: a bi-center study. *Cancers (Basel)*. 2020;12(8):2319. doi:10.3390/cancers12082319
18. Mahmood SS, Fradley MG, Cohen JV, et al. Myocarditis in patients treated with immune checkpoint inhibitors. *J Am Coll Cardiol*. 2018;71(16):1755-1764. doi:10.1016/j.jacc.2018.02.037
19. Bonaca MP, Olenchock BA, Salem JE, et al. Myocarditis in the setting of cancer therapeutics: proposed case definitions for emerging clinical syndromes in cardio-Oncology. *Circulation*. 2019;140(2):80-91. doi:10.1161/circulationaha.118.034497
20. Kumar S, Dispenzieri A, Lacy MQ, et al. Revised prognostic staging system for light chain amyloidosis incorporating cardiac biomarkers and serum free light chain measurements. *J Clin Oncol*. 2012;30(9):989-995. doi:10.1200/jco.2011.38.5724
21. Barrett CD, Dobos K, Liedtke M, et al. A changing landscape of mortality for systemic light chain amyloidosis. *JACC Heart Fail*. 2019;7(11):958-966. doi:10.1016/j.jchf.2019.07.007
22. Connors LH, Sam F, Skinner M, et al. Heart failure resulting from age-related cardiac amyloid disease associated with wild-type transthyretin: a prospective, observational cohort study. *Circulation*. 2016;133(3):282-290. doi: 10.1161/circulationaha.115.018852
23. Gillmore JD, Damy T, Fontana M, et al. A new staging system for cardiac transthyretin amyloidosis. *Eur Heart J*. 2018;39(30):2799-2806. doi:10.1093/eurheartj/ehx589
24. Alvarez-Cardona Jose A, Zhang Kathleen W, Mitchell Joshua D, Zaha Vlad G, Fisch Michael J, Lenihan Daniel J. Cardiac biomarkers during cancer therapy. *JACC CardioOncol*. 2020;2(5):791-794. doi:10.1016/j.jaccao.2020.08.014
25. Balanescu DV, Donisan T, Deswal A, et al. Acute myocardial infarction in a high-risk cancer population: outcomes following conservative versus invasive management. *Int J Cardiol*. 2020;313:1-8. doi:10.1016/j.ijcard.2020.04.050

16 MRI Techniques to Monitor Cardiac Safety During and After Cancer Treatment

Srilakshmi Vallabhaneni, Pamela K. Woodard, Gregory M. Lanza, and Daniel J. Lenihan

- **Cardiovascular imaging tools** utilized in patients undergoing active cancer therapy, as well as survivors of cancer treatment, are a mainstay in the armamentarium for clinicians **to monitor for cardiac damage**. Recognizing potential cardiotoxicity of chemotherapeutic drugs, identifying metastatic disease, and enhanced detection of specific infiltrative cardiomyopathies such as cardiac amyloidosis are all important goals of imaging.[1] Table 16-1 describes **characteristics of imaging modalities and their strengths and weaknesses** for detecting important abnormalities.
- Cardiac magnetic resonance (CMR), with its relatively high spatial and excellent contrast resolution, can provide qualitative and **quantitative assessment of cardiac structure, function, perfusion, and tissue characterization in a single study** and aid in the diagnosis of cancer therapy–related cardiac dysfunction (CTRCD) (Fig. 16-1).
- **As noted in the sections that follow, there are several important clinical indications for the use of CMR in cardio-oncology.**

TABLE 16-1 Comparison of Commonly Used Cardiac Imaging Modalities in Cardio-Oncology and Important Imaging Characteristics

	Echocardiography	CMR	CT
Advantages	• First line for diagnosis and follow-up • Widely available • Easily repeatable • Portability	• Highly reproducible and reference standard for both anatomic and functional information • Independent from acoustic window • No exposure to radiation • Ability for myocardial tissue characterization	• Excellent anatomic evaluation • Best visualization of extracardiac structures • Highly sensitive to define coronary anatomy and vascular structures • Ability to detect pericardial calcification • Preoperative planning for surgical/percutaneous procedures
Temporal resolution	++++	+++	++

(*continued*)

TABLE 16-1	Comparison of Commonly Used Cardiac Imaging Modalities in Cardio-Oncology and Important Imaging Characteristics (*continued*)		
	Echocardiography	**CMR**	**CT**
Spatial resolution	+++	+++	++++
Contrast to noise ratio	++	++++	+++
Tissue characterization	++	++++	+++
Chamber dimensions	+++	++++	++++
LV function	+++	++++	+++
Myocardial viability	++	++++	–
Modalities	• 2D/3D echocardiography • M-mode • Spectral/tissue Doppler • Contrast echocardiography • Speckle tracking/strain	• Black blood images • Bright blood SSFP • Cine imaging • LGE • Strain	• Non-contrast (coronary calcium scoring) • Contrast imaging (CT angiography)
Disadvantages	• Poor quality imaging • Operator dependent • Acoustic window dependent • Limited tissue characterization	• Contraindication with certain devices (AICD, pacemakers) • Need for breath hold • Gadolinium not recommended in patients with ESRD patients/acute renal insufficiency • Cannot be used in hemodynamically unstable patients	• Limited functional assessment • Use of radiation limits utility with serial studies (1-4 mSv with modern scanners) • Need for breath hold • Use of iodinated contrast • Patients with arrhythmias/hemodynamically unstable patients

2D, two-dimensional; 3D, three-dimensional; AICD, automatic implantable cardioverter defibrillator; CMR, cardiovascular magnetic resonance; CT, computed tomography; ESRD, end stage renal disease; LGE, late gadolinium enhancement; LV, left ventricle; SSFP, Steady-state free precession.

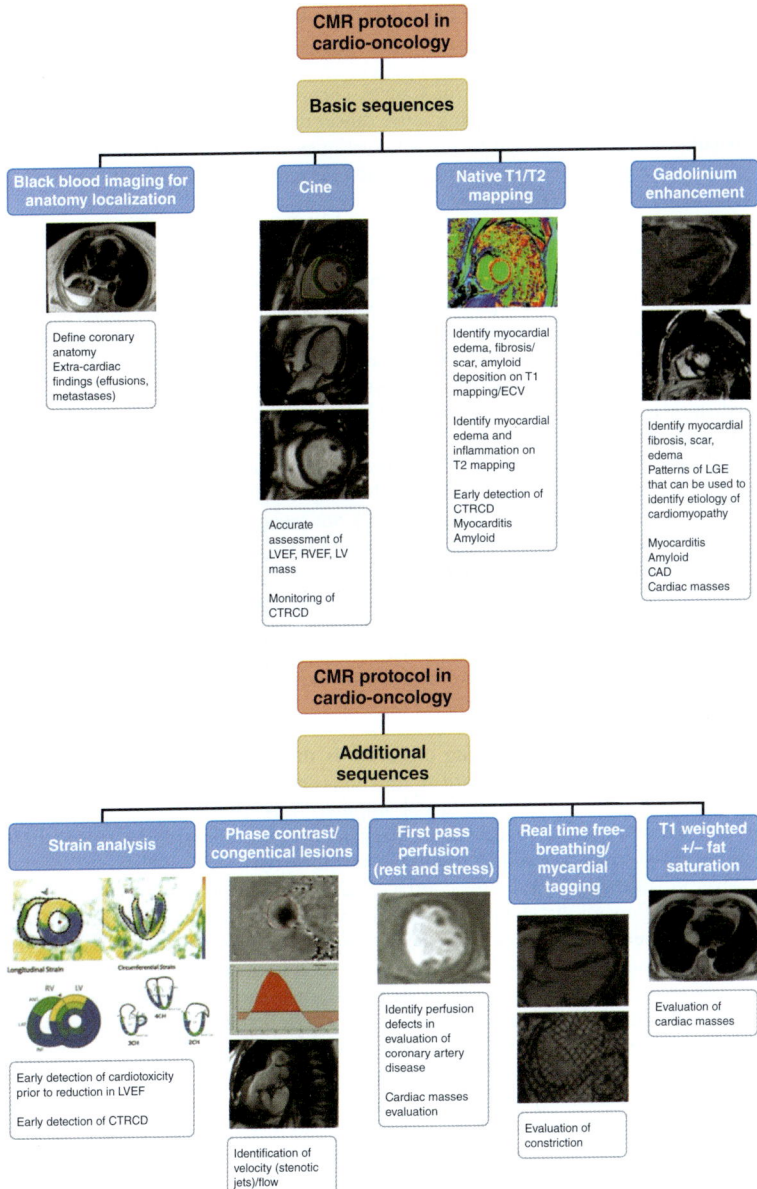

Figure 16-1. Role of CMR in cardio-oncology. CAD, coronary artery disease; CMR, cardiovascular magnetic resonance; CTRCD, cancer therapy–related cardiac dysfunction; ECV, extracellular volume; LGE, late gadolinium enhancement; LV, left ventricle; LVEF, left ventricular ejection fraction; RVEF, right ventricular ejection fraction.

CANCER THERAPY–RELATED CARDIAC DYSFUNCTION

Functional Assessment

- The most common indication of Cancer Therapy–Related Cardiac Dysfunction (CTRCD) in patients undergoing active cancer therapy is a **reduction in left ventricular function**, especially with anthracyclines and human epidermal receptor (HER-2) targeted therapies. This **is typically detected as a drop in left ventricular ejection fraction (LVEF).**
- Echocardiography (Echo) remains the mainstay of diagnosing CTRCD, with drop in LVEF defining cardiotoxicity, as cited in multiple consensus statements. **However, interobserver variability is high in evaluating LVEF by Echo** using modified Simpson's biplane and three-Dimensional echocardiography (3-DE) at 6.5% and 3%, respectively, compared to 2.5% with CMR.[2] Echo also relies on good acoustic windows, which can be limited by body habitus, prior lung disease, or recent chest wall procedures.
- **CMR is the reference standard for assessment of ventricular volumes and LVEF** when there is discordance in evaluating LVEF with different imaging modalities or limited acoustic windows.[3]
- **CMR can reliably measure LVEF,** calculated from a short-axis series of 2D cine slices acquired from the base of the heart through the apex. A bright blood sequence such as balanced steady-state free precession (bSSFP) cine imaging is used because of its high signal to noise ratio (SNR) and better contrast to noise ratio (CNR) between myocardium and blood pool. **CMR can detect a drop in LVEF with improved accuracy and minimize inappropriate interruptions of chemotherapy**. It can also be used for serial monitoring of cardiac function in patients receiving potentially cardiotoxic agents. In addition to drop in LVEF, LV mass index (LVMI) has been found to be an important predictor of future cardiovascular events in patients receiving anthracyclines.[4]

Myocardial Strain

- The **main limitation of relying on LVEF is that reduction in LVEF is a late manifestation** of decline in cardiac function, and that, as a result, the potential for full recovery is reduced.[5] To further improve the sensitivity of early detection of cardiotoxicity, the focus in cardio-oncology has been to investigate the **utility of LV myocardial strain as a robust marker of cardiotoxicity.**[6]
- Myocardial strain quantifies the contractile properties of the myocardium by direct measure of myocardial deformation during contraction. **The changes in myocardial function via strain can be detected despite normal or preserved LVEF.** This allows for the application of early cardioprotection in these patients.
- CMR strain methods measure **tissue deformation in the longitudinal, radial, and circumferential dimensions** (Fig. 16-2). They perform better than echo, are highly reproducible, can be used to assess segmental function, and can be used in combination with other techniques for tissue characterization with T1/T2 mapping.[7]
- **CMR feature tracking strain can be done** as part of **routine CMR** protocol with standard cine sequences and some additional postprocessing. **Myocardial tagging, strain-encoded CMR (SENC),** and displacement encoding with stimulated echoes (DENSE) requires acquisition of additional imaging sequences and postprocessing software. **All of these techniques are performed without contrast.**[8]
- **CMR strain analysis has demonstrated utility in detection of early changes and subclinical deterioration of LVEF in patients receiving potentially cardiotoxic chemotherapy.**[9,10]

   However, **CMR strain techniques are not widely clinically** available, and future studies are needed to help define the role of CMR strain/regional variation in strain in

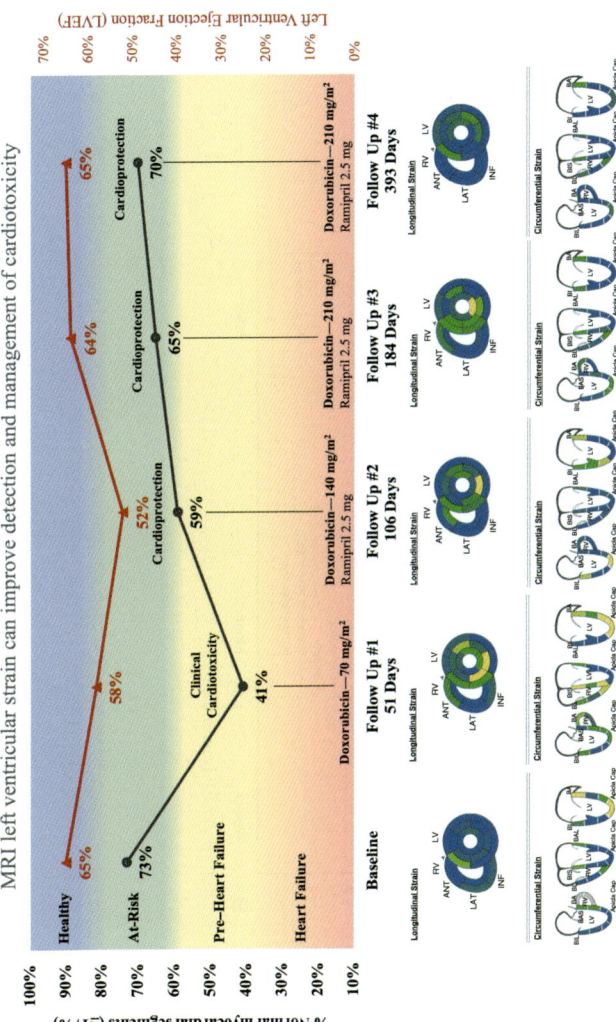

Figure 16-2. Utility of CMR strain in early detection of cancer therapy–related cardiac dysfunction (CTRCD). (A) Actual CMR measurements with LV strain in a patient undergoing anthracycline-based chemotherapy. Note the initial reduction in % normal segments after just one dose of anthracycline. Once cardioprotective therapy with Ramipril was started, the LV strain values improved even during subsequent dosing with anthracycline. (B) Schematic of the utility of LV strain for the early detection of CTRCD. Once the LVEF is reduced below normal, the chances of LV recovery are less, especially without cardioprotective therapy. CTRCD, cancer therapy–related cardiac dysfunction; LVEF, left ventricular ejection fraction; NYHA, New York Heart Association; LV, left ventricular; ACEI/ARB, renin angiotensin system inhibitors; GDMT, Guideline-directed optimal medical therapy. Modified from Teske AJ, Linschoten M, Kamphuis JAM, et al. Cardio-oncology: an overview on outpatient management and future developments. *Neth Heart J.* 2018;26:521-532.)

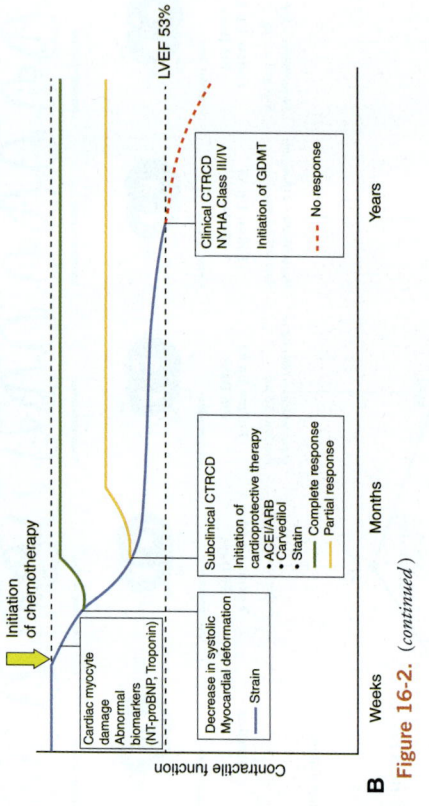

Figure 16-2. (*continued*)

identifying patients at risk of developing cardiotoxicity. Once we can identify actual cardiac injury in a reliable fashion, we can then optimize cardioprotection to ultimately improve clinical outcomes.

Tissue Characterization

Tissue characterization with **T1/T2 mapping** can help our current understanding of chemotherapy-induced cardiotoxicity and help **ascertain if the myocardial injury is acute (T2 mapping) and subacute or chronic (T1 mapping).** It can potentially help in the implementation of preventive strategies.

Myocardial Edema

- **Myocardial edema can be assessed with use of T2-weighted imaging** and should be performed prior to administration of contrast. Detection of myocardial edema and inflammation is important in the assessment of patients with new onset cardiomyopathy.
- Quantitative assessment with T2 relaxation time can also be done to evaluate for myocardial edema (myocardial T2 mapping). Normal myocardial T2 is around 55 ms for a 1.5T scanner and 51 ms for a 3T scanner, but the numbers can vary depending on the normal for a particular scanner.[11] **Myocardial edema will prolong T2 values.**
- There are several ongoing clinical trials on the utility of myocardial edema detected on T2 imaging with cancer therapy. A carefully done animal model showed an increase in T2 relaxation time with doxorubicin toxicity.[12] For now, the usefulness of monitoring patients undergoing cancer therapy is still under investigation.

Myocardial T1 Mapping

- **Native and postcontrast T1 mapping and extracellular volume (ECV) have better sensitivity for tissue characterization.**[13] Native T1/ECV values are influenced by the field strength used, pulse sequence used, cardiac phase (diastole versus systole), and region of measurement. Thus, the normal native T1 values are specific to local setup.
- **Myocardial edema and increase in interstitial space secondary to fibrosis or infiltration increase native T1 values** and help identify etiology of cardiotoxicity. Postcontrast T1 mapping is used to calculate **ECV and is a marker of myocardial tissue remodeling.**
- In cardio-oncology, there is conflicting evidence regarding the utility of tissue characterization with T1 mapping and/or ECV. Studies have shown elevated native T1 relaxation time and postcontrast ECV in patients with prior anthracycline chemotherapy.[9,14] This can occur as early as three months after initiation of therapy. However, other studies have shown acute decrease in T1 values when measured 48 hours after anthracycline administration.[15]

Gadolinium-Based Imaging

- **Late gadolinium enhancement (LGE) imaging helps recognize both myocardial scar and replacement fibrosis and also helps assess myocardial fibrosis burden.** Gadolinium-based agents do not distribute into intact myocardial cells and accumulate in areas of interstitial expansion (acute necrosis as well as scar and focal fibrosis) or in leaky myocytes. Normal washout period from the myocardium for these agents is 10 to 20 minutes after intravenous administration, but expansion of extracellular matrix with replacement fibrosis or deposition diseases like amyloidosis will delay washout. Delayed imaging (10 minutes after gadolinium-based injection) can identify regions of hyperintensity on T1-weighted sequences.
- **The pattern of LGE can be used to distinguish ischemic from nonischemic etiologies** (Fig. 16-3). LGE is not typically seen in patients with anthracycline-induced

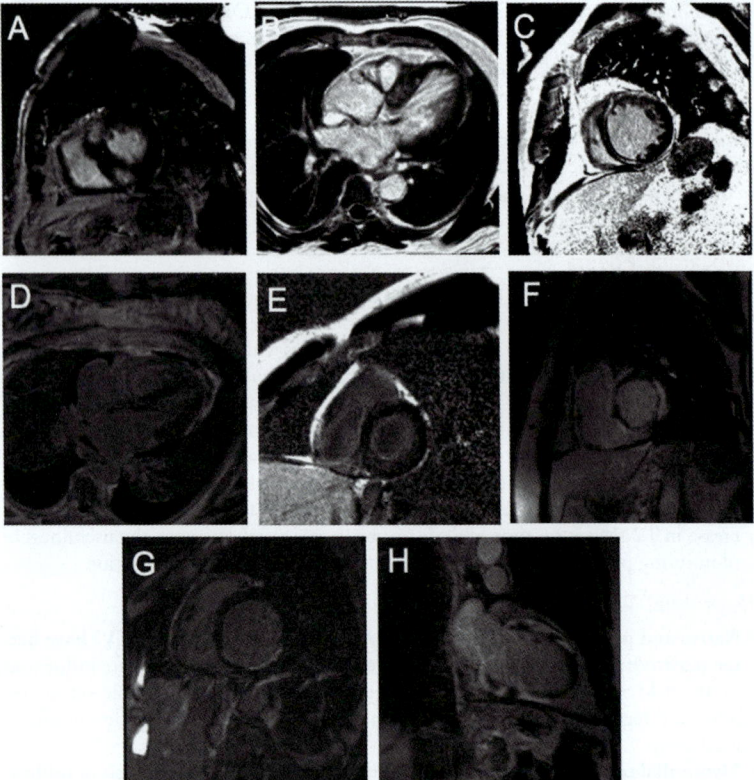

Figure 16-3. Tissue characterization: edema/fibrosis: *Delayed gadolinium enhancement.* Used to identify myocardial fibrosis, scar, edema. Patterns of late gadolinium enhancement (LGE) can be used to identify etiology of cardiomyopathy. (A, B) LGE at the right ventricle insertion point, basal interventricular septum suggestive of hypertrophic cardiomyopathy in a patient with newly diagnosed multiple myeloma referred to cardio-oncology for heart failure with preserved ejection fraction. (C) Midmyocardial LGE in the interventricular septum suggestive of dilated nonischemic cardiomyopathy. (D) Pericardial LGE in a patient with constrictive pericarditis with metastatic pulmonary carcinoid tumor treated with chemoradiation. (E) Diffuse subendocardial LGE suggestive of cardiac involvement in a patient with light chain amyloidosis. (F, H) Patchy multifocal subepicardial involving multiple segments of the left ventricle in a noncoronary distribution, transmural LGE of the lateral wall on short axis in a patient with sarcoidosis. (G) Subendocardial LGE in the inferior/inferolateral wall suggestive of myocardial ischemia in a patient treated with 5-fluorouracil–based chemotherapy.

cardiotoxicity[4] and is uncommonly seen in HER2-related cardiotoxicity.[16] Lack of LGE in anthracycline-induced cardiotoxicity is thought to be related to diffuse myocardial involvement with lack of normal myocardium. If there is diffuse fibrosis, it may be difficult to differentiate between normal tissue and fibrosis based on LGE because there will not be high-contrast areas to compare.

- **Specific cardio-oncology conditions and the characteristics of Echo, CMR, and CT imaging for diagnosing these conditions are summarized in** Table 16-2.

TABLE 16-2 Characteristic Findings with Specific Imaging Tools for Commonly Encountered Conditions in Cardio-Oncology

Common conditions encountered in cardio-oncology

	echo	CMR	CT
Cancer therapy–related cardiac dysfunction (CTRCD)	• Dilated LV • Reduced LVEF • Diastolic dysfunction • Reduced LV GLS • Mitral regurgitation (MR)	• Dilated LV • Increased LV volume and mass • Elevated T1/T2 relaxation times • Abnormal LV/RV strain	• Dilated LV with increased volumes • Reduced LV systolic function • Absence of significant CAD
Coronary artery disease	• Reduced LVEF • Regional wall motion abnormalities • Abnormal diastolic dysfunction	• Reduced LVEF • Regional wall motion • Perfusion defects with stress CMR • Subendocardial LGE suggestive of ischemic in the coronary distribution • Transmural LGE suggestive of myocardial scar with minimal viability • Microvascular disease	• Direct visualization of coronary arteries • Functional coronary physiology with CT-derived fractional flow reserve (FFR$_{CT}$) • Stress perfusion cardiac CT with perfusion defects
Cardiac amyloidosis	• Concentric LV hypertrophy • Preserved LVEF, mild to severe reduction in LVEF in advanced disease • Diastolic dysfunction • Biatrial enlargement • Small pericardial effusion • Relative apical sparing of LV longitudinal strain	• Concentric LV wall hypertrophy • Small pericardial effusion • With gadolinium-based imaging—simultaneous nulling of the myocardium and blood pool • LGE—subendocardial/transmural • Increased native T1/T2 • T2 is higher in untreated AL • T1 prolongation and ECV elevation seen earlier than LGE	• Increased LV wall thickness with subtle lower attenuation on arterial phase cardiac CT
Myocarditis	• Reduced LVEF • Regional wall motion abnormalities	• Regional or global wall motion abnormalities • Myocardial edema on T2-weighted imaging/increased T2 relaxation time • Increased T1/ECV	• Midwall or subepicardial delayed enhancement on delayed phase cardiac CT • Absence of significant CAD

(continued)

TABLE 16-2 Characteristic Findings with Specific Imaging Tools for Commonly Encountered Conditions in Cardio-Oncology *(continued)*

Common conditions encountered in cardio-oncology echo CMR CT

	echo	CMR	CT
Cardiac tumors/thrombi	<ul><li>Abnormal diastolic parameters with normal LVEF</li><li>New pericardial effusion</li><li>With use of ultrasound enhancing agents</li><li>Malignant tumors—greater contrast enhancement than surrounding myocardium due to high vascularity</li><li>Benign tumors—lower perfusion compared to surrounding myocardium</li><li>Cardiac tumors—avascular, complete absence of perfusion</li></ul>	<ul><li>LGE</li><li>Pericardial effusion or abnormal LGE/T2 or T1 findings in pericardium</li><li>Malignant tumors</li><li>Location and size of the tumor</li><li>Ill-defined margins</li><li>Hemorrhagic pericardial effusion</li><li>Heterogeneous signal on T1- and T2-weighted imaging</li><li>First-pass perfusion enhancement</li><li>Heterogeneous LGE</li><li>Cardiac metastasis— Iso/hypointense on T1, Iso/hyperintense on T2, heterogeneous LGE</li><li>Benign tumors—Myxoma—Isointense on T1, hyperintense on T2, heterogeneous LGE</li><li>Lipoma—Hyperintense on T1/T2, no LGE</li><li>Hemangioma—Isointense on T1, hyperintense on T2, intense LGE</li><li>Acute thrombus: Hyperintense on T1/T2-weighted imaging</li><li>Chronic thrombus: Hypointense on T1/T2-weighted imaging</li><li>Dark, without early or late gadolinium enhancement (>600 ms)</li></ul>	<ul><li>Malignant tumors—hypo-attenuated masses surrounded by enhancing intracardiac blood</li><li>Benign tumors—hypo-attenuated masses surrounded by enhancing intracardiac blood, hyperenhancement in areas of focal calcification</li><li>Hemangiomas—heterogeneous on precontrast CT, intensely enhanced post contrast</li><li>Extracardiac disease in the chest</li></ul>

AICD, automatic implantable cardioverter defibrillator; AL, amyloid light chain; CAD, coronary artery disease; CMR, cardiovascular magnetic resonance; CT, computed tomography; ECV, extracellular volume; Echo, echocardiography; ESRD, end stage renal disease; GLS, global longitudinal strain; LGE, late gadolinium enhancement; LV, left ventricle; LVEF, left ventricular ejection fraction; MR, mitral regurgitation; RV, right ventricle; SSFP, steady-state free precession.

INFILTRATIVE CARDIOMYOPATHY/AMYLOIDOSIS

- Key features seen on CMR with patients suspected to have cardiac amyloidosis[17] are (Fig. 16-4):
  - Increased concentric LV wall thickness with preserved ejection fraction
  - LGE—either subendocardial or transmural. Diffuse subendocardial LGE with failure to null the myocardium is highly specific for cardiac amyloidosis, and transmural can be seen in advanced disease.

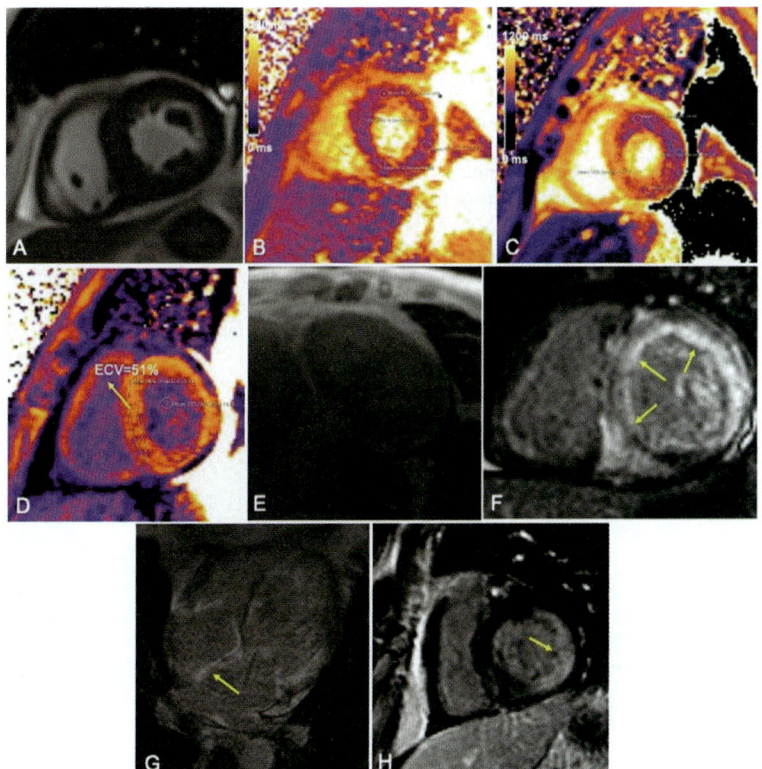

Figure 16-4. CMR findings in cardiac amyloidosis. (A) Cine imaging showing concentric left ventricular hypertrophy, small pericardial effusion. (B) T2 mapping showing normal T2 values (normal < 50 ms). (C) T1 mapping showing diffusely elevated T1 values at 1100 to 1335 ms (normal—950-1050 ms). (D) Postcontrast T1 mapping and calculated ECV, which is markedly elevated at 51% (normal < 30%). (E) T1-weighted postcontrast short-axis imaging showing absence of contrast in the blood pool on LGE imaging, which is a common and specific imaging feature in cardiac amyloidosis. Other LGE patterns: T1-weighted inversion recovery (IR) showing diffuse subendocardial LGE of the left and right ventricle (F), also seen along the atrial walls on the apical four-chamber view (G), transmural LGE of the entire lateral wall on short axis (H). CMR, cardiovascular magnetic resonance; ECV, extracellular volume; LGE, late gadolinium enhancement.

- Elevated myocardial T2 suggestive of myocardial edema, higher in untreated AL amyloidosis compared to those treated, and this finding is a predictor of prognosis.
- Elevated T1 times and ECV
- A small pericardial effusion may also be present

IMMUNE CHECKPOINT INHIBITOR–RELATED MYOCARDITIS

- **CMR can aid in the diagnosis of myocarditis related to immune checkpoint inhibitors (ICI).**
- Modified Lake Louise Criteria with positive T1 and T2–based criterion are routinely used (Fig. 16-5).[14]
  - **Myocardial edema**
    - standard T2 sequences: **Regional or global increase of T2 signal intensity**
    - T2 mapping: regional or global increase of T2 relaxation times
  - Nonischemic myocardial injury
    - **late enhancement imaging: nonischemic (subepicardial or midmyocardial) late enhancement**
    - native T1 mapping: **increased T1 relaxation times** or ECV
  - Supportive criteria:
    - signs of pericarditis—effusion or pericardial late enhancement
    - systolic LV dysfunction—regional or global wall motion abnormalities

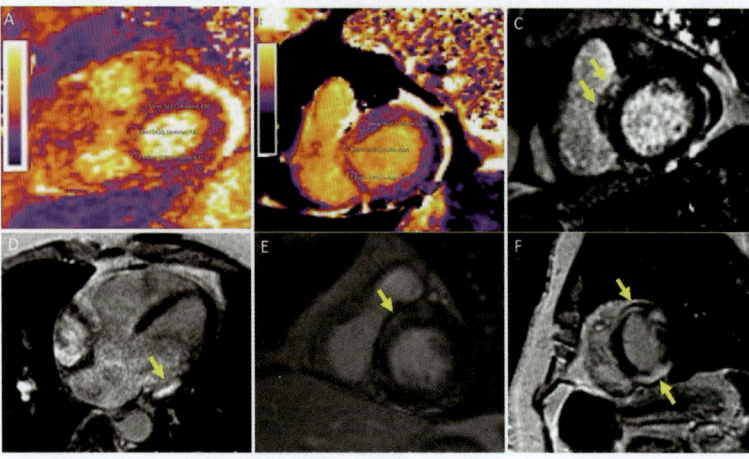

Figure 16-5. CMR findings in myocarditis due to immune checkpoint inhibitors. (A) T2 mapping showing high-signal intensity in the interventricular septum at 55 ms (normal < 50 ms), suggesting edema in the anterior septum. (B) Native T1 mapping showing increased T1 values in the septum at 1262 ms (normal 950-1050 ms). (C) T1-weighted postcontrast short-axis imaging showing epicardial to midmyocardial LGE in the basal anteroseptum. Other patterns of LGE can also be seen—(D) transmural LGE of the basal lateral wall, (E) midmyocardial LGE of the anterior wall, (F) midmyocardial LGE of the anterior wall, transmural LGE of the inferior wall on short axis. LGE, late gadolinium enhancement.

- However, LGE is not always present in patients with suspected ICI-associated myocarditis. Incorporating native T1 relaxation times/ECV improve the diagnostic accuracy of myocarditis on CMR.[18,19]
- A normal CMR does not exclude ICI-myocarditis, and a high index of suspicion is needed in patients presenting with elevation of cardiac biomarkers while on ICI and treatment for myocarditis started without delay.

CARDIAC TUMORS

- CMR is very useful in the evaluation of **cardiac masses, specifically, to help differentiate from a thrombus, determine tissue invasion and potential etiologies**[20,21] (Fig. 16-6).

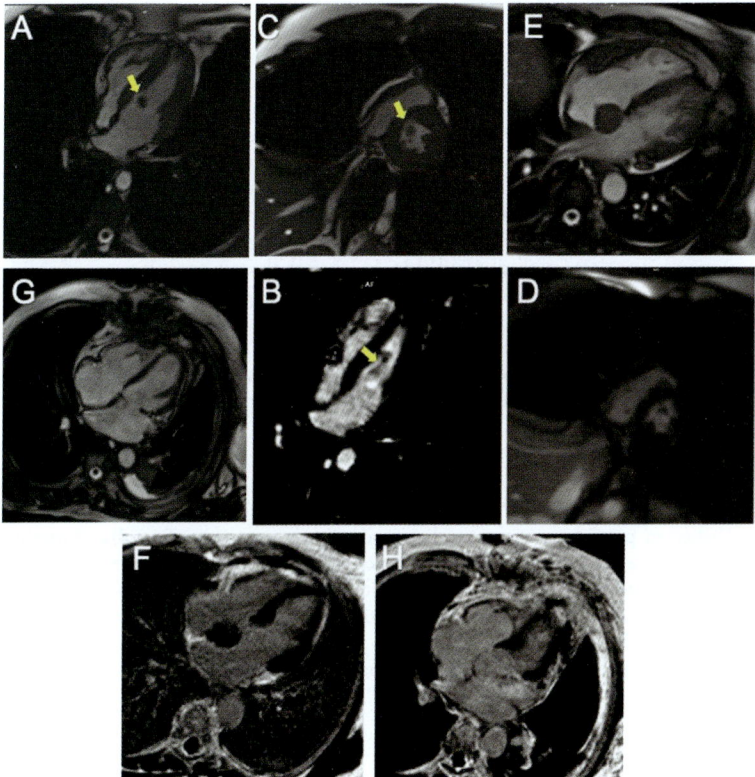

Figure 16-6. CMR in evaluation of cardiac tumors. (A, C) Cine imaging sequence showing a well-defined mass in the cavity of the left ventricle in a 29 years old male with cerebrovascular accident. (B, D) There was no enhancement of the mass on prolonged T1-weighted inversion recovery (IR) (>500 ms) suggestive of thrombus, which was confirmed on biopsy on excision. (E, F) Metastatic Merkel cell carcinoma with involvement of the interatrial septum with rim of LGE but mostly with no enhancement. (G, H) Pericardial metastasis with no LGE in a patient with metastatic lung cancer.

- Tissue characterization (T1 and T2 weighted imaging), first-pass perfusion, LGE, postcontrast long inversion time imaging can help differentiate tumor from thrombus.
- **Tumors are heterogeneous with potentially greater contrast uptake on first-pass perfusion.**
- **Thrombi are mostly homogeneous** and appear as a **very low-signal-intensity mass** (owing to absence of contrast uptake and presence of hemosiderin) surrounded by high-signal-intensity (contrast enhanced) structures such as cavity blood or surrounding myocardium with delayed imaging. An inversion time set to >600 ms can enhanced thrombus conspicuity.

CMR IN RADIATION-INDUCED HEART DISEASE

- Radiation therapy is an integral part of cancer therapy and is commonly used in intrathoracic malignancies such as breast, lung, esophageal, and thyroid cancers, and, historically, Hodgkin's lymphoma. RT-induced heart disease manifests late and can affect the heart valves, pericardium, and coronary vasculature.[22,23] It can also cause accelerated atherosclerosis in a dose-dependent manner. CMR can detect myocardial infarctions and its complications. **CMR is very helpful in differentiating viable from nonviable myocardium** and guide management strategies.
- Pericardial manifestations with acute pericarditis or constrictive pericarditis can occur years after therapy. **CMR can help identify pericardial inflammation (via LGE), ventricular interdependence (on cine imaging).** Active pericardial inflammation is associated with pericardial LGE, whereas chronic constrictive pericarditis does not enhance after contrast. This can be helpful in identifying patients with active pericarditis who may benefit from aggressive anti-inflammatory therapy and may also assist in guiding duration of treatment.
- **CMR acts as an important adjunct to echo in the assessment of valvular heart disease when echo assessment is inadequate or uncertain.**

SUMMARY AND FUTURE DIRECTIONS

In summary, the main advantages of CMR in cardio-oncology are the following:
- **Ability to provide accurate and reproducible assessment of cardiac function without the need for ionization radiation owing to its high-contrast resolution**
- **Early detection of CTRCD**, especially with the developing use of **Strain techniques**
- **Identification of myocardial inflammation related to myocarditis** and for evaluation of etiology of cardiomyopathy
- **Accurate identification of cardiac tumors or thrombi**

REFERENCES

1. Harries I, Liang K, Williams M, et al. Magnetic resonance imaging to detect cardiovascular effects of cancer therapy. *JACC CardioOncol.* 2020;2(2):270-292.
2. Bellenger NG, Davies LC, Francis JM, Coats AJS, Pennell DJ. Reduction in sample size for studies of remodeling in heart failure by the use of cardiovascular magnetic resonance. *J Cardiovasc Magn Reson.* 2000;2(4):271-278.
3. Mooij CF, De Wit CJ, Graham DA, Powell AJ, Geva T. Reproducibility of MRI measurements of right ventricular size and function in patients with normal and dilated ventricles. *J Magn Reson Imaging.* 2008;28(1):67-73.

4. Neilan TG, Coelho-Filho OR, Shah RV, et al. Myocardial extracellular volume by cardiac magnetic resonance imaging in patients treated with anthracycline-based chemotherapy. *Am J Cardiol.* 2013;111(5):717-722.
5. Cardinale D, Colombo A, Torrisi R, et al. Trastuzumab-induced cardiotoxicity: clinical and prognostic implications of troponin I evaluation. *J Clin Oncol.* 2010;28(25):3910-3916.
6. Houbois CP, Nolan M, Somerset E, et al. Serial cardiovascular magnetic resonance strain measurements to identify cardiotoxicity in breast cancer: comparison with echocardiography. *JACC Cardiovasc Imaging.* 2020;14(5):962-974.
7. Erley J, Genovese D, Tapaskar N, et al. Echocardiography and cardiovascular magnetic resonance based evaluation of myocardial strain and relationship with late gadolinium enhancement. *J Cardiovasc Magn Reson.* 2019;21(1):46.
8. Bucius P, Erley J, Tanacli R, et al. Comparison of feature tracking, fast-SENC, and myocardial tagging for global and segmental left ventricular strain. *ESC Hear Fail.* 2020;7(2):523-532.
9. Jordan JH, Vasu S, Morgan TM, et al. Anthracycline-associated T1 mapping characteristics are elevated independent of the presence of cardiovascular comorbidities in cancer survivors. *Circ Cardiovasc Imaging.* 2016;9(8):e004325.
10. Thavendiranathan P, Negishi T, Somerset E, et al. Strain-guided management of potentially cardiotoxic cancer therapy. *J Am Coll Cardiol.* 2021;77(4):392-401.
11. Granitz M, Motloch LJ, Granitz C, et al. Comparison of native myocardial T1 and T2 mapping at 1.5T and 3T in healthy volunteers: reference values and clinical implications. *Wien Klin Wochenschr.* 2019;131(7-8):143-155.
12. Galán-Arriola C, Lobo M, Vílchez-Tschischke JP, et al. Serial magnetic resonance imaging to identify early stages of anthracycline-Induced cardiotoxicity. *J Am Coll Cardiol.* 2019;73(7):779-791.
13. Haaf P, Garg P, Messroghli DR, Broadbent DA, Greenwood JP, Plein S. Cardiac T1 mapping and extracellular volume (ECV) in clinical practice: a comprehensive review. *J Cardiovasc Magn Reson.* 2016;18(1):89.
14. Ferreira VM, Schulz-Menger J, Holmvang G, et al. Cardiovascular magnetic resonance in nonischemic myocardial inflammation: expert recommendations. *J Am Coll Cardiol.* 2018;72(24):3158-3176.
15. Muehlberg F, Funk S, Zange L, et al. Native myocardial T1 time can predict development of subsequent anthracycline-induced cardiomyopathy. *ESC Hear Fail.* 2018;5(4):620-629.
16. Fallah-Rad N, Walker JR, Wassef A, et al. The utility of cardiac biomarkers, tissue velocity and strain imaging, and cardiac magnetic resonance imaging in predicting early left ventricular dysfunction in patients with human epidermal growth factor receptor II-positive breast cancer treated with adjuvant trastuzumab therapy. *J Am Coll Cardiol.* 2011;57(22):2263-2270.
17. Fontana M, Ćorović A, Scully P, Moon JC. Myocardial amyloidosis: The exemplar interstitial disease. *JACC Cardiovasc Imaging.* 2019;12(11 pt 2):2345-2356.
18. Mahmood SS, Fradley MG, Cohen JV, et al. Myocarditis in patients treated with immune checkpoint inhibitors. *J Am Coll Cardiol.* 2018;71(16):1755-1764.
19. Zhang L, Awadalla M, Mahmood SS, et al. Cardiovascular magnetic resonance in immune checkpoint inhibitor-associated myocarditis. *Eur Heart J.* 2020;41(18):1733-1743.
20. Fussen S, De Boeck BWL, Zellweger MJ, et al. Cardiovascular magnetic resonance imaging for diagnosis and clinical management of suspected cardiac masses and tumours. *Eur Heart J.* 2011;32(12):1551-1560.
21. Pazos-López P, Pozo E, Siqueira ME, et al. Value of CMR for the differential diagnosis of cardiac masses. *JACC Cardiovasc Imaging.* 2014;7(9):896-905.
22. Desai MY, Windecker S, Lancellotti P, et al. Prevention, diagnosis, and management of radiation-associated cardiac disease: JACC scientific expert panel. *J Am Coll Cardiol.* 2019;74(7):905-927.
23. Lancellotti P, Nkomo VT, Badano LP, et al. Expert consensus for multi-modality imaging evaluation of cardiovascular complications of radiotherapy in adults: a report from the European Association of Cardiovascular Imaging and the American Society of Echocardiography. *Eur Heart J Cardiovasc Imaging.* 2013;14(8):721-740.

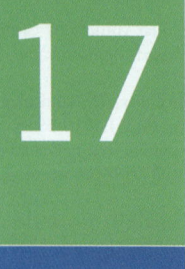

17 Cancer Survivorship: Adverse Outcomes and Other Long-term Cardiovascular Considerations

Jeannette Wong-Siegel, Debra Spoljaric, and Daniel J. Lenihan

GENERAL PRINCIPLES

- There are 16.9 million adult cancer survivors in the United States. It is estimated that by 2040, 73% of cancer survivors will be 65 years old or older and that there will be 22 million expected cancer survivors by 2030.[1]
- More than 11,000 children <15 years in the United States will be diagnosed with cancer in 2020, given the slightly increasing trend in annual incidence rates over the past few decades.[2]
  - Survival rates have improved significantly secondary to advances in treatment and diagnostics. The overall probability of five-year survival has improved from <30% in 1960 to >70% in 1990.[3] Almost 80% of adolescents and young adults aged 15 to 39 years will survive >5 years after their cancer diagnosis.[4]
- Survival rates vary in response to many factors, including cancer diagnosis, demographic characteristics (age, gender, and race), and by tumor characteristics, as well as genetic alterations. More intensive therapeutic protocols have been developed to improve survival rates in the poor prognosis groups, and this in turn may increase the risk of long-term adverse outcomes.

STANDARDS OF SURVIVORSHIP CARE

GENERAL PRINCIPLES

- **Obtain an accurate and complete cancer history, including initial diagnosis and staging if applicable, detailing any treatments received and any complications that may have occurred during treatment course** (Table 17-1).
- Childhood cancer survivors are especially vulnerable to having **limited information about their cancer and subsequent treatment**, mostly as a result of the young age at diagnosis. In addition, the pediatric medical institution may not be integrated into an adult care institution.
- Lack of accurate and complete information typically has a negative impact on the survivor's ability to seek and receive appropriate long-term care, which may further contribute to psychosocial complications (Table 17-2).

TABLE 17-1	Long-Term Physical Issues in Cancer Survivors

Secondary malignant neoplasms

Cardiovascular disease
- Coronary
- Valvular
- Pericardial
- Myocardial dysfunction

Cardiovascular risk factors

Adverse hormonal effects

Reproductive consideration

Lymphedema

Pain

Exercise limitation

TABLE 17-2	Long-Term Psychological/Social Issues in Cancer Survivors

Psychiatric issues

Cognitive function

Fatigue

Educational achievement

CARDIAC COMPLICATIONS

GENERAL PRINCIPLES

- **Cardiovascular (CV) toxicity from cancer therapies may not be evident for many years following treatment.** The resulting CV complications can have a significant, and sometimes fatal, impact on patients. As a result, there is a compelling need for continued surveillance in hopes of early detection of CV disease with effective interventions among cancer survivors.
- **Patients who have been treated with certain chemotherapeutic agents or any chest/mediastinal radiation have the greatest risk for developing CV complications**, but all survivors should be routinely screened for other comorbidities that may increase their risk for CV disease.
- Next to secondary malignancies, **childhood cancer survivors are most likely to die secondary to cardiac events.**[5] Because they are already at increased risk for developing adverse cardiac outcomes, survivors should be routinely screened for other comorbidities that **may increase their risk for developing CV disease** (tobacco use, obesity, diabetes, hypertension, and dyslipidemia), and **regular exercise should be encouraged.**[6]

VASCULAR COMPROMISE

- Radiation therapy is an associated risk factor for development of atherosclerosis in cancer survivors.[7] Specifically, **chest/mediastinal radiation has been associated with the development of coronary artery disease and atherosclerosis in all vessels that are exposed to radiation** (Fig. 17-1).[8,9]
  - Neck radiation also increases risk for carotid disease.
  - Optimize CV risk factor management with early detection and initiation of appropriate pharmacotherapy (aspirin, statin-based lipid, and/or antiplatelet therapy) for atherosclerosis if identified.

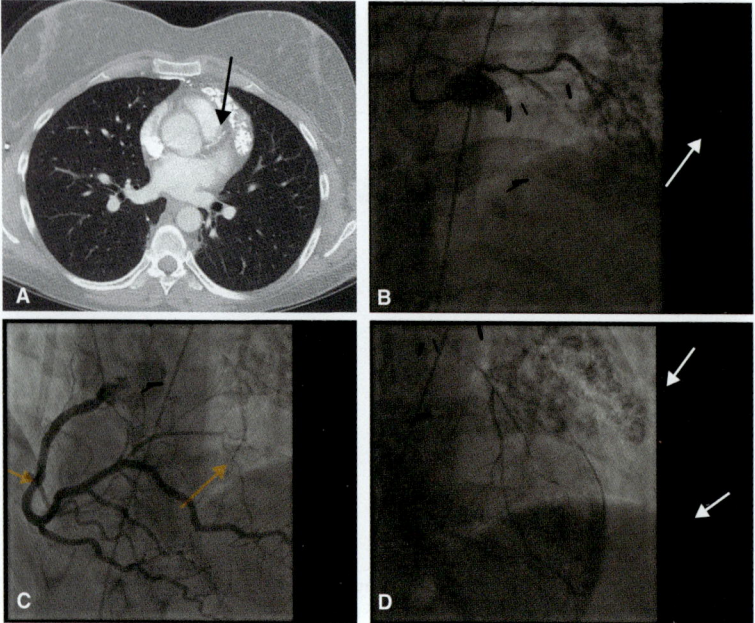

Figure 17-1. Atherosclerosis in an area exposed to radiation is at major risk for a cancer survivor. Case description: **A 38-year-old female with refractory Hodgkin disease.** Prior Tx: Adriamycin, bleomycin, vinblastine, dacarbazine (×6) cycles; etoposide, solumedrol, cytarabine, cisplatin (×2) cycles; mediastinal radiation for bulky disease all at age 24. Autologous SCT + BEAM chemotherapy at age 25, with relapse; allogeneic matched unrelated donor allogeneic SCT + fludarabine, busulfan, thymoglobulin at age 26. Graft versus host disease (GVHD) for several years involving the muscles, skin (scleroderma), and gastrointestinal (GI) tract. Previously treated with ibrutinib and currently on mycophenylate 500 mg daily, Jakafi, prednisone 7 mg daily, sirolimus 1mg daily, and photopheresis. (A) Computed tomography (CT) images show calcified residual bulky disease and coronary calcification in close proximity (black arrow). (B) Left anterior descending (LAD) subtotal occlusion near residual bulky disease (white arrow). (C) Right coronary artery without major disease but collaterals to L system (2 yellow arrows). (D) LAD fills by retrograde collaterals (2 white arrows). Note: Radiation promotes accelerated atherosclerosis in any vessels exposed, and a young patient who is a cancer survivor is at high risk.

- **Hypertension is also a long-term consequence of some chemotherapeutic agents**, such as cis-platinum and, more recently, antiangiogenic therapy.
  - Prompt and effective antihypertensive treatment is important for minimizing further complications, such as stroke, heart failure, or sudden death.[10]
- Formation of thrombosis is thought to be multifactorial, related to the malignancy itself, applied therapies, as well as chronic history of intravenous access for chemotherapy and blood transfusions.
- The classic Virchow triad of **promotion of thrombosis is typically all abnormal in a survivor of cancer therapy: (a) stasis (lack of exercise), (b) hypercoagulability (resulting from cancer), and (c) endothelial dysfunction,** thought to be secondary to venous injury in the past owing to catheter placement or prior deep vein thromboses.

STRUCTURAL ABNORMALITIES

Valvular

- **Valvular degeneration with calcification is a recognized complication** following chest/mediastinal radiation and can be further exacerbated by hyperlipidemia and hypertension (Fig. 17-2).
- **Most patients are asymptomatic.** Routine physical examination is important for monitoring valvular disease progression, because sudden progression of aortic stenosis or regurgitation may result in sudden death or acute heart failure.
- There are usually multiple valves affected by radiation, so mitral, tricuspid, and pulmonic valve dysfunction should be considered.[11]

Pericardial

- Patients may also experience pericardial effusion during treatment for their cancer, especially those with esophageal cancer.
- Constrictive pericarditis can infrequently be a late manifestation secondary to radiotherapy.

Conduction Disease

- There is increased frequency of a variety of arrhythmias in cancer survivors, including atrial fibrillation, bradycardia, heart block, or ventricular tachycardia, occurring among survivors previously treated with anthracyclines.[12]

MYOCARDIAL DYSFUNCTION, HEART FAILURE

- **Cardiotoxicity, specifically left ventricular dysfunction, as detected by imaging or natriuretic peptides, is a major adverse outcome in cancer survivors.**
- **Anthracyclines** have been studied extensively in regard to their known cardiotoxic effect. Previous investigations reported that the cardiotoxic effects from anthracycline therapy were considered irreversible. However, newer data confirm that if there is prompt intervention when cardiotoxicity is detected, the toxicity is mostly reversible.[13]
- **Cardiac dysfunction and heart failure have been reported with human epidermal growth factor receptor (HER2) blocking therapies in breast cancer**, as well as several other classes of targeted agents, especially therapies that have profound antiangiogenic activity.[14,15]

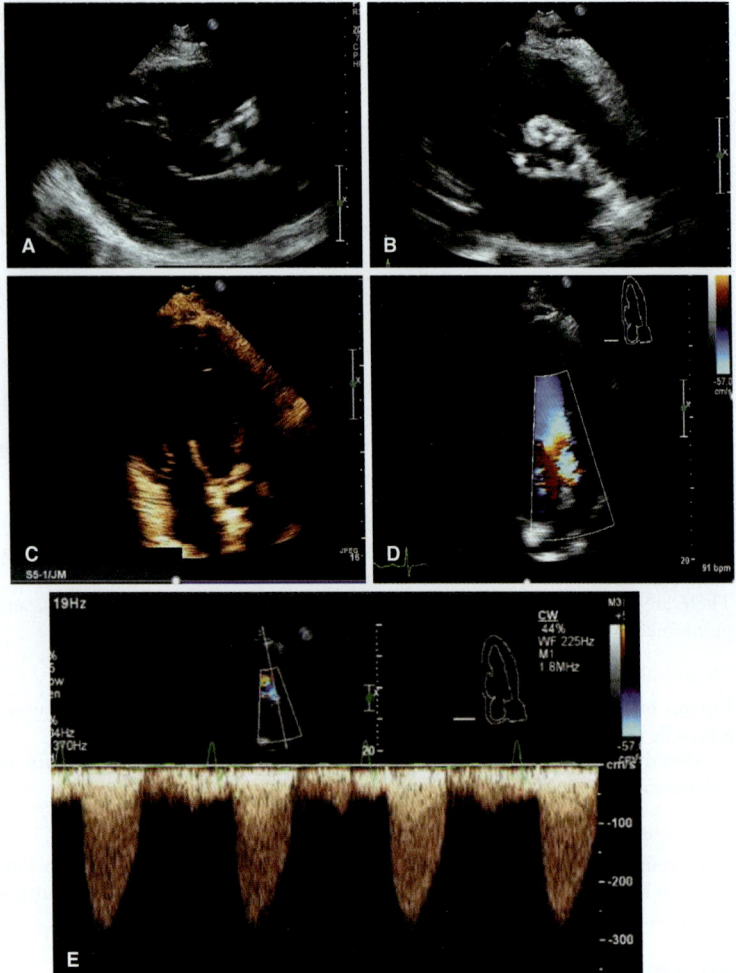

Figure 17-2. Typical valvular disease encountered in cancer survivors. Case description: 47 years old F, with recently diagnosed breast cancer undergoing chemotherapy with trastuzumab and pertuzumab, presents to assess her cardiac status while she receives treatment. She reports shortness of breath after walking even up to just 100 ft. She denies paroxysmal nocturnal dyspnea (PND) or orthopnea. She does have some lower extremity edema but denies any chest pain. PMH: Stage IIA Hodgkin lymphoma at age 27 treated with mantle radiation, relapsed disease treated with MOPP-ABVD. Current stage IIA (T2N0M0) R-sided breast cancer (3 cm), ER 3+ (99%), PR 3+ (99%), human epidermal growth factor receptor (HER2)–amplified by fluorescence in situ hybridization) FISH (3+) s/p R total mastectomy with 0/6 SLNs at age 45. (A, B) Arrow indicates aortic valve calcification. (C-E) left, aortic calcification, aortic insufficiency (middle panel arrow), and aortic stenosis (right panel arrow). Note: Previous radiation results in valvular calcification and both stenosis and regurgitation, most commonly of the aortic valve, although all valves can be affected.

OTHER MEDICAL COMPLICATIONS

Secondary Malignant Neoplasms
- Childhood cancer survivors are at increased risk for developing subsequent malignancies, attributed to association with initial cancer diagnosis (eg, Hodgkin disease or soft tissue sarcoma) and therapies (eg, radiation exposure and chemotherapy agents, specifically alkylating agents).[16]
- Female gender has also been reported to be an independent risk factor for development of subsequent malignancies, most likely related to the increased risk of breast cancer following exposure to ionizing radiation.
- **Bone, breast, central nervous system, and thyroid cancers were the most common subsequent malignancies among childhood cancer survivors.**[16]

Adverse Hormonal Effects
- Systemic chemotherapy and radiation affecting the ovaries can result in menopause. The resulting hot flashes can have a negative impact on a woman's quality of life.
- Men may also experience hot flashes after undergoing androgen deprivation therapy for prostate cancer.
- In addition to behavior modifications and supportive measures, moderate to severe hot flashes can be treated with pharmacotherapy, including antidepressants (serotonin and norepinephrine reuptake inhibitor [SNRI] and selective serotonin reuptake inhibitor [SSRI]), gabapentin, and clonidine.
- Consideration for hormonal treatment should be made in conjunction with a patient's oncology provider.

Reproductive Considerations
- **Common issues affecting women's sexual health include vaginal dryness, decreased libido, and dyspareunia. Common issues affecting men include erectile dysfunction, which may include inability to maintain an erection, inability to penetrate partner, or problems with ejaculation; as well as decreased libido.**[17]
- Review oncologic history and obtain lab work to evaluate for endocrine abnormalities. Determine whether any other past medical history (depression, hypertension, diabetes) or pharmacotherapy (SSRI, beta blocker) is a contributing factor.
- Consider referring patient to a sexual health specialist, psychotherapy, couples counseling, urology, gynecologic care, and/or pelvic floor therapy.
- Given long-term consequences of cancer therapies, fertility is a significant issue, especially among childhood and young adult cancer survivors. Although the risk of miscarriage has been reported to be higher among women whose ovaries were in or near the radiation therapy field, male survivors also had significantly fewer live births when compared to their siblings.[16,18]
- Although chemotherapy, overall, does not appear to negatively affect pregnancy outcomes, all children and young adults who have been diagnosed with cancer must undergo further discussions regarding fertility preservation.

Lymphedema
- **Lymphedema can occur anytime in survivorship.** Initial symptoms may include a sensation of heaviness, full or tightness of the skin, or pain.[19] Decreased range of motion or strength may also be present.

- Increased swelling can predispose a patient to localized infections, requiring hospitalization for IV antibiotic administration.
- Early detection allows for more effective intervention. Patients maintain improved mobility and independence with adequate pain control and access to physical therapy. Certified therapists can also provide more targeted therapies, such as compression garments. Physical activity and strength training are not a contraindication and should be encouraged.

Pain

- Patients with chronic pain may not exhibit any overt physical signs.
- Additional symptoms may include tachycardia, hypertension, hyperventilation, facial grimace, and verbalizations.
- **Pain may also be secondary to neuropathies, which is associated with certain chemotherapeutic agents such as vincristine.**
- New onset and acute pain should include cancer recurrence in the differential diagnosis.[17]
- After a comprehensive pain assessment and evaluation, consider initiation of supportive care first (heat/cold, massage, occupational/physical therapy). Nonopioids should be used primarily for pain relief and opioids prescribed for short periods of time as needed to treat breakthrough pain.
- Educate patients on dosing, side effects, and differences between addiction, tolerance, and physical dependence if using opioid therapies for pain.

PSYCHOLOGICAL AND SOCIAL COMPLICATIONS

PSYCHIATRIC ISSUES

- **Cancer survivors are at increased risk for mental health issues, especially in the setting of fear of recurrence. Distress, anxiety, and depression may persist for many years after their cancer diagnosis.**[20]
- Diagnosis and treatment can be challenging. Patients may complain of physical and somatic manifestations. Referral to psychiatry and psychology may be necessary for further evaluation.
- Treatment is focused on first addressing any contributable factors, such as pain or sleep.
- Social work referral may be useful for any financial needs, including transportation and housing concerns.
- In addition to counseling with oncologic psychologists, pharmacologic interventions may be necessary. Patients should expect to see some effect 4 to 6 weeks after initiation of antidepressant, SNRI or SSRI, 8 to 12 weeks for full effect.

COGNITIVE FUNCTION

- **Cancer-related cognitive impairment is not limited to those survivors treated with chemotherapy.**[21] Screen patients for potentially reversible factors that may be contributing to their impairment, such as sleep disturbance, fatigue, and depression. There are, unfortunately, no approved pharmacologic agents to improve cognition.[21]

- Consider neuroimaging based on primary cancer diagnosis and risk for metastatic disease. Evaluate for other factors such as medication side effects, substance use, vitamin deficiencies, and endocrinopathies.[17]
- Refer patients to cognitive rehabilitation, which includes occupational and speech therapies and referrals to neuropsychology and psychotherapy.

FATIGUE

- Cancer-related fatigue is defined as a distressing, persistent, subjective sense of physical, emotional, and/or cognitive tiredness or exhaustion related to cancer or cancer treatment that is not proportional to recent activity and that interferes with usual functioning.[22]
- **Fatigue can also be an indication of a treatable condition, such as cardiac or pulmonary dysfunction, endocrinopathy, anemia, or deconditioning secondary to prolonged cancer therapy course**. Review patient's current medications, sleep behaviors, nutritional status, and overall emotional well-being to determine other contributing factors to fatigue.
- Reinforce healthy lifestyle behaviors, discussed further on. Refer to psychology, physical therapy, exercise programs, and other resources as appropriate.
  - Encourage patients to eat a healthy diet, high in vegetables, fruits, and whole grains but low in sugars and fats. Limit red and processed meats.
  - Maintain a healthy weight by promoting vigorous exercise and strength/resistance training.[6]
  - Practice safe sun exposure by using broad-spectrum sunscreen with SPF ≥ 30 and limiting time spent in the sun. Wear appropriate ultraviolet (UV)-protective clothing. Avoid tanning beds.
  - Avoid tobacco, marijuana, and vaping products.
  - No alcohol is best, otherwise, limit alcohol intake: 1 drink per day for women and 2 drinks per day for men.
  - Ensure adequate sleep with good sleep hygiene. For patients experiencing chronic insomnia, consider referral to cognitive behavioral therapy and medications (trazodone vs. mirtazapine).
- **Follow up with primary care provider regularly.**

Educational Achievement

- **Educational achievement is an important predictor of social outcome**. Significant academic disruptions are unfortunately common for children diagnosed with cancer.
- Childhood cancer survivors report a significantly higher use of special education services and rate of not completing high school compared to their siblings. This, in turn, affects their ability to achieve employment and then live independently.
- Chronic medical conditions after cancer therapy have also been shown to increase risk for unemployment.
- Early intervention is key to improving psychosocial well-being among childhood cancer survivors to reduce risk of long-term adverse outcomes.

IMMUNIZATION CONSIDERATIONS

- Providers should encourage immunizations as recommended by the Centers for Disease Control (CDC).
- Vaccines may not trigger protective immune response in actively immunocompromised individuals or in survivors with residual immune deficits.
- Vaccinations should be delayed for at least 6 months after receiving anti-B cell antibody therapy.[17]

TRANSITIONING TO ADULT-CENTERED CARE

- **Delays in transition from pediatric-focused to adult-focused care may result in adverse long-term physical and psychological outcomes**, as highlighted previously.
- Successful transition involves a multidisciplinary team of physicians, therapists, and social workers to provide developmentally appropriate and specialty care while promoting the patient's autonomy, personal responsibility, and self-reliance.[23]

SUMMARY

- **Advances in therapies and management have decreased cancer mortality and increased survival rates.** The cancer survivorship population continues to grow, and routine screening for long-term complications secondary to their cancer therapies cannot be emphasized enough. The burden of CV complications specifically contributes to significant morbidity and mortality among cancer survivors. **Active screening and early intervention are necessary to prevent these secondary complications** (Fig. 17-3). Although CV complications carry a significant burden among cancer survivors, other complications, both physical and psychosocial, warrant continued screening and management as well.

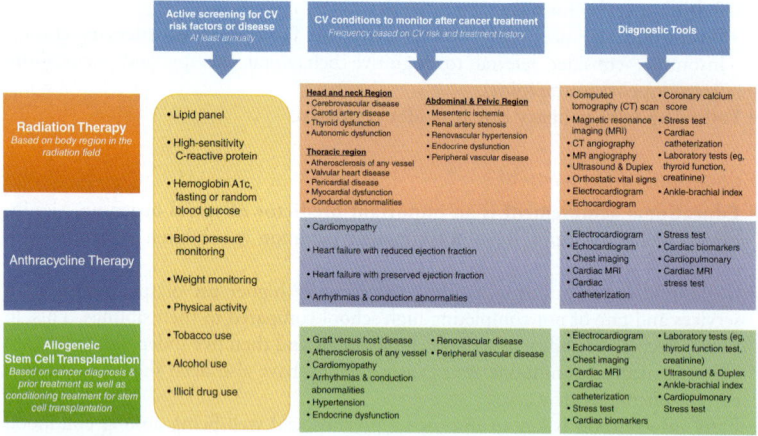

Figure 17-3. Overall recommendations cardiac monitoring and treatment in cancer survivors.

REFERENCES

1. American Cancer Society, *Cancer treatment and survivorship facts and figures 2019-2021*. American Cancer Society; 2019.
2. American Cancer Society. Key statistics for childhood cancers. 2021. https://www.cancer.org/cancer/cancer-in-children/key-statistics.html.
3. Linet MS, Ries LA, Smith MA, Tarone RE, Devesa SS. Cancer surveillance series: recent trends in childhood cancer incidence and mortality in the United States. *J Natl Cancer Inst*. 1999;91(12):1051-1058.
4. Henley SJ, Ward EM, Scott S, et al. Annual report to the nation on the status of cancer, part I: National Cancer Statistics. *Cancer*. 2020;126(10):2225-2249.
5. Mertens AC, Yasui Y, Neglia JP, et al. Late mortality experience in five-year survivors of childhood and adolescent cancer: the Childhood Cancer Survivor Study. *J Clin Oncol*, 2001;19(13):3163-3172.
6. Scott JM, Li N, Liu Q, et al. Association of exercise with mortality in adult survivors of childhood cancer. *JAMA Oncol*. 2018;4(10):1352-1358.
7. Lenihan DJ, Cardinale DM. Late cardiac effects of cancer treatment. *J Clin Oncol*. 2012;30(30):3657-3664.
8. Desai MY, Jellis CL, Kotecha R, Johnston DR, Griffin BP. Radiation-associated cardiac disease: a practical approach to diagnosis and management. *JACC Cardiovasc Imaging*. 2018;11(8):1132-1149.
9. Atkins KM, Chaunzwa TL, Lamba N, et al. Association of left anterior descending coronary artery radiation dose with major adverse cardiac events and mortality in patients with non-small cell lung cancer. *JAMA Oncol*. 2020;7(2):206-219.
10. Gibson TM, Li Z, Green DM, et al. Blood pressure status in adult survivors of childhood cancer: a report from the St. Jude Lifetime Cohort Study. *Cancer Epidemiol Biomarkers Prev*. 2017;26(12):1705-1713.
11. Bijl JM, Roos MM, van Leeuwen-Segarceanu EM, et al. Assessment of valvular disorders in survivors of Hodgkin's lymphoma treated by mediastinal radiotherapy $\pm$ chemotherapy. *Am J Cardiol*. 2016;117(4):691-696.
12. Mazur M, Wang F, Hodge DO, et al. Burden of cardiac arrhythmias in patients with anthracycline-related cardiomyopathy. *JACC Clin Electrophysiol*. 2017;3(2):139-150.
13. Cardinale D, Colombo A, Bacchiani G, et al. Early detection of anthracycline cardiotoxicity and improvement with heart failure therapy. *Circulation*. 2015;131(22):1981-1988.
14. Slamon D, Eiermann W, Robert N, et al., Adjuvant trastuzumab in HER2-positive breast cancer. *N Engl J Med*. 2011;365(14):1273-1283.
15. Hall PS, Harshman LC, Srinivas S, Witteles RM. The frequency and severity of cardiovascular toxicity from targeted therapy in advanced renal cell carcinoma patients. *JACC Heart Fail*. 2013;1(1):72-78.
16. Robison LL. Treatment-associated subsequent neoplasms among long-term survivors of childhood cancer: the experience of the childhood cancer survivor study. *Pediatr Radiol*. 2009;39(suppl 1):S32-S37.
17. National Comprehensive Cancer Network. Survivorship version 2. NCCN clinical practice guidelines in oncology. 2020. https://www.nccn.org/professionals/physician_gls/pdf/survivorship.pdf.
18. Green D, Galvin H, Horne B. The psycho-social impact of infertility on young male cancer survivors: a qualitative investigation. *Psychooncology*. 2003;12(2):141-152.
19. National Cancer Institute. Lymphedema (PDQ)-health professional version. 2019. https://www.cancer.gov/about-cancer/treatment/side-effects/lymphedema/lymphedema-hp-pdq.
20. Lu D, Andersson TM, Fall K, et al. Clinical diagnosis of mental disorders immediately before and after cancer diagnosis: a nationwide matched cohort study in Sweden. *JAMA Oncol*. 2016;2(9):1188-1196.

21. Lange M, Joly F, Vardy J, et al. Cancer-related cognitive impairment: an update on state of the art, detection, and management strategies in cancer survivors. *Ann Oncol.* 2019;30(12):1925-1940.
22. National Comprehensive Cancer Network. Cancer-related fatigue. Version 2. NCCN clinical practice guidelines in oncology. 2020. https://www.nccn.org/professionals/physician_gls/pdf/fatigue.pdf.
23. Henderson TO, Friedman DL, Meadows AT. Childhood cancer survivors: transition to adult-focused risk-based care. *Pediatrics.* 2010;126(1):129-136.

18 Hematopoietic Cell Transplantation

Tushar Tarun,* Michael Kramer,* and Iskra Pusic

Hematopoietic cell transplantation (HCT) is a potentially curative therapy for a variety of disorders including hematologic malignances, bone marrow failure disorders, hemoglobinopathies, immunodeficiencies, autoimmune conditions, and selected solid tumors. It involves the administration of high-dose chemotherapy and/or radiation, followed by the infusion of previously collected autologous or allogeneic hematopoietic cells. More than 65,000 HCTs are performed annually worldwide. Advancement in HCT strategies and supportive care has led to a significant improvement in survival of HCT recipients.[1,2] As patients survive longer, however, they are at risk for developing late side effects, including cardiovascular (CV) complications.[3] This chapter summarizes the principles of HCT, pre-HCT cardiac assessment, and CV complications after HCT.

OVERVIEW OF HEMATOPOIETIC CELL TRANSPLANTATION

Types of Hematopoietic Cell Transplantation

HCT is classified based on the source of the hematopoietic cells to be infused.
- **Autologous HCT (auto-HCT) involves mobilization, collection, and cryopreservation of a patient's own hematopoietic cells.** These cells are then reinfused as "rescue" of hematopoiesis after the administration of high-dose chemotherapy and/or radiation.
- **Allogeneic HCT (allo-HCT) involves collection of hematopoietic cells from a healthy person (donor) followed by infusion into the patient (recipient), after the administration of chemotherapy and/or radiation.** A certain degree of matching between donor and recipient for the human leukocyte antigen (HLA) loci is necessary to ensure successful allo-HCT. The donor may be a fully HLA-matched sibling, half HLA-matched relative (haploidentical), fully HLA-matched unrelated donor, or partially HLA-matched unrelated donor. Recipients of allo-HCT require immunosuppression for a period of time posttransplant to ensure successful engraftment and to prevent both rejection and graft-versus-host disease (GVHD).

Indications for Hematopoietic Cell Transplantation

The most common indications for auto-HCT are multiple myeloma and lymphoma. The most common indications of allo-HCT are acute leukemia, myelodysplastic syndrome, and aplastic anemia (Table 18-1).

---

*These authors contributed equally to this chapter.

TABLE 18-1	Indications for Hematopoietic Cell Transplantation

Autologous transplant
Multiple myeloma
Light chain amyloidosis
Hodgkin and non-Hodgkin lymphoma
Neuroblastoma
Germ cell tumors

Allogeneic transplant
Leukemia
Myelodysplastic syndrome and myeloproliferative neoplasms
Hodgkin and non-Hodgkin lymphoma
Aplastic anemia and other bone marrow failure syndromes
Hemoglobinopathies (thalassemia, sickle cell disease)
Immunodeficiency syndromes
Inborn errors of metabolism
Autoimmune conditions

Adapted from Govindan R, Morgensztern D. *The Washington Manual of Oncology*. 4th ed. Wolters Kluwer; 2020.

Hematopoietic Cell Transplantation Procedures and Techniques

Collection of Hematopoietic Cells

- Hematopoietic cells may be harvested directly from bone marrow by performing a series of marrow biopsies on an anesthetized donor/patient or from peripheral blood via apheresis. Although hematopoietic cells can be detected in the blood at very low levels, their yield is increased ~1000-fold using hematopoietic growth factors, typically granulocyte colony-stimulating factor (G-CSF) and/or plerixafor, in a process called hematopoietic cell mobilization. These mobilized hematopoietic cells can then be harvested from the blood via apheresis. Mobilized blood hematopoietic cells are used for all auto-HCT. Both bone marrow and mobilized blood hematopoietic cells may be used for allo-HCT, each with its own advantages and disadvantages, and practices vary among centers.

Conditioning

- **Prior to HCT, a conditioning regimen (multiple chemotherapy agents and/or radiation) is given to eradicate any remaining malignant cells.** In allo-HCT, conditioning also serves to "make space" in the recipient marrow for the donor cells by incapacitating the recipient immune system, which would otherwise reject donor cells. Types of conditioning include *myeloablative conditioning (MAC), reduced intensity conditioning (RIC),* and *non-myeloablative (NMA)* (Table 18-2).
  - MAC regimens are more intense and cause long-lasting cytopenias. The patient's marrow is unlikely to recover without HCT.

TABLE 18-2 Common Conditioning Regimens and Toxicities

Myeloablative regimens	HCT type	Significant toxicities
Cy/TBI Cyclophosphamide Total Body Irradiation	Allo-HCT	Arrhythmia, heart failure, cardiac tamponade, restrictive cardiomyopathy, arrhythmia, pericarditis, pneumonitis, pulmonary fibrosis
Flu/Bu4 Fludarabine Busulfan (4 days)	Allo-HCT	Chest pain, arrhythmia, edema, interstitial lung disease
BEAM Carmustine (BCNU) Etoposide Cytarabine (Ara-C) Melphalan	Auto-HCT (lymphoma)	Seizures, chest pain, peripheral neuropathy, cerebellar toxicity edema, gastrointestinal (GI) toxicity
High-dose melphalan	Auto-HCT (multiple myeloma)	Edema, GI toxicity
Reduced Intensity (RIC)		
Flu/Bu2 Fludarabine Busulfan (2 days)	Allo-HCT	Chest pain, arrhythmia, edema, interstitial lung disease
Flu/Cy Fludarabine Cyclophosphamide	Allo-HCT	Chest pain, arrhythmia, edema, heart failure, cardiac tamponade
Nonmyeloablative regimens		
Flu/TBI	Allo-HCT	Chest pain, arrythmia, edema, restrictive cardiomyopathy, congestive heart failure, pericarditis, pneumonitis, pulmonary fibrosis
TLI/ATG Total Lymphocyte Irradiation Anti-thymocyte globulin	Allo-HCT	Infusion reactions, bradycardia, chest pain

Allo-HCT, allogeneic hematopoietic cell transplantation; auto-HCT, autologous hematopoietic cell transplantation.

- RIC and NMA regimens are significantly less toxic and the marrow will recover even in the absence of hematopoietic cell infusion. However, these regimens are less likely to completely destroy any residual malignant cells. RIC and NMA regimens rely on graft-versus-tumor effect for additional elimination of malignant cells. Use of RIC and NMA has expanded the availability of allo-HCT to less fit and older patients, who are less likely to tolerate standard MAC.

Infusion of Hematopoietic Cells

After the patient undergoes conditioning, the harvested hematopoietic cell product is infused through the central venous catheter. Close patient observation, including cardiac monitoring, is mandatory during the infusion.

Engraftment

After HCT, the patient is closely monitored and supported with transfusions and antibiotics while awaiting engraftment of the new hematopoietic system (engraftment is the process by which hematopoietic cells make their way to bone marrow niches and proliferate). G-CSF is usually started several days after HCT and continued until the absolute neutrophil count exceeds 1500 cells/mm^3 (usually 10-20 days after HCT).

Immunosuppression

Short-term immunosuppression is used after allo-HCT to prevent acute GVHD. Acute GVHD is caused by allo-reactive donor T cells in the hematopoietic cell product (graft) that recognize recipient (host) antigens as foreign. The most commonly affected organs are skin, gastrointestinal system, and liver. Standard immunosuppressant regimens use an antimetabolite (ie, methotrexate, mycophenolate mofetil) in combination with a calcineurin inhibitor (ie, tacrolimus, cyclosporine). The use of cyclophosphamide early after allo-HCT has enabled the use of haploidentical donors, revolutionizing the transplant world.[4]

PRETRANSPLANT CARDIOVASCULAR EVALUATION

Cardiovascular Screening

- Many patients being considered for HCT have previously received cardiotoxic cancer therapy (ie, anthracyclines, cyclophosphamide, chest radiation) and are at increased risk for cardiac dysfunction. Certain HCT indications (ie, light chain amyloidosis, thalassemia, systemic sclerosis) are associated with CV disease.[5] With improvement in HCT techniques over the last decade, more patients aged >60 years are undergoing HCT.[6] These older patients are more likely to have CV comorbidities including hypertension, hyperlipidemia, arteriosclerosis, and diabetes.
- **All patients should be screened with clinical history, 12-lead electrocardiography, transthoracic echocardiography, and chest x-ray. Patients with high-risk features** (Table 18-3) **should be referred to a cardio-oncologist for further evaluation and risk factor modification.**

Cardiovascular Optimization

- All patients with known coronary artery disease should be on statin therapy peri-HCT.
- Patients suspected of having unstable angina should undergo pre-HCT stress testing and/or cardiac catheterization, assuming that HCT can safely be delayed, to allow for a period of dual antiplatelet therapy after coronary revascularization.

TABLE 18-3 Risk Factors for Cardiovascular Complications After Hematopoietic Cell Transplantation

1. Signs or symptoms of angina and/or heart failure
2. Significant abnormalities on electrocardiography (arrhythmias, heart block, Q waves)
3. Left ventricular dysfunction (left ventricular ejection fraction <40%)
4. Abnormal cardiac biomarkers (troponin, brain natriuretic peptide)
5. Prior cardiotoxic cancer therapy (anthracyclines, proteasome inhibitors, cyclophosphamide, chest radiation)
6. History of heart failure, cardiomyopathy, or at least grade II diastolic dysfunction
7. History of myocardial infarction within 30 days
8. History of unexplained syncope
9. History of aortic or mitral valve stenosis
10. History of pulmonary hypertension

- Arrhythmias should be well controlled on medical therapy prior to HCT.
- Patients with heart failure should be on optimal guideline-directed heart failure therapy, including beta-blockers, angiotensin-converting enzyme (ACE) inhibitors, angiotensin receptor blockers, mineralocorticoid receptor antagonists, and/or angiotensin receptor-neprilysin inhibitors. Volume status should be optimized using loop diuretics.
- The risks and benefits of HCT for patients with left ventricular ejection fraction (LVEF) <40% should be discussed by a multidisciplinary care team.

CARDIOVASCULAR COMPLICATIONS OF HEMATOPOIETIC CELL TRANSPLANTATION

Early Cardiovascular Complications
- Several early post-HCT complications may lead to increased cardiac stress and CV complications.
  - Bacteremia, pneumonia, septic shock, and multiorgan failure are not uncommon in the early post-HCT period.
  - Cytokine release syndrome is an acute systemic inflammatory syndrome that may occur after allo-HCT, particularly haploidentical HCT. Severe cases are characterized by hypotension, circulatory collapse, vascular leakage, peripheral and pulmonary edema, renal failure, and cardiac dysfunction. Steroids and tocilizumab are used for treatment.
- **Heart failure, arrhythmias, and pericardial effusion may occur.**
  - Loop diuretics should be used to manage volume status in patients with decompensated heart failure. Beta-blockers and/or ACE inhibitors can be used in patients with new-onset systolic dysfunction when blood pressure will tolerate.
  - Atrial fibrillation and atrial flutter are the most common arrhythmias.[7] Short-term antiarrhythmic therapy with amiodarone may be necessary, because of concomitant hypotension and acute renal injury in the early post-HCT period.

- Asymptomatic pericardial effusion can be monitored with serial echocardiograms and/or intravenous fluid administration. For patients with cardiac tamponade, pericardiocentesis should be performed under echocardiography guidance and with platelet count >50,000.
- Cyclophosphamide, which may be used for pre-HCT conditioning, is associated with acute CV toxicities including heart failure, pericarditis, and hemorrhagic myocarditis occurring within 3 weeks of cyclophosphamide administration.
- Acute cardiac GVHD is extremely rare, but there are reports of patients with acute GVHD (or acute flare of chronic GVHD) who developed bradycardia (including sinus node failure or complete heart block); all those patients responded to increased immunosuppression.[8]

Late Cardiovascular Complications

- **The prevalence of all CV risk factors, such as hyperlipidemia, diabetes, hypertension, and abdominal obesity, is increased in HCT survivors compared with the general population.** These patients are at 4 times higher risk of developing CV disease with onset ~14 years earlier as compared to the general population. The cumulative incidence of CV complications after HCT is 5% to 10% at 10 years, and CV deaths account for 2% to 4% of mortality in long-term HCT survivors.[9-11]
  - The cumulative incidence of congestive heart failure is 5% at 5 years and up to 10% at 15 years.
  - After allo-HCT, the cumulative incidence of arterial vascular events (coronary artery disease, peripheral vascular disease, stroke) is 10% at 15 years and >20% at 20 years.
  - Risk of arrhythmias increases over time and is highest in older populations. Cumulative incidence of conduction abnormalities approaches 10% at 10 years.
  - Prevalence of chronic health conditions is higher after allo-HCT than after auto-HCT.[12]
  - Several risk factors specific to cancer therapy and HCT contribute to increased risk of late CV complications after HCT.
    - Pre-HCT anthracycline therapy increases the risk of heart failure, whereas chest radiation is associated with restrictive cardiomyopathy and heart failure, conduction abnormalities, arrhythmias, coronary artery disease, pericarditis, and autonomic dysfunction.[13]
    - Total body irradiation, used as part of HCT conditioning regimens, leads to endothelial damage, which raises the risk of arterial vascular disease (coronary artery disease, peripheral vascular disease, and cerebrovascular disease).
    - Patients who develop GVHD require prolonged immunosuppression with calcineurin inhibitors, corticosteroids, and/or mTOR inhibitors. These medications are associated with hyperlipidemia, hypertension, and diabetes mellitus, all of which are risk factors for CV disease.
    - Frequent blood transfusions raise the risk for iron overload, which may lead to cardiomyopathy.

Hematopoietic Cell Transplantation Survivorship Considerations

- Currently, there is no universal strategy for monitoring long-term transplant survivors for CV complications. Efforts should focus on prevention and early treatment of CV risk factors.[9,10]

- Routine clinical assessment for all HCT survivors is recommended on an annual basis.
- **Aggressive CV risk factor modification should be implemented (smoking cessation, blood pressure control, lipid management, weight control, glycemic control, therapeutic lifestyle modification).**
- Patients should receive counseling and education regarding regular exercise and a heart-healthy diet.
- CV symptoms should be thoroughly investigated with cardiac biomarkers, transthoracic echocardiography, Holter monitoring, and/or stress testing as clinically indicated.
- In patients requiring frequent blood transfusions, measures should be taken to avoid iron overload.

CARDIAC COMPLICATIONS OF CHRONIC GRAFT-VERSUS-HOST DISEASE

- Chronic GVHD is the leading cause of non-relapse morbidity and mortality after allo-HCT, occurring in 40% to 60% of long-term survivors. It is characterized by immune dysregulation and associated with increased morbidity, risk of infections, and reduction of functionality, resulting both from the disease itself and long-term immunosuppression. The most commonly involved organ systems are skin, eyes, mouth, musculoskeletal system, gut, liver, and lungs.
- Although chronic "cardiac" GVHD is rare and not clearly defined, there are important indirect CV effects of chronic GVHD.
  - All of the immunosuppressant medications used to treat chronic GVHD have CV adverse effects (Table 18-4), which predispose to adverse CV events.
  - Increased LV mass and impaired diastolic function have been reported in patients with chronic GVHD.[14]

TABLE 18-4 Immunosuppressant Drugs and Side Effects

Drugs	Significant adverse effects
Corticosteroids	Hypertension, diabetes, myopathy, obesity, adrenal suppression
Calcineurin inhibitors (tacrolimus, cyclosporine)	Hypertension, nephrotoxicity, tremor, diabetes, hyperlipidemia, squamous cell skin cancer, arrhythmias, congestive heart failure
Methotrexate	Hepatotoxicity, pulmonary toxicity, nephrotoxicity, prothrombotic state, diabetes
Mycophenolate mofetil	Hypertension, edema, tachycardia, hyperlipidemia, diabetes, gastrointestinal toxicity, liver toxicity
Sirolimus	Edema, prothrombotic state, hypertension, hyperlipidemia, diabetes

- Chronic, systemic inflammation results in increased risk of arterial vascular disease (coronary artery disease, peripheral vascular disease, cerebrovascular disease) in patients with chronic GVHD.
- **Aggressive CV risk factor modification and prompt investigation of symptoms suggestive of arterial vascular disease are necessary for patients with chronic GVHD.**

REFERENCES

1. Bhatia S, Francisco L, Carter A, et al. Late mortality after allogeneic hematopoietic cell transplantation and functional status of long-term survivors: report from the Bone Marrow Transplant Survivor Study. *Blood*. 2007;110(10):3784-3792. doi:10.1182/blood-2007-03-082933
2. Bhatia S, Robison LL, Francisco L, et al. Late mortality in survivors of autologous hematopoietic-cell transplantation: report from the Bone Marrow Transplant Survivor Study. *Blood*. 2005;105(11):4215-4222. doi:10.1182/blood-2005-01-0035
3. Armenian SH, Chemaitilly W, Chen M, et al. National Institutes of Health hematopoietic cell transplantation late effects initiative: the cardiovascular disease and associated risk factors working group report. *Biol Blood Marrow Transplant*. 2017;23(2):201-210. doi:10.1016/j.bbmt.2016.08.019
4. Fuchs EJ. Haploidentical transplantation for hematologic malignancies: where do we stand? *Hematology Am Soc Hematol Educ Program*. 2012;2012:230-236. doi:10.1182/asheducation-2012.1.230
5. Coghlan JG, Handler CE, Kottaridis PD. Cardiac assessment of patients for haematopoietic stem cell transplantation. *Best Pract Res Clin Haematol*. 2007;20(2):247-263. doi:10.1016/j.beha.2006.09.005
6. Majhail NS, Tao L, Bredeson C, et al. Prevalence of hematopoietic cell transplant survivors in the United States. *Biol Blood Marrow Transplant*. 2013;19(10):1498-1501. doi:10.1016/j.bbmt.2013.07.020
7. Tonorezos ES, Stillwell EE, Calloway JJ, et al. Arrhythmias in the setting of hematopoietic cell transplants. *Bone Marrow Transplant*. 2015;50(9):1212-1216. doi:10.1038/bmt.2015.127
8. Rackley C, Schultz KR, Goldman FD, et al. Cardiac manifestations of graft-versus-host disease. *Biol Blood Marrow Transplant*. 2005;11(10):773-780.
9. Majhail NS, Rizzo JD, Lee SJ, et al. Recommended screening and preventive practices for long-term survivors after hematopoietic cell transplantation. *Bone Marrow Transplant*. 2012;47(3):337-341. doi:10.1038/bmt.2012.5
10. Armenian SH, Chow EJ. Cardiovascular disease in survivors of hematopoietic cell transplantation. *Cancer*. 2014;120(4):469-479. doi:10.1002/cncr.28444
11. Tichelli A, Bhatia S, Socie G. Cardiac and cardiovascular consequences after haematopoietic stem cell transplantation. *Br J Haematol*. 2008;142(1):11-26. doi:10.1111/j.1365-2141.2008.07165.x
12. Sun CL, Francisco L, Kawashima T, et al. Prevalence and predictors of chronic health conditions after hematopoietic cell transplantation: a report from the Bone Marrow Transplant Survivor Study. *Blood*. 2010;116(17):3129-3139; quiz 3377. doi:10.1182/blood-2009-06-229369
13. Ratosa I, Ivanetic Pantar M. Cardiotoxicity of mediastinal radiotherapy. *Rep Pract Oncol Radiother*. 2019;24(6):629-643. doi:10.1016/j.rpor.2019.09.002
14. Dogan A, Dogdu O, Ozdogru I, et al. Cardiac effects of chronic graft-versus-host disease after stem cell transplantation. *Tex Heart Inst J*. 2013;40(4):428-434.

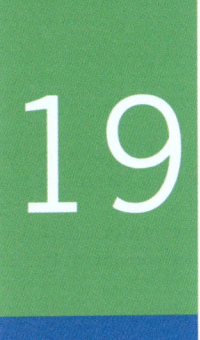

19 Drug-Drug Interactions and the Importance of a PharmD

Marissa Olson

GENERAL PRINCIPLES

- Cancer treatment has vastly improved over the past 10 years, leading to an increased life span of patients with cancer.
- More patients being treated for a malignancy are concurrently being treated for chronic medical conditions. Specifically, many patients face cardiac complications and are on multiple medications to manage heart failure, coronary artery disease, atrial fibrillation, hypertension, etc.[1]
- Cancer therapy and many medications used to manage cardiac conditions are metabolized and/or affect the cytochrome P (CYP) 450 monooxygenase system and other drug transporters, resulting in a high frequency of drug-drug interactions.
- The availability of oral antineoplastics has also increased substantially and nearly a quarter of drugs in development are oral medications. One study found that nearly 50% of patients on oral chemotherapy experienced a drug interaction related to their treatment.[2,3]
- Drug-drug interactions can lead to either increased drug exposure and toxicity or decreased drug exposure and efficacy. The narrow therapeutic index of most antineoplastics and many cardiac medications makes this particularly concerning.
- Management of drug interactions is vital to improving patient outcomes and quality of life.

Definitions

- **Pharmacokinetic drug-drug interactions are the result of changes in absorption, distribution, metabolism, or elimination of a combination of drugs. Metabolism through the CYP450 system is an example of a pharmacokinetic interaction.**[2,4]
- The CYP450 system is a family of >100 genetically similar enzymes located primarily in the liver that are responsible for drug metabolism.[5]
  - A CYP450 substrate is a drug that is metabolized by the CYP450 system.
  - A CYP450 inducer increases the enzymatic activity of the system and often results in a reduction in efficacy of a substrate.
  - A CYP450 inhibitor decreases the enzymatic activity of the system.[6,7]
    - A strong inhibitor is defined by its ability to produce a >5-fold increase in the plasma area under the curve (AUC) of a substrate and/or an 80% reduction in drug clearance.
    - A 2- to 5-fold increase in plasma AUC of a substrate and/or 50% to 80% decrease in clearance is referred to as a moderate inhibitor.

- A weak inhibitor results in a 1.25- to 2-fold increase in plasma AUC of a substrate and/or 20% to 50% decrease in drug clearance.
- P-glycoprotein (p-gp) is an efflux pump most commonly found in the intestine, liver, kidney, and around the blood-brain barrier. It can alter the absorption and elimination of drugs.[8]
- **Pharmacodynamic drug interactions may also occur when medications exert synergistic, additive, or antagonistic effects because of similar mechanisms of action.**[4]

Cytochrome P450 3A4 Pathway

- CYP3A4 is the most common CYP450 enzyme in humans that is responsible for metabolizing 45% to 60% of drugs in use.[5]
- **A significant number of antineoplastic and anti-infective agents commonly utilized in treating patients with cancer inhibit or induce CYP3A4.** Examples include:
  - Antineoplastic CYP3A4 inhibitors[6]:
    - Strong: Ceritinib, idelalisib, tucatinib
    - Moderate: Crizotinib, duvelisib, imatinib, nilotinib, ribociclib
  - Antineoplastic CYP3A4 inducers: Enzalutamide, dabrafenib[6]
  - Anti-infective CYP3A4 inhibitors[6]
    - Moderate: Fluconazole, isavuconazole, letermovir
    - Strong: Posaconazole, voriconazole
- These medications can have significant effects on CYP3A4 substrates used to manage cardiac conditions including the following medications in each class[6]:
  - Direct oral anticoagulants (DOACs): Apixaban and rivaroxaban
    - Dabigatran and edoxaban are not metabolized by the CYP3A4 and may be preferred in the appropriate clinical setting when CYP3A4 inhibitors/inducers are necessary. See Table 19-1 for guidance on managing drug interactions with DOACs.
    - Alternatively, enoxaparin may be utilized to avoid significant drug interactions.
  - Hydroxymethylglutaryl-CoA (HMG-CoA) reductase inhibitors (statins): Atorvastatin, lovastatin, and simvastatin
    - Fluvastatin, pravastatin, pitavastatin, and rosuvastatin are not significantly metabolized by CYP3A4 and may be preferred when CYP3A4 inhibitors/inducers are necessary. See Table 19-2 for guidance on management of drug interactions with statins.
  - Antiarrhythmics: Amiodarone, dronedarone, dofetilide
    - Flecainide and sotalol are not substrates of CYP3A4 and would not be impacted by CYP3A4 inhibitors/inducers.
  - Calcium channel blockers (CCBs): Dihydropyridines (amlodipine, nicardipine, nifedipine) and nondihydropyridines (diltiazem and verapamil)
    - Clevidipine is not a CYP3A4 substrate.
  - Additional examples: eplerenone, ivabradine, ranolazine, and ticagrelor
- Tables 19-1, 19-2, and 19-3 summarize monitoring and recommendations for managing potential drug interactions.
- Diltiazem and verapamil are moderate inhibitors of CYP3A4. Many antineoplastics and immunosuppressants used to manage patients undergoing allogeneic hematopoietic cell transplant are CYP3A4 substrates. Examples and drug interaction management strategies are summarized in Tables 19-4 and 19-5.[6,9]

TABLE 19-1 Managing Drug Interactions With Direct Oral Anticoagulants

	Apixaban	Rivaroxaban	Dabigatran	Edoxaban
Substrate	CYP3A4, P-gp (minor)	CYP3A4, P-gp (minor)	P-gp	P-gp
CYP3A4 inducers (dabrafenib, enzalutamide)	May DECREASE concentration and result in therapy failure. Avoid if possible.	May DECREASE concentration and result in therapy failure. Avoid if possible.	—	—
Moderate CYP3A4 inhibitors (crizotinib, duvelisib, imatinib, nilotinib, ribociclib)	May INCREASE concentration and risk of bleeding. Monitor therapy.	May INCREASE concentration and risk of bleeding. Monitor therapy.	—	—
Strong CYP3A4 inhibitors (ceritinib, idelalisib)				
P-gp inducers (lorlatinib)	May DECREASE concentration and result in therapy failure. Monitor for reduced efficacy.	May DECREASE concentration and result in therapy failure. Monitor for reduced efficacy.	May DECREASE concentration and result in therapy failure. Avoid combination.	May DECREASE concentration and result in therapy failure. Monitor for reduced efficacy.
P-gp inhibitors (capmatinib, lapatinib, neratinib, osimertinib, vemurafenib)	May INCREASE concentration. No action needed.	May INCREASE concentration. No action needed.	May INCREASE concentration of and risk of bleeding. Monitor therapy.	

CYP, cytochrome P; P-gp, P-glycoprotein.

From Lexicomp Online. Web applications access. Accessed December 3, 2020. https://online.lexi.com/lco/action/home; Asnani A, Manning A, Mansour M, et al. Management of atrial fibrillation in patients taking targeted cancer therapies. Cardio-Oncol. 2017;3:2-10.

TABLE 19-2 Managing HMG-CoA Reductase Inhibitor (Statin) Drug-Drug Interactions

	Atorvastatin	**Lovastatin**	**Simvastatin**
Major substrate	CYP3A4, OATP1B1/1B3	CYP3A4	CYP3A4
Strong CYP3A4 inhibitors *Antineoplastics*: ceritinib, idelalisib, tucatinib; *Anti-infectives*: posaconazole, voriconazole	Avoid use.	Avoid use.	Avoid use.
Moderate CYP3A4 inhibitors *Antineoplastics*: crizotinib, duvelisib, imatinib, nilotinib, ribociclib; *Anti-infectives*: fluconazole, isavuconazole	Monitor for increased risk of toxicity.	Monitor for increased risk of toxicity.	Monitor for increased risk of toxicity.
Dual inhibitor of OATP1B1/1B3 and CYP3A4 *Anti-infective*: letermovir	Use is not recommended. If used, limit dose to 20 mg. Use is contraindicated if coadministered with cyclosporine.	Monitor for increased risk of toxicities. Use is not recommended if coadministered with cyclosporine.	Use is not recommended. Use is contraindicated if coadministered with cyclosporine.
Inhibitor of OATP1B1/1B3, BCRP, P-gp, CYP2C9, CYP3A4 *Immunosuppressant*: cyclosporine	Use is not recommended. Limit dose to 10 mg daily.	Use is not recommended.	Use is contraindicated.
CYP3A4 inducers *Antineoplastics*: enzalutamide, dabrafenib	Avoid use.	Avoid use.	Avoid use.

	Fluvastatin	**Pitavastatin**	**Pravastatin**	**Rosuvastatin**
Major substrate	CYP2C9, OATP1B1/1B3	OATP1B1/1B3, UGT1A3, UGT2B7	OATP1B1/1B3	BCRP/ABCG2, OATP1B1/1B3
Moderate CYP2C9 inhibitors *Anti-infective:* fluconazole	Monitor for increased risk of toxicity. Do not exceed 20 mg daily.	—	—	—
Dual inhibitor of OATP1B1/1B3 and CYP3A4 *Anti-infective:* letermovir	Monitor for increased risk of toxicities.	Use is not recommended. Contraindicated if coadministered with cyclosporine.	Monitor for increased risk of toxicities.	Monitor for increased risk of toxicities.
Dual BCRP and OATP1B1/1B3 *Antineoplastics:* darolutamide and enasidenib	—	—	—	Monitor for increased risk of toxicity. In patients taking darolutamide limit dose to 5 mg daily.
BCRP inhibitors *Antineoplastic:* regorafenib	—	—	—	Monitor for increased risk of toxicity. Limit dose to 10 mg daily.
Inhibitor of OATP1B1/1B3, BCRP, P-gp, CYP2C9, CYP3A4 *Immunosuppressant:* cyclosporine	Monitor for increased risk of toxicity. Limit dose to 20 mg twice daily.	Use is contraindicated.	Monitor for increased risk of toxicity. Initiate at 10 mg daily and limit the max dose to 20 mg daily.	Monitor for increased risk of toxicity. Limit dose to 5 mg daily.

CYP, cytochrome P; HMG-CoA, hydroxymethylglutaryl-CoA; P-gp, P-glycoprotein.
From Lexicomp Online. Web applications access. Accessed December 3, 2020. https://online.lexi.com/lco/action/home

TABLE 19-3 Managing Drug Interactions of Antiarrhythmics and CCBs Metabolized by CYP3A4

	Recommendations for use with strong CYP3A4 inhibitors (*Antineoplastics*: ceritinib, idelalisib, tucatinib; *Antifungals*: posaconazole, voriconazole)	Recommendations for use with moderate CYP3A4 inhibitors (*Antineoplastics*: crizotinib, duvelisib, imatinib, nilotinib, ribociclib; *Anti-infectives*: fluconazole, isavuconazole, letermovir)
Amiodarone, dronedarone	May increase drug concentration. Use is contraindicated.	May increase drug concentration. Carefully monitor for increased risk of toxicity. Avoid use with moderate CYP3A4 inhibitors with a risk of QT prolongation.
Dofetilide	May increase concentration. Use is contraindicated with posaconazole and voriconazole because of risk of QT prolongation. May be administered cautiously with other strong CYP3A4 inhibitors.	May increase concentration of dofetilide. Carefully monitor for increased risk of toxicity. Avoid use with moderate CYP3A4 inhibitors with a risk of QT prolongation.
Dihydropyridine CCBs (amlodipine, felodipine, nicardipine, nifedipine)	May increase drug exposure and adverse events. Avoid use if possible.	May increase drug concentration. Dose reductions may be needed. Monitor for increased effects and toxicity.
Non-dihydropyridine CCBs (diltiazem, verapamil)	May increase concentration and enhance inotropic properties. Avoid use if possible.	May increase drug concentration. Dose reductions may be needed. Monitor for increased effects and toxicity.

	Recommendations for use with strong CYP3A4 inhibitors	Recommendations for use with moderate CYP3A4 inhibitors
Eplerenone	Will increase serum concentration. Use is contraindicated.	May increase drug concentration. For the treatment of heart failure limit dose to 25 mg daily. For the treatment of hypertension limit dose to 25 mg twice daily.
	Spironolactone is preferred when there is a concern for concomitant use with CYP3A4 inhibitors.	
Ivabradine	Will increase serum concentration. Use is contraindicated.	Will increase serum concentration. Avoid if possible. May consider initiation in patients with resting heart rate >70 beats/min at 2.5 mg twice daily.
Ranolazine	May result in significant increases in drug exposure. Use is contraindicated.	May increase serum concentration. Limit dose to 500 mg twice daily and monitor for increased toxicities.
Ticagrelor	May result in significant increases in ticagrelor exposure. Use is contraindicated.	May increase ticagrelor exposure. Monitor for increased toxicity (ie, bleeding).

CCB, calcium channel blocker; CYP, cytochrome P.

From Lexicomp Online. Web applications access. Accessed December 3, 2020. https://online.lexi.com/lco/action/home; Asnani A, Manning A, Mansour M, et al. Management of atrial fibrillation in patients taking targeted cancer therapies. *Cardio-Oncol.* 2017;3:2-10.

TABLE 19-4 Managing Antineoplastics That Are Substrates of CYP3A4 or P-gp

	Moderate CYP3A4 inhibitors (eg, Diltiazem, verapamil)	P-gp inhibitors (eg, amiodarone)
Avoid use	Bosutinib, ivosidenib	Doxorubicin, pazopanib, topotecan
Monitor for increased risk of toxicity	Axitinib, bortezomib, cabozantinib, copanlisib, dasatinib, erlotinib, gilteritinib, ibrutinib (for GVHD), imatinib, midostaurin, palbociclib, pazopanib, ruxolitinib, sunitinib, trabectedin, vemurafenib, vincristine	Etoposide
Dose adjustments	Acalabrutinib: Reduce to 100 mg daily.	Afatinib: Reduce dose to 10 mg daily.
	Ibrutinib for B-cell malignancies: Reduce to 280 mg daily.	Venetoclax: Reduce dose by 50%.
	Olaparib tablets: Reduce to 150 mg twice daily.	—
	Olaparib capsules: Reduce to 200 mg twice daily.	
	Venetoclax: Reduce dose by 50%.	—
	Zanubrutinib: Reduce dose to 80 mg BID.	—
Monitor for reduced therapeutic effects	Cyclophosphamide, ifosfamide (CYP3A4 is responsible for converting these agents to their active metabolite.)	—

CYP, cytochrome P; GVHD, graft-versus-host disease; P-gp, P-glycoprotein.

From Lexicomp Online. Web applications access. Accessed December 3, 2020. https://online.lexi.com/lco/action/home; Asnani A, Manning A, Mansour M, et al. Management of atrial fibrillation in patients taking targeted cancer therapies. *Cardio-Oncol*. 2017;3:2-10.

TABLE 19-5 — Managing Immunosuppression

	Cyclosporine, Tacrolimus, Sirolimus	Ruxolitinib
Substrate	CYP3A4 and P-gp	CYP3A4
Moderate CYP3A4 inhibitors (diltiazem, verapamil)	May increase drug exposure. Increase monitoring of serum drug levels.	May increase drug exposure. Monitor for an increase in cytopenias and adjust dose as clinically indicated per package insert.
P-gp inhibitors (amiodarone, dronedarone)	May increase drug exposure. Increase monitoring of serum drug levels.	–

CYP, cytochrome P; P-gp, P-glycoprotein.
From Lexicomp Online. Web applications access. Accessed December 3, 2020. https://online.lexi.com/lco/action/home; Asnani A, Manning A, Mansour M, et al. Management of atrial fibrillation in patients taking targeted cancer therapies. *Cardio-Oncol.* 2017;3:2-10.

Cytochrome P450 2C19 Pathway

- **The most pertinent cardiac medication that requires CYP2C19 metabolism is clopidogrel. It is a prodrug that requires CYP2C19 to be converted to its active metabolite.**[5,6]
- Fluconazole and voriconazole are inhibitors of CYP2C19 metabolism. Both should be avoided with concurrent clopidogrel use because of potential reduced concentrations of the active metabolite and diminished activity.[6]

Cytochrome P450 2C9 Pathway

- Warfarin is a major substrate of the CYP2C9 pathway. It is also a minor substrate of CYP1A2, CYP2C19, and CYP3A4.[4,6]
- **Managing the variability in warfarin pharmacokinetics is of increased importance in patients undergoing treatment for cancer because of an inherent increased risk for thromboembolic events. Conversely, thrombocytopenia and bleeding are common.**
  - CYP2C9 inducers that can decrease the therapeutic effect of warfarin include alpelisib, bicalutamide, and enzalutamide. Increased international normalized ratio (INR) monitoring is recommended when initiating or discontinuing these medications.[4,6]
  - CYP2C9 inhibitors that can increase warfarin exposure and potential toxicity are capecitabine, 5-fluorouracil, fluconazole, sorafenib, tamoxifen, and voriconazole. Increased INR monitoring is recommended.[4,6]
  - Warfarin is contraindicated with tamoxifen (a potent inhibitor of CYP2C9) that can increase warfarin concentrations by up to 60%.[6]
  - Warfarin is not recommended for use in combination with capecitabine because of the sporadic dosing schedule of capecitabine, leading to unpredictable INR changes.

- This is only a summary of antineoplastics that can alter warfarin metabolism. Prior to initiating warfarin therapy, it is important to consult the package insert and tertiary resources to assess for drug interactions.

P-glycoprotein
- Digoxin is a major substrate for the p-gp drug transporter system. Examples of antineoplastics that can inhibit p-gp include capmatinib, lapatinib, osimertinib, neratinib, and tucatinib, and vemurafenib. Lorlatinib is an inducer of p-gp.[6]
  - Measure serum digoxin concentrations prior to initiation of the p-gp inhibitors. Reduce digoxin dosage by 15% to 30% and continue monitoring serum concentrations.[6]
  - Reduce digoxin dosage by 30% to 50% prior to the initiation of lapatinib or vemurafenib.
  - Increase digoxin dosage by 20% to 40% prior to the initiation of lorlatinib.[6]
- DOACs are also substrates of p-gp. Table 19-1 describes appropriate management of these drug interactions.[9]
- Amiodarone is an inhibitor of the p-gp drug transporter system. It can inhibit the metabolism of the following:[6]
  - Antineoplastics: Afatinib, doxorubicin, etoposide, pazopanib, topotecan
  - Immunosuppressants: Cyclosporine, tacrolimus, sirolimus
- Tables 19-4 and 19-5 describe the management of clinically significant drug interactions involving p-gp in more detail.

PHARMACODYNAMIC DRUG INTERACTIONS

- Bleeding: Ibrutinib, acalabrutinib, zanubrutinib, and dasatinib have inhibitory effects on platelets. Use these agents with caution in patients receiving antiplatelet or anticoagulant therapy as they may increase the risk of bleeding.[4,6]
- Hyperkalemia: Cyclosporine and tacrolimus can cause hyperkalemia. This adverse event can be potentiated by concurrent use with angiotensin-II receptor blockers, angiotensin-II-converting enzyme inhibitors, and potassium-sparing diuretics.[6]
- Rhabdomyolysis: HMG-CoA reductase inhibitors may enhance the myopathic effect of trabectedin. Use with caution and increase creatine phosphokinase monitoring.[6]
- Bradycardia: Avoid ceritinib and crizotinib in combination with other agents that can cause bradycardia (ie, beta-blockers, diltiazem, verapamil, digoxin) as the bradycardic effect may be exacerbated. Refer to the package insert for dose adjustments because of symptomatic bradycardia if concomitant use cannot be avoided.[5,6]

RESOURCES

- **It is vital to use clinical judgment and work as part of a multidisciplinary team to prospectively identify and manage drug-drug interactions when dealing with this complex patient population.**
- The package insert for each medication and tertiary drug resources (Lexicomp, Micromedex, Facts and Comparisons) should be consulted to identify and manage drug interactions.[4]
- Appropriate identification and analysis of drug interactions will help to improve medication efficacy, reduce the potential for adverse events, and improve overall patient quality of life.

REFERENCES

1. Parsad S, Ratain M. Drug-drug interactions with oral antineoplastic agents. *JAMA Oncol.* 2017;3:736-738.
2. Van Leeuwen RWF, Brundel DHS, Neef C, et al. Prevalence of potential drug-drug interactions in cancer patients treated with oral anticancer drugs. *Br J Cancer.* 2013;108:1071-1078.
3. Solomon J, Ajewole V, Schneider A, Sharma M, Bernicker E. Evaluation of the prescribing pattern, adverse effects, and drug interactions of oral chemotherapy agents in an outpatient cancer center. *J Oncol Pharm Pract.* 2019;25:1564-1569.
4. Rogala B, Charpentier M, Nguyen M, et al. Oral anticancer therapy: management of drug interactions. *J Oncol Pract.* 2019;15:81-90.
5. Fatunde O, Brown, SA. The role of CYP450 drug metabolism in precision cardio-oncology. *Int J Mol Sci.* 2020;21:604.
6. Lexicomp Online. Web applications access. Accessed December 3, 2020. https://online.lexi.com/lco/action/home
7. Segal E, Flood M, Mancini R, et al. Oral chemotherapy food and drug interactions: a comprehensive review of the literature. *J Oncol Pract.* 2014;10:e255-e268.
8. Van Leeuwen RWF, Van Gelder T, Mathijssen RHJ, Jansman FGA. Drug-drug interactions with tyrosine-kinase inhibitors: a clinical perspective. *Lancet Oncol.* 2014;15:e315-e326.
9. Asnani A, Manning A, Mansour M, et al. Management of atrial fibrillation in patients taking targeted cancer therapies. *Cardio-Oncol.* 2017;3:2-10.

20 Permissive Cardiotoxicity

Brandon W. Lennep and Joshua D. Mitchell

- **Cancer therapy–related cardiotoxicity** (CTRC) has been variously defined in prior research, often with a focus on myocardial dysfunction (Table 1-1, Chapter 1). However, the adverse cardiovascular effects of cancer therapies are broad and may also include arrhythmia/conduction abnormalities, hypertension, venous thromboembolism (VTE), pericardial disease, and vascular toxicity.
- **Permissive cardiotoxicity** is the principle that cancer treatment can often be continued when the benefits of further cancer treatment outweigh the risks of further cardiac deterioration. Cardioprotective medications and comanagement with a cardio-oncologist can help reduce the risk of cardiac deterioration in the setting of ongoing treatment.

GENERAL PRINCIPLES

Definition
- The suspicion of CTRC should always trigger a prompt and thorough cardiovascular evaluation. Situations have been identified, though, in which **cancer treatment may be safely continued despite diagnosis of CTRC**.
- Relatedly, patients may also be found to have baseline cardiovascular disease on pretreatment screening. These patients may also be safely treated under similar circumstances.
- A **thorough upfront cardiovascular evaluation** (ideally prior to initiation of cancer therapy) can help identify those patients at highest risk who may benefit from further cardiovascular optimization and/or initiation of cardioprotective medications.
- When either baseline cardiac dysfunction or CTRC is diagnosed, effective **multidisciplinary** discussions among the cardio-oncologist, hematologist/oncologist, radiation oncologist, and other treating specialists are paramount to ensure **clear communication** of the **overall risk-benefit profile** of any proposed alteration to the patient's treatment plan (Fig. 20-1).
- **Etiologies of cardiotoxicity** other than cancer therapy must also be kept in mind, as there is significant overlap between traditional risk factors for cardiovascular disease and for various forms of malignancy. Further, the presence of active malignancy often results in an inflammatory, prothrombotic state that may subject the patient to further incremental cardiovascular risk independent of the cancer treatment (eg, takotsubo cardiomyopathy and VTE).
- The severity of left ventricular (LV) dysfunction, or cardiotoxicity in general, will certainly influence management decisions. There is growing evidence that cancer therapy can usually be continued with milder forms of cardiotoxicity, such as

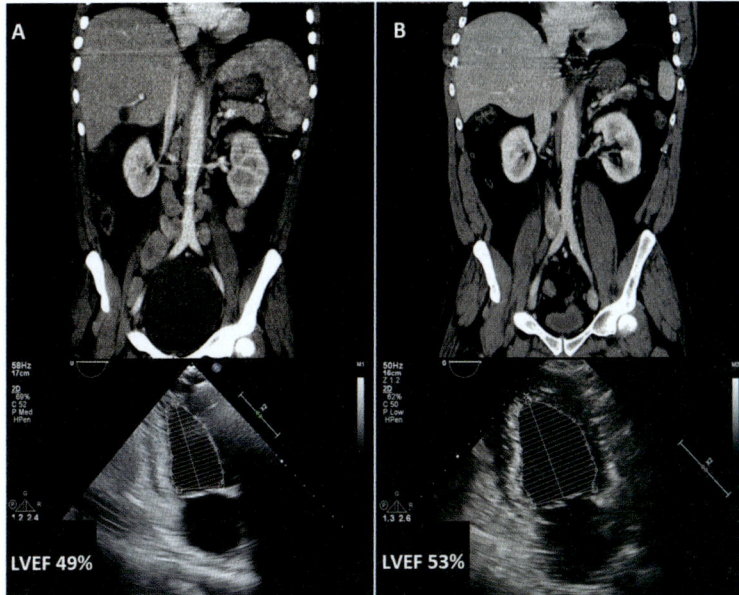

Figure 20-1. A 40-year-old male with newly diagnosed stage IVb classical Hodgkin lymphoma. Prior to treatment, CT shows extensive paraaortic and inguinal (as well as mediastinal and supraclavicular) lymphadenopathy and baseline echocardiogram reveals borderline LV function with LVEF 49% (A). He is started on carvedilol and losartan, then treated with A+AVD (doxorubicin component of the first round was held) with significant clinical improvement. Follow-up CT imaging after cycle 3 (B) shows drastic improvement in the lymphadenopathy and repeat echocardiogram shows LVEF 53%. He remains on treatment with no heart failure decompensation. A+AVD, brentuximab vedotin, doxorubicin, vinblastine, dacarbazine; CT, computed tomography; LV, left ventricular; LVEF, left ventricular ejection fraction.

human epidermal growth factor receptor 2 (HER2) antagonists in the setting of mild LV dysfunction.[1] A careful **risk-benefit analysis** should be employed as the severity of cardiotoxicity increases.
- **Optimal screening and close monitoring** can potentially diagnose cardiotoxicity early, allowing prompt initiation of treatment to mitigate toxicity and reduce need for treatment pauses or discontinuation. Even in the setting of mild LV dysfunction, **cardioprotective medications and optimal cardiovascular management** can often allow the **continuation of cardiotoxic cancer treatment** including anthracyclines and HER2 antagonists (see section that follows).

PREVENTION

- Any "permissive cardiotoxicity" strategy begins with prevention, as **preventing cardiotoxicity will always be the most effective option, when possible**, at enabling maximal cancer therapy to be administered.

- Extensive efforts have thus been made to identify upfront treatments capable of preventing the development or further worsening of cancer therapy–related cardiac dysfunction (CTRCD), especially with anthracycline chemotherapy, and research is ongoing (Table 20-1).
- Administration of **dexrazoxane** alongside anthracyclines has demonstrated perhaps the strongest beneficial effect (see "Selected Specific Drugs/Therapies" section). Although its widespread use has been hindered by previous, unfounded concerns over potential decreased antitumor efficacy, these concerns have not borne out in further research. In a recent study in sarcoma, dexrazoxane allowed for the use of high doses of doxorubicin (up to nearly 3 g/m^2) with minimal cardiotoxicity and significant improvement in progression-free survival compared to historical controls.[2]
- **Neurohormonal antagonism** with β-blockers, angiotensin-converting enzyme inhibitors (ACEi), and angiotensin receptor blockers (ARBs) has also been a focus of research interest. Small sample sizes and differences in study populations and methodology have limited the generalizability of findings to date. However, in aggregate, the results of several studies have suggested that **patients at increased risk for cardiotoxicity receiving anthracycline chemotherapy likely benefit from cardioprotective therapy**, with weaker evidence in patients receiving HER2-targeted therapy. At a minimum, an argument can certainly be made that patients who already require antihypertensive therapy may benefit from preferential use of antihypertensives that have cardioprotective properties.
- Among the β-blockers, **carvedilol** has been suggested to confer a stronger protective effect potentially because of its antioxidant properties, whereas trials of metoprolol have overall been disappointing. There are no sufficient data to suggest preferential use of any specific **ACEi or ARB** over the others. Research is ongoing regarding the benefit of combination angiotensin receptor blockade and neprilysin inhibition via sacubitril/valsartan. Whether this combination drug will outperform the ACEi/ARB classes in the CTRCD arena (as it did in the treatment of chronic heart failure [HF] with reduced ejection fraction) remains to be seen.
- With regard to **atherosclerosis**, **statins** (or equivalent) and/or **aspirin** can be used to reduce the risk of atherosclerotic cardiovascular events in patients with increased baseline cardiovascular risk. Available computed tomographic (CT) imaging can be reviewed for the presence of **coronary calcifications** to target more aggressive preventive therapy (see Chapter 6).

EARLY IDENTIFICATION AND SUBCLINICAL LEFT VENTRICULAR DYSFUNCTION

- CTRC **exists on a spectrum** ranging from asymptomatic changes in serum biomarkers to florid cardiogenic shock. Monitoring for subclinical LV dysfunction may allow early detection of patients at higher risk for subsequent deterioration,[3] and thus who are more likely to benefit from **initiation of cardioprotective medications before more significant dysfunction develops**.
- Asymptomatic elevation in serum troponin levels at or shortly after administration of chemotherapy has been shown to be a predictor of poor cardiovascular outcomes. Among patients with such **elevated troponin levels**, administration of **ACEi** has demonstrated a reduction in incidence of significant decline in left ventricular ejection fraction (LVEF).[4]

TABLE 20-1 Selected Studies Suggesting Benefit of Cardioprotective Medical Therapy

Trial	Study group	Treatment	Follow-up	Primary outcome	Results
ACEi/ARB					
Cardinale et al (2006)[4]	$n = 114$. Various malignancies and chemotherapies with elevated troponin I early after chemotherapy	Enalapril vs. placebo	12 months	Absolute decrease in LVEF >10 percentage points to <50%	Enalapril group: 0/56 Placebo group: 25/58
Janbabai et al 2017[19]	$n = 69$. Various malignancies (primarily breast cancer and lymphoma) treated with anthracyclines	Enalapril vs. placebo	6 months	Change in LVEF from baseline	Enalapril pre/post-LVEF: 59.4%/59.9% Placebo pre/post-LVEF: 59.6%/46.3%
β-blocker					
Kaya et al 2013[20]	$n = 45$. Breast cancer patients treated with anthracyclines	Nebivolol vs. placebo	6 months	Change in LVEF from baseline	Nebivolol pre/post-LVEF: 65.6%/63.8% Placebo pre/post-LVEF: 66.6%/57.5%
Kalay et al 2006[21]	$n = 50$. Primarily breast cancer and lymphoma patients undergoing anthracycline therapy	Carvedilol vs. placebo	6 months	Change in LVEF from baseline	Carvedilol pre/post-LVEF: 70.5%/69.7% Placebo pre/post-LVEF: 68.9%/52.3%

(continued)

TABLE 20-1 Selected Studies Suggesting Benefit of Cardioprotective Medical Therapy (continued)

Nabati et al 2017[22]	n = 91. Breast cancer patients undergoing anthracycline therapy	Carvedilol vs. placebo	6 months	Change in LVEF from baseline	Carvedilol pre/post-LVEF: 58.7%/57.4% Placebo pre/post-LVEF: 61.1%/51.7%

Dexrazoxane

Swain et al 1997[9]	n = 534 (two studies). Breast cancer patients treated with anthracyclines	Dexrazoxane vs. placebo	Median 397–532 days in the two studies	Fall in LVEF **or** development of CHF	Hazard ratios of placebo to dexrazoxane were 2.63 and 2.00 for the two studies.

Strain vs. LVEF-guided use of ACEi and β-blocker

Thavendiranathan et al 2021[5]	n = 331. Primarily breast cancer and lymphoma patients undergoing anthracycline therapy	Initiation of ACEi, β-blocker with drop in GLS (early) vs. initiation after drop in LVEF (delayed)	12 months	Fall in LVEF or development of CTRCD	Absolute change in LVEF was −3% in EF-guided group vs. −2.7% in GLS-guided group overall. Incidence of CTRCD was 13.7% in the EF-guided group vs. 5.8% in GLS-guided group.

ACEi, angiotensin-converting enzyme inhibitor; ARB, angiotensin receptor blocker; CTRCD, cancer therapy–related cardiac dysfunction; GLS, global longitudinal strain; LVEF, left ventricular ejection fraction.

- **Global longitudinal strain (GLS)** has also been shown to represent a potentially useful method of identifying patients with subclinical LV dysfunction during or after cancer therapy.
- In the **SUCCOUR trial**, cardioprotective medicines (ACEi or ARB, followed by β-blocker) initiated after a **relative drop in GLS of 12%** prevented subsequent decline in LVEF in patients treated with anthracyclines at increased risk for HF.[5]
- Patients with an abnormal baseline GLS with planned cardiotoxic cancer therapy should also be considered for cardioprotective medications.
- **GLS** has a significant advantage of **reduced variability and improved inter-reader reliability** relative to LVEF measurement. **Inter-vendor variability** in measurements do exist and should be taken into account if a patient has a follow-up examination using different equipment.
- It is important to note that **subclinical LV dysfunction**, regardless of the modality by which it is detected, **does not constitute grounds for discontinuation of chemotherapy**.

RISK-BENEFIT ANALYSIS

- As is true in most situations in the practice of medicine, the decision whether to modify or even discontinue cancer therapies because of more significant cardiovascular toxicity must be made in the context of careful considerations of risks and benefits of said therapies.
- Central to this decision is the consideration of cardiovascular disease caused by factors other than cancer therapeutic agents, particularly in light of the fact that there is a high incidence of cardiovascular disease in cancer patients at baseline because of overlap between risk factors for cardiovascular disease and various forms of malignancy. **The mere presence of cardiovascular disease, even when newly diagnosed during cancer treatment, should not be immediately construed as CTRCD.**
- The **tremendous benefit in cancer-related outcomes associated with certain antineoplastic agents must also be considered** when deciding how to proceed with cancer therapy in light of concurrent cardiovascular disease.
  - For example, the **checkpoint inhibitors have revolutionized care of multiple forms of cancer** previously associated with dismal prognosis. In cases where mild cardiotoxicity is diagnosed, the patient may stand to benefit from continued cancer treatment under the attentive care of a cardio-oncologist.
  - **Anthracyclines** are another drug class associated with **significant cancer benefits**, albeit their potential for adverse cardiovascular side effects. In any such situation, careful assessment of the severity of cardiotoxicity and vigilant ongoing monitoring are of paramount importance.
- In the general population, substantial reductions in cardiovascular morbidity and mortality can be achieved through **initiation and aggressive uptitration of guideline-directed medical therapies**. Although many of these therapies have not been extensively studied in patients with active malignancy, it is reasonable to expect some degree of cardiovascular benefit for this patient population as well. This becomes particularly pertinent for patients treated with cancer therapeutics not commonly known to cause cardiotoxicity, and the option to optimize cardiovascular medical therapies while continuing cancer therapies with close cardiovascular monitoring should not be overlooked (Fig. 20-2).

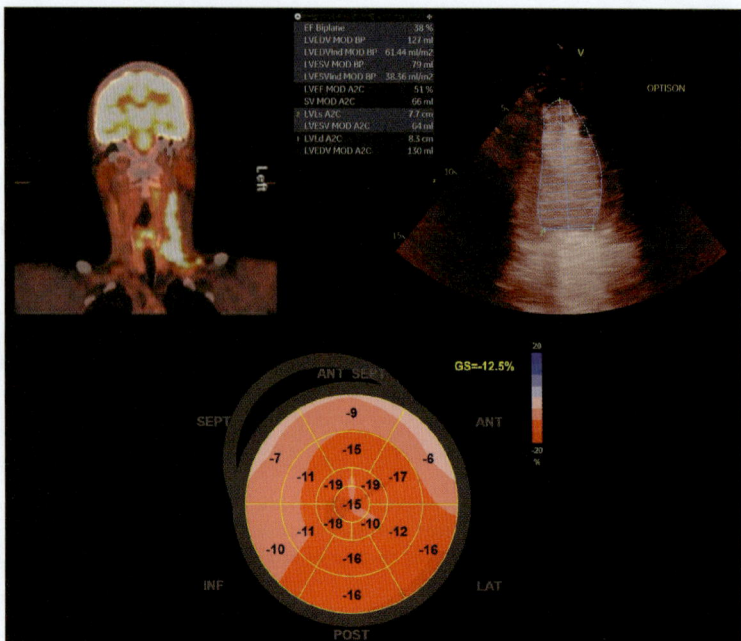

Figure 20-2. A 51-year-old male with history of Hodgkin lymphoma 6 years ago presents with relapse with extensive, FDG-avid, left cervical lymphadenopathy. Previously treated with ABVD for six cycles, he is started on ICE for two cycles and then transitioned to immunotherapy as he is evaluated for stem cell transplant. Pretransplant echocardiogram shows LVEF of 38% (GLS −12.5%). He is overall asymptomatic from a cardiovascular standpoint and is started on guideline-directed medical therapy. Repeat echocardiogram shows LVEF of 40% to 45% (not shown) and he undergoes cardiopulmonary stress test during which he achieves VO_2 max of 24.70 mL/kg/min. He proceeds forward with an autologous stem cell transplant, which he tolerates well with stable cardiac function 1 year later. ABVD, adriamycin, bleomycin, vinblastine, dacarbazine; ANT, anterior; FDG, ^{18}F-fluorodeoxyglucose; GLS, global longitudinal strain; ICE, ifosfamide, carboplatin, etoposide; INF, inferior; LAT, lateral; LVEF, left ventricular ejection fraction; POST, posterior; SEPT, septal; VO_2 max, maximum rate of oxygen used during exercise.

INDICATIONS TO STOP THERAPY

- The decision to withhold or discontinue a particular form of cancer therapy should always include **multidisciplinary discussion** regarding cardiovascular risk, cancer prognosis, availability of alternative treatments, and patient goals of care.
- Regardless of the degree of LV dysfunction, the development of signs and/or symptoms of the clinical syndrome of **decompensated congestive HF should generally prompt temporary cessation** of causative cancer therapies in order to reestablish a compensated state. After a patient is optimized, they can be clinically reevaluated for reinitiation of therapy.
- The development of **severely reduced LV function** portends a high risk of adverse cardiovascular outcomes irrespective of cancer diagnosis or treatment, and

thus in many cases will necessitate withholding of cancer therapies that risk continued exacerbation. **Management will vary depending on the agent being used**, however. Patients with LVEF as low as 20% may be able to be continued on bevacizumab therapy (a more mildly cardiotoxic agent) for some time with optimal guideline-directed medical therapy (Fig. 20-3), even though they usually would not be able to tolerate further treatment with anthracyclines.
- Progression to **cardiogenic shock** represents the extreme of this spectrum, at which point the short-term mortality risk is quite high and continuation of cardiotoxic cancer therapies is rarely justifiable.
- **Ventricular arrhythmias** also confer a high short-term risk of morbidity and mortality if left untreated. When these are suspected because of cancer therapies, said therapies should be discontinued in the vast majority of cases.
- **Acute myocardial infarctions** will require short-term cessation of therapy and appropriate treatment, though decisions on discontinuation of therapy should be made on a case-by-case basis, especially given the often multifactorial etiology.

SELECTED SPECIFIC DRUGS/THERAPIES

- Note that the following is not intended to represent a comprehensive list of all potentially cardiotoxic drugs/classes, but rather a summary of some of the more commonly encountered treatments in clinical practice.

Anthracyclines
- Despite their high efficacy in treatment of many forms of malignancy, the use of anthracyclines is limited by a dose-dependent risk of cardiotoxicity, which is further elevated by the presence of underlying heart disease.[6,7]

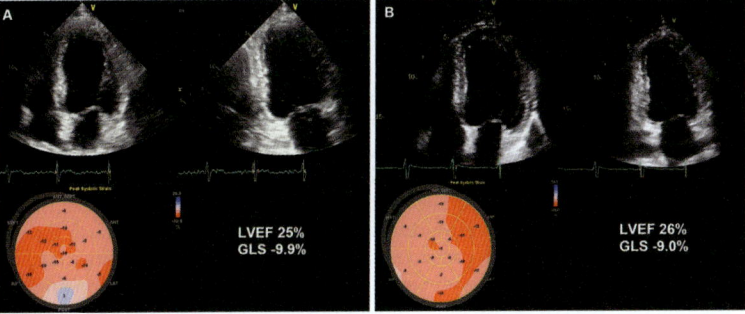

Figure 20-3. A 69-year-old with metastatic rectal adenocarcinoma being treated with FOLFORI and bevacizumab. Screening echocardiogram after cycle 8 of FOLFORI showed LVEF of 25%, GLS −9.9% (A). Patient referred to cardio-oncology and was noted to be hypervolemic (JVP 12-14 cm H$_2$O, no edema) with increased dyspnea and he was started on low doses of sacubitril/valsartan, carvedilol, and furosemide with rapid improvement in symptoms. Once compensated, he shortly resumed on FOLFIRI with bevacizumab with stability of his LVEF and GLS 7 months later (B). The patient eventually succumbed to cancer progression 17 months after his initial screening echocardiogram with no further heart failure exacerbations. FOLFORI, leucovorin calcium (folinic acid), fluorouracil, irinotecan hydrochloride; GLS, global longitudinal strain; JVP, jugular venous pressure; LVEF, left ventricular ejection fraction.

- Dexrazoxane has been demonstrated to have cardioprotective effect specifically in anthracycline exposure,[8,9] however its widespread use has been delayed by early concerns for possible reduced tumor response rate which were not supported by followup studies.[9] A Cochrane meta-analysis found that dexrazoxane successfully reduced incident HF without affecting progression-free or overall survival.[10]
- In a systematic review and meta-analysis of randomized controlled trial data, the use of liposomal doxorubicin versus conventional formulation and the use of continuous infusion versus bolus dosing have been associated with decreases in risk of clinical or subclinical cardiotoxicity.[11] It should be noted that most of the studies in the meta-analysis specifically excluded patients with baseline cardiac dysfunction, but given the higher risk of cardiotoxicity in such patients, these treatment modalities should be considered nonetheless.
- Limited data suggest that with concurrent administration of dexrazoxane and guideline-directed HF therapy, anthracyclines can be safely administered to anthracycline-naive patients with asymptomatic reduction in LVEF at baseline.[7]
- When a significant drop in LVEF occurs during anthracycline treatment, involved clinicians must carefully consider the risks and benefits of continuing the treatment. Keys to these considerations are the presence/absence of clinical congestive HF, degree of LV dysfunction, and alternative cancer therapies available. In cases of asymptomatic mild LV dysfunction, it is reasonable to continue anthracycline therapy with concurrent cardioprotective measures and close monitoring. This is particularly pertinent in diseases for which anthracycline therapy is associated with high cure rates, such as some forms of lymphoma.

Human Epidermal Growth Factor Receptor 2 Antagonists

- Breast cancer is the most common cancer among women, and approximately 20% of cases demonstrate amplification of the HER2 gene.[12] In many such cases, treatment with HER2-targeted therapies such as trastuzumab, pertuzumab, lapatinib, T-deruxtecan, and ado-trastuzumab emtansine (T-DM1) can improve outcomes.
- HER2-targeted therapies have been shown to cause decline in LVEF that is generally reversible with discontinuation of therapy and is thought to represent a distinct clinical entity separate from the cardiotoxicity caused by anthracyclines (with which they are frequently coadministered).[13,14]
- Food and Drug Administration (FDA)-approved package inserts for trastuzumab, pertuzumab, and T-DM1 recommend holding these drugs in the presence of either pretreatment or treatment-associated declines in LVEF (Table 1-1, Chapter 1).
- Based on data from retrospective reviews[14,15] suggesting that trastuzumab therapy can be safely continued with concurrent administration of cardioprotective medications in the setting of mild, asymptomatic decline in LVEF, two single-arm prospective studies have been carried out with similar results. See Table 20-2.

Checkpoint Inhibitors

- Immune checkpoint inhibitors have tremendously improved prognosis for many forms of malignancy, but have also been associated with immune-related adverse cardiovascular events including myocarditis, cardiomyopathy, pericarditis, and arrhythmia.[16]
- The incidence of immune checkpoint inhibitor–associated myocarditis has been reported to be around 1%, with a higher risk among patients treated with combination checkpoint inhibitor therapy.[17]

TABLE 20.2	Evidence for Safe Continuation of HER2 Therapy Despite Mild Cardiotoxicity	
	SAFE-HEaRt[1]	**SCHOLAR**[23]
n	30	20
Key Inclusion Criteria	• Stage I-IV breast cancer either currently receiving or planning to receive HER2-targeted therapy (trastuzumab, pertuzumab, or T-DM1) • LVEF 40%-49% at baseline	• Stage I-III, HER2-positive breast cancer treated with trastuzumab • LVEF 40%-54%, or >54% with absolute fall >15% from baseline
Key Exclusion Criteria	• Symptomatic HF • HF hospitalization within prior 12 months	• NYHA functional class III or IV • Systolic BP <90 mm Hg
Intervention	• β-blocker initiation and up-titration followed by ACEi if tolerated, with continuation of HER2-targeted therapy • Echocardiography at 6 weeks, 3/6/9/12 months	• ACEi/ARB and β-blocker initiation, with continuation of trastuzumab • Echocardiography at 6 weeks, 3/6/12/24 months
Primary Endpoint	Asymptomatic worsening of LVEF >10% points and/or LVEF <35%, occurrence of symptomatic HF, cardiac arrhythmia requiring treatment, MI, or death because of cardiac cause	Occurrence of cardiovascular death, LVEF <40% with any HF symptoms, or LVEF <35% regardless of symptoms
Result	• 90% of patients (27/30) were able to complete therapy; two patients developed symptomatic HF and 1 patient had asymptomatic decline in LVEF <35%. • No cardiac deaths on study	• 90% (18/20) patients were able to complete trastuzumab therapy; two patients developed LVEF <40% with HF symptoms. • No patient died of a cardiovascular complication.

ACEi, angiotensin-converting enzyme inhibitor; ARB, angiotensin receptor blocker; BP, blood pressure; HER, human epidermal growth factor receptor; HF, heart failure; LVEF, left ventricular ejection fraction; MI, myocardial infarction; NYHA, New York Heart Association; T-DM1, ado-trastuzumab emtansine.

- Although permanent discontinuation of therapy is appropriate for severe cases, those patients with mildly abnormal screening tests (electrocardiogram [ECG], echocardiogram) and no symptoms may be monitored off therapy until resolution or demonstrated stability of said abnormalities. Pending no clinical worsening, resumption of immune checkpoint inhibitor therapy under close monitoring can be considered in many such cases.[18]

In asymptomatic patients with mildly abnormal biomarkers and otherwise normal evaluation, it should be clear that there are no data to suggest how likely these patients are to develop future fulminant myocarditis. Decisions on changes in cancer therapy should be made deliberately with a true risk-versus-benefit, multidisciplinary discussion.

REFERENCES

1. Lynce F, Barac A, Geng X, et al. Prospective evaluation of the cardiac safety of HER2-targeted therapies in patients with HER2-positive breast cancer and compromised heart function: the SAFE-HEaRt study. *Breast Cancer Res Treat.* 2019;175:595-603.
2. Van Tine BA, Hirbe AC, Oppelt P, et al. Interim analysis of the phase II study: noninferiority study of doxorubicin with upfront dexrazoxane plus olaratumab for advanced or metastatic soft-tissue sarcoma. *Clin Cancer Res.* 2021;27(14):3854-3860.
3. Nicol M, Baudet M, Cohen-Solal A. Subclinical left ventricular dysfunction during chemotherapy. *Card Fail Rev.* 2019;5:31-36.
4. Cardinale D, Colombo A, Sandri MT, et al. Prevention of high-dose chemotherapy-induced cardiotoxicity in high-risk patients by angiotensin-converting enzyme inhibition. *Circulation.* 2006;114:2474-2481.
5. Thavendiranathan P, Negishi T, Somerset E, et al. Strain-guided management of potentially cardiotoxic cancer therapy. *J Am Coll Cardiol.* 2021;77:392-401.
6. Pai VB, Nahata MC. Cardiotoxicity of chemotherapeutic agents: incidence, treatment and prevention. *Drug Saf.* 2000;22:263-302.
7. Ganatra S, Nohria A, Shah S, et al. Upfront dexrazoxane for the reduction of anthracycline-induced cardiotoxicity in adults with preexisting cardiomyopathy and cancer: a consecutive case series. *Cardiooncology.* 2019;5:1.
8. Lipshultz SE, Rifai N, Dalton VM, et al. The effect of dexrazoxane on myocardial injury in doxorubicin-treated children with acute lymphoblastic leukemia. *N Engl J Med.* 2004;351:145-153.
9. Swain SM, Whaley FS, Gerber MC, et al. Cardioprotection with dexrazoxane for doxorubicin-containing therapy in advanced breast cancer. *J Clin Oncol.* 1997;15:1318-1332.
10. van Dalen EC, Caron HN, Dickinson HO, Kremer LC. Cardioprotective interventions for cancer patients receiving anthracyclines. *Cochrane Database Syst Rev.* 2011;CD003917.
11. Smith LA, Cornelius VR, Plummer CJ, et al. Cardiotoxicity of anthracycline agents for the treatment of cancer: systematic review and meta-analysis of randomised controlled trials. *BMC Cancer.* 2010;10:337.
12. Wolff AC, Hammond ME, Schwartz JN, et al. American Society of Clinical Oncology/College of American Pathologists guideline recommendations for human epidermal growth factor receptor 2 testing in breast cancer. *J Clin Oncol.* 2007;25:118-145.
13. Nowsheen S, Viscuse PV, O'Sullivan CC, et al. Incidence, diagnosis, and treatment of cardiac toxicity from trastuzumab in patients with breast cancer. *Curr Breast Cancer Rep.* 2017;9:173-182.
14. Ewer MS, Vooletich MT, Durand JB, et al. Reversibility of trastuzumab-related cardiotoxicity: new insights based on clinical course and response to medical treatment. *J Clin Oncol.* 2005;23:7820-7826.
15. Yu AF, Yadav NU, Eaton AA, et al. Continuous trastuzumab therapy in breast cancer patients with asymptomatic left ventricular dysfunction. *Oncologist.* 2015;20:1105-1110.
16. Heinzerling L, Ott PA, Hodi FS, et al. Cardiotoxicity associated with CTLA4 and PD1 blocking immunotherapy. *J Immunother Cancer.* 2016;4:50.
17. Mahmood SS, Fradley MG, Cohen JV, et al. Myocarditis in patients treated with immune checkpoint inhibitors. *J Am Coll Cardiol.* 2018;71(16):1755-1764.
18. Ball S, Ghosh RK, Wongsaengsak S et al. Cardiovascular toxicities of immune checkpoint inhibitors: JACC review topic of the week. *J Am Coll Cardiol.* 2019;74:1714-1727.
19. Janbabai G, Nabati M, Faghihinia M, Azizi S, Borhani S, Yazdani J. Effect of enalapril on preventing anthracycline-induced cardiomyopathy. *Cardiovasc Toxicol.* 2017;17:130-139.

20. Kaya MG, Ozkan M, Gunebakmaz O, et al. Protective effects of nebivolol against anthracycline-induced cardiomyopathy: a randomized control study. *Int J Cardiol.* 2013;167:2306-2310.
21. Kalay N, Basar E, Ozdogru I, et al. Protective effects of carvedilol against anthracycline-induced cardiomyopathy. *J Am Coll Cardiol.* 2006;48:2258-2262.
22. Nabati M, Janbabai G, Baghyari S, Esmaili K, Yazdani J. Cardioprotective effects of carvedilol in inhibiting doxorubicin-induced cardiotoxicity. *J Cardiovasc Pharmacol.* 2017;69:279-285.
23. Leong Darryl P, Cosman T, Alhussein Muhammad M, et al. Safety of continuing trastuzumab despite mild cardiotoxicity. *JACC: CardioOncol.* 2019;1:1-10.

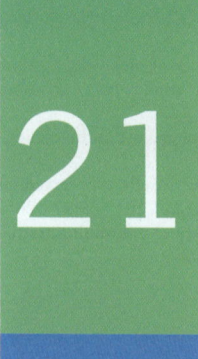

Multidisciplinary Approach to Cardio-Oncology and the Use of Advanced Practice Provider

Molly Rater, Holly Wiesehan, Ann Mahoney, and Karen Sneed

The discipline of cardio-oncology (C-O) is a new field of medicine that is committed to the idea of collaboration and cooperation to achieve many things, but first and foremost, to provide optimal cardiac care to those patients being treated for cancer. By definition this would require intensive **collaboration from a multidisciplinary team to optimally treat two major medical conditions.**

MULTIDISCIPLINARY TEAM

Definition
- A multidisciplinary team is a group of heath care workers who are experts in different areas with different professional backgrounds, united as a team for the purpose of planning and implementing treatment programs for complex medical conditions (Fig. 21-1).
- The members of the C-O team may include:
  - Cardio-oncologist(s)
  - Trainees (students, residents, and fellows)
  - Advanced practice providers (NP and PA)
  - Nurses
  - Research staff
  - Pharmacists
  - Exercise physiologists
  - Administration
- Multidisciplinary teams provide a **seamless and complete continuity of care**. Ideally, these teams should meet regularly to develop optimal treatment plans and share expert opinions on complex patients. The motivation of a cardio-oncologist is to provide optimal cardiovascular (CV) care to allow the best possible cancer care to be delivered. It should be emphasized that **C-O practitioners are on the same team as the cancer treatment specialists with the patient as the focal point.**[1]

COLLABORATION WITH OTHER DISCIPLINES

- **Hematology/Oncology.** The hematologist/oncologist formulates the cancer treatment plan and may need help from a C-O provider when cardiology problems arise or have the potential to arise. Some common needs for **referral to C-O include heart failure, pericardial effusion, thromboembolism, pulmonary hypertension, or cardiac dysrhythmias.** It is common in the case of breast cancer for an

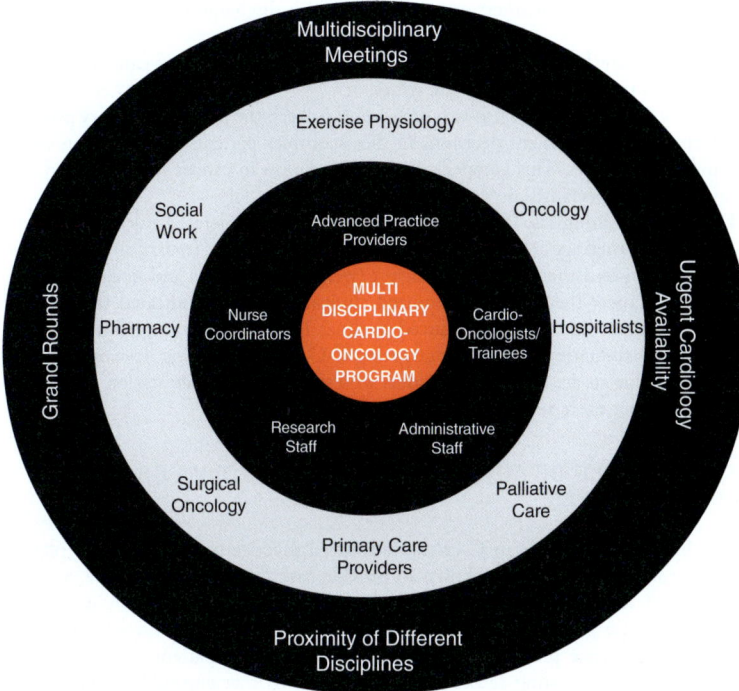

Figure 21-1. The cardio-oncology multidisciplinary team. There are many members of the cardio-oncology Team all with the common goal of optimal cardiovascular care and risk factor modification in patients undergoing cancer treatment. (American Association of Nurse Practitioners. Quality of nurse practitioner practice. https://www.aanp.org/advocacy/advocacy-resource/position-statements/quality-of-nurse-practitioner-practice)

oncologist to seek the opinion of a C-O provider to discuss continuation of human epidermal growth factor receptor 2 (HER2)-targeted therapies or anthracyclines. In some cases, the use of a **C-O provider may prevent premature discontinuation of a cancer treatment**, leading to better chance of overall survival. Ideally the hematology/oncology and C-O **centers are in close proximity to one another**.
- **Surgical Oncology.** A C-O provider may be called upon to provide perioperative risk assessment and postsurgical CV management.
- **Pharmacy.** Pharmacists play an essential role as medication experts who improve the quality of care through optimization of pharmacotherapy. Several well-conducted randomized controlled trials have documented benefits of pharmacist-led interventions within a multidisciplinary team setting.[2] Many cancer drugs have important drug interactions and side effects that are not commonly known to most providers, especially with the tremendous influx of targeted therapies.
- **Hospitalists.** These providers are on the front lines of taking care of complex medical patients in the hospital setting. They are responsible for the day-to-day management of patient care and coordinating communication with the various specialists involved.

- **Social Work.** Social workers assist the team with discharge planning, placement, and counseling.
- **Palliative Care/Hospice.** In some cases, the services of palliative care and hospice are needed to help with end-of-life issues.
- **Primary Care Providers.** It is very important to keep the patients' primary provider informed of management decisions in these complex patients that are often seeing multiple specialists. This is especially true in relation to cancer survivors who may not be seeing specialists any longer.
- **Exercise Physiologists.** Patients with cancer have an accelerated risk of CV disease related to normal age-related pathologies coupled with direct (radiation, chemotherapy, and targeted therapies) and indirect (weight gain or loss and deconditioning) effects of cancer therapies. Randomized clinical trials have indicated that exercise may attenuate the treatment-induced declines in cardiorespiratory fitness (CRF). Cardiac rehabilitation specifically targeting C-O patients is being developed.[3] Exercise physiologists are often the providers who staff cardiac rehabilitation centers and design various exercise prescriptions.

CRITICAL ROLE OF ADVANCED PRACTICE PROVIDERS ON THE C-O TEAM

It has been clear to those in C-O that advanced practice providers (APPs) play an integral role. APPs have been shown to provide care that is safe, equitable, and evidence based, resulting in excellent outcomes and high patient satisfaction. APPs bring a comprehensive perspective to health care, blending clinical expertise with an added emphasis on disease prevention, health management, and patient education. They often develop long-lasting relationships with patients that engender superior communication and compliance. APPs have been shown to lower the overall cost of health care. Patients who regularly seek primary care services from an APP have fewer visits to the emergency department, fewer readmissions, and shorter hospital stays.[4] The APP role varies from institution to institution, but some of the benefits of having an APP on the multidisciplinary team are:

- **Networking.** APPs can develop relationships and network with other APPs to communicate the need for C-O, increase the visibility of the program, and increase referrals. By making themselves available and responsive to other disciplines, especially other areas that are not frequented by C-O providers, awareness of the program increases as well as enhanced collaboration.
- **APP collaboration groups.** Multicenter APP groups can be formed to network and share resources. In-person or virtual meetings can be held on regular intervals to promote communication.
- **Support groups.** The APP can facilitate or lead support groups for patients and families.
- **Patient, family, and staff education.** APPs should participate in nursing continuing education and grand rounds to educate other providers. Teaching tools and in-person teaching of patients and families can occur during office visits. It is especially important for the APP to counsel patients on their CV risk factors. There are an increasing number of Food and Drug Administration (FDA)-approved anticancer agents with potential cardiotoxic effects, making CV risk factor modification even more important.[5] One study found nurse practitioners to be at least as successful as physicians when counseling patients on CV risk factors.[6]

- **Improved continuity of care.** Increased clinic availability and use of satellite locations provides continuity of care and improved clinical flow. Many patients have multiple appointments with various providers, making it more convenient to have a provider available multiple days per week at different locations. Patients being treated for cancer have frequent changes in status, so an APP who can be flexible is invaluable. Telemedicine visits have become a new option for care and can be utilized well by APPs. Continuity can also be improved on the inpatient service if the APP is a consistent presence with attending MDs and fellows that rotate weeks on service.
- **Collaborative practice.** Physicians who work with APPs generally report that APPs allow each physician more time to see complicated patients and enhance the capacity to do teaching and research. The APP and MD bring shared and unique knowledge and skill that should complement one another. The advantages of collaborative practice are decreased cost of care and increased quality and access of care.[7]

ROLE OF NURSE COORDINATORS FOR THE CARDIO-ONCOLOGY MULTIDISCIPLINARY TEAM

The role of the nurse coordinator is invaluable in any C-O team. **Advanced cardiac and oncologic clinical knowledge and experience are critical skill sets for the nurse in this role** as an integral part of the collective collaboration among other providers. Other members of the interprofessional team utilize nurse coordinators to establish high-quality clinical care for the C-O service. This is accomplished through ongoing, active interaction and care coordination across all disciplines.

- Nurse coordinators serve as educators, collaborators, coordinators, clinic managers, and important resources of emotional support for patients/families (Table 21-1).
- Nurse coordinators are usually the first point of contact for patients and families to discuss plan of care, referral of care, care concerns, symptoms, medication issues, testing interpretation, etc. This provides timely care management strategies because they also have direct, ongoing communication with the providers.
- To help minimize provider office visits and hospital admissions, cardiopulmonary monitoring is common in the home setting. A nurse coordinator is typically responsible for obtaining appropriate clinical updates regarding vital sign readings or symptoms in response to treatment changes.
- Coordinators commonly facilitate the arrangement of diagnostic tests and procedures such as cardiac catheterizations, endomyocardial biopsies, electrical cardioversions, cardiac magnetic resonance imaging (MRI), all echo imaging, as well as stress tests.
- Coordinators consolidate needed blood work between C-O and other clinical services in an effort to reduce phlebotomy frequency and improve patient safety.
- C-O nurse coordinators possess a vast knowledge base of disease processes and are often called upon to be resources and advocates for patients dealing with complex medical conditions.
- Health care access often presents challenges in C-O in regard to obtaining specialty medications or treatments that are often denied by insurance. Nurse coordinators are responsible for completing the first line of prior authorizations for insurance approval. Even with insurance approval, recommended treatment is often cost-prohibitive because of patients' income, insurance restrictions, or both. By

TABLE 21-1	The Myriad Roles of the Nurse Coordinator for the Cardio-Oncology Team[a]
Disease and medication education	The four most common complications in this population are cardiac ischemia, thromboembolism, heart failure, and arrhythmias. The nurse is able to listen to patient symptoms and has to be able to recognize what needs immediate attention and what can wait. The nurse also educates patients about symptoms to call for, what to watch for, what is normal, and when to be concerned.
Home monitoring	The nurse is often called upon to monitor patient's vital signs, weights, symptoms, and responses to patient intervention. The nurse is often the contact for home health nurse to call with concerns and questions.
Health Care Access	Health Care Access is often a challenge for patients for a variety of reasons such as availability, accessibility, and affordability. Nurses can help with obtaining costly mediations and arranging transportation to provider visits.
Family support	It is important for the nurse to clarify the patient's support system. The nurse coordinator often develops close relationships with caregivers and is considered a trusted, helpful advocate. They are often the first person to speak with the patient or family to discuss symptoms, concerns, or issues.
Collaboration with other specialties	The RN on the cardio-oncology team bridges the cardiologist, oncologist, oncology nurses, hospitalists, trainees, and advanced practice providers to provide cohesive care.
Clinic flow management	Nurses help with placing orders during clinic and can help with the general flow. They often have to obtain records before the visit. They can provide valuable information to the provider before the visit based on phone conversations or contacts they have had with the patient.
Coordination of testing and results	Nurses are often required to assist with ordering and scheduling testing. They are usually responsible for calling patients with test results and answering questions about those results.
Assistance with specialty medications	Many of the drugs used in cardio-oncology require specialty pharmacies, preauthorization, and financial assistance programs. The nurse is usually the person who provides that service.

RN, registered nurse.
[a]The nurse coordinator is an integral part of the team carrying out several essential tasks required for a successful program.

assisting patients with locating, applying, and submitting applications for financial assistance, patients are often able to receive recommended therapies that are otherwise cost-prohibitive.

CARDIO-ONCOLOGY RESEARCH: MULTIDISCIPLINARY APPROACH

C-O research is focused on improving the lives and overall survival of cancer patients and survivors. The priorities are to:
- **Develop and implement clinical research protocols** to promote precision medicine
- **Develop evidence-based guidelines** with predictor models to improve overall survival
- **Disseminate evidence-based knowledge** that displays evidence of CV effects related to cancer and the various treatment modalities of cancer.

The Essential Components for C-O Research (Fig. 21-2) summarizes the multidisciplinary approach to research including, but not limited to, cardiologists and oncologists, research administrators, and research coordinators who are often nurses.

The development of clinical research in C-O has been identified as a top 10 priority for the discipline.[8] Understanding how to integrate disciplined research into clinical care is a very important strategy for improving C-O patient care.[9]

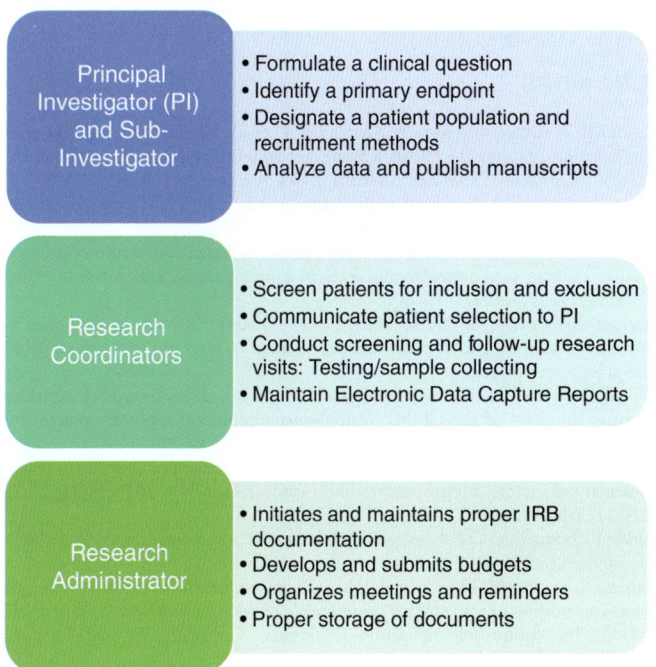

Figure 21-2. The collaborative research team. Several members of a research team, all with different roles and specific tasks, are necessary to implement a successful research project. IRB, institutional review board; PI, principal investigator.

THE ROLE OF ADMINISTRATIVE SUPPORT IN CARDIO-ONCOLOGY

Administrative support comes in many forms in the discipline of C-O: from the day-to-day operations to broader institutional support. It is well known that a lack of institutional support will hinder the growth and success of any C-O program.[10]

Administrative professionals to facilitate day-to-day operations:
- **Coordinating** meetings, public outreach, and CMEs
- **Managing schedules** of providers
- Support and orientation for trainees
- Document management (ongoing meetings, research)
- Obtaining final reports and outside testing
- **Enhance communication** between services
- Help develop order sets, educational tools, and presentations

Institutional administration to support growth of the program:
- Approve salary support for new team members
- **Evaluate need for new clinical sites/locations for expansion**
- Assess financials/budgets
- Assist with public relations activities
- Billing/compliance
- Promote referrals
- **Raise awareness of services**
- Build/monitor website communication

REFERENCES

1. Adusumalli S, Alvarez-Cardona J, Khatana SM, et al. Clinical practice and research in cardio-oncology: finding the "Rosetta Stone" for establishing program excellence in cardio-oncology. *J Cardiovasc Transl Res.* 2020;13(3):495-505. doi: 10.1007/s12265-020-10010-x
2. Hwang AY, Smith SM. Partnering with pharmacists to reduce cardiovascular risk in outpatient settings. *J Am Heart Assoc.* 2019;8:22.
3. Gilchrist SC, Barac A, Ades PA, et al. AHA scientific statement: cardio-oncology rehabilitation to manage cardiovascular outcomes in cancer patients and survivors. *Circulation.* 2019;139(21):e997-e1012.
4. American Association of Nurse Practitioners. Quality of nurse practitioner practice. https://www.aanp.org/advocacy/advocacy-resource/position-statements/quality-of-nurse-practitioner-practice
5. Fadol AP, Palaskas NL, Ewer MS, et al. An overview of a different type of cardio-oncology gathering: summary of the COMP (cardio-oncology multidisciplinary practice) meeting held in Houston Texas, January 2020. *Cardiooncology.* 2020;6:20.
6. Klemenc-Ketis Z, Terbovc A, Gomiscek B, et al. Role of nurse practitioners in reducing cardiovascular risk factors: a retrospective cohort study. *J Clin Nurs.* 2015;24(21-22):3077-83. doi:10.1111/jocn.12889
7. Resnick B, Bonner A. Collaboration: foundation for a successful practice. *J Am Med Dir Assoc.* 2003; 4(6):344-349.
8. Lenihan DJ, Fradley M, Dent S, et al. Proceedings from the global cardio-oncology summit: the top 10 priorities to actualize for cardiooncology. *JACC: CardioOncol.* 2019;1:256-272.
9. Pudil R. The future role of cardio-oncologists. *Card Fail Rev.* 2017;3(2):140-142. doi:10.15420/cfr.2017:16:1
10. Austin-Mattison C. Joining forces: establishing a cardio-oncology clinic. *J Adv Pract Oncol.* 2018;9(2):222-229.

22 Cardiac Amyloidosis: General Diagnostic Approach

Walter B. Schiffer and Kathleen W. Zhang

GENERAL PRINCIPLES

- Previously thought to be a rare and untreatable condition, cardiac amyloidosis is now recognized as a treatable disease that is underdiagnosed,[1] especially among the elderly.
- Findings of cardiac amyloidosis on history, physical examination, and routine diagnostic testing can be nonspecific.
- Diagnostic delays of up to 36 months from symptom onset are common, and one-third of patients are evaluated by ≥5 specialists prior to being diagnosed.[2]
- Integration of all clinical and diagnostic findings and a high index of suspicion for the diagnosis are necessary when assessing patients for cardiac amyloidosis.

BACKGROUND AND EPIDEMIOLOGY

- Amyloidosis is a systemic illness that results from the deposition of misfolded protein aggregates as amyloid fibrils in tissue, causing organ dysfunction.
- **Over 30 amyloid proteins have been associated with human disease. However, the vast majority of cardiac amyloidosis (>95%) is associated with either transthyretin amyloidosis (ATTR) or light chain amyloidosis (AL).**
  - ATTR results from misfolding of transthyretin, a serum transport protein for thyroxine and retinol. Transthyretin misfolding may occur as a wild-type variant or because of a point mutation in the transthyretin gene.
  - AL results from overproduction of clonal immunoglobulins by a plasma cell neoplasm, leading to misfolding and deposition of light chain fragments as amyloid fibrils.
- Less common types of cardiac amyloidosis include secondary amyloidosis (AA) and ApoA1 amyloidosis (AApoA1).
  - AA is caused by deposition of amyloid fibrils composed of serum amyloid A, an inflammatory protein. AA is associated with chronic inflammatory conditions such as rheumatoid arthritis, juvenile inflammatory arthritis, intravenous drug use, and familial periodic fever syndromes. The kidney is the primary organ affected by AA.
  - AApoA1 is a hereditary condition that results from misfolding of the apolipoprotein A1 protein because of gene mutation. The kidneys and liver are primarily affected.

Epidemiology

Light Chain Amyloidosis
- **AL is a rare disease with an estimated incidence of 14 cases per million in the United States**.[3]

- Single-center studies indicate that AL typically affects older patients (median age 65 years) with a slight male predominance (~60%), although age at diagnosis can be highly variable.[4]
- Although 10% to 15% of patients with multiple myeloma develop AL, the majority of patients with AL do not meet diagnostic criteria for multiple myeloma.
- Monoclonal gammopathy of undetermined significance is a known precursor of AL and progresses to AL in 1% of cases.[5]

Transthyretin Amyloidosis
- **Wild-type ATTR, previously known as senile amyloidosis, is a disease of the elderly that predominantly affects Caucasian men with median age of 76 at diagnosis.**[6]
    - Wild-type transthyretin cardiac amyloidosis (ATTR-CM) has been found in 13% of those hospitalized for heart failure with preserved ejection fraction, and in 13% of patients with severe aortic stenosis referred for transcatheter aortic valve replacement.[7,8]
    - Prevalence of carpal tunnel syndrome may be as high as 25% among patients with wild-type ATTR-CM, and transthyretin amyloid deposits have been detected in 7% of unselected patients undergoing carpal tunnel release surgery.[9,10]
- **Hereditary ATTR is a rare, autosomal dominant disease with incomplete penetrance that leads to a familial cardiomyopathy, polyneuropathy, or both.**
    - Age of onset is highly variable and depends on the mutation involved.
    - Val122Ile is the most common genetic variant found in the United States and presents in individuals of African descent as a restrictive cardiomyopathy and/or polyneuropathy. It is estimated that 3% to 4% of African Americans are carriers for the Val122Ile mutation.[6]
    - Thr60Ala is the second most common genetic variant in the United States and causes a mixed cardiomyopathy and polyneuropathy in patients of Irish descent.[6]

CLINICAL EVALUATION

- The presenting symptoms of cardiac amyloidosis (dyspnea, lower extremity edema, and fatigue) are fairly nonspecific.
- "Red flag" findings on history, physical examination, and diagnostic testing can raise clinical suspicion for cardiac amyloidosis (Table 22-1).

History

Light Chain Cardiac Amyloidosis
- **Heart failure is the most prominent manifestation of AL cardiac amyloidosis (AL-CM), especially findings of right heart failure. Atrial fibrillation and atrial flutter are commonly seen.**
- **Renal involvement is common with AL and manifests as proteinuria, which may lead to diffuse anasarca.**
- Neurologic manifestations include numbness and tingling as well as orthostatic hypotension.
- Gastrointestinal manifestations include unintentional weight loss, early satiety, nausea, constipation, and diarrhea.

Transthyretin Cardiac Amyloidosis
- **Heart failure is the most prominent manifestation of ATTR-CM.**
- Dysrhythmias are common and include atrial fibrillation, atrial flutter, and (particularly with wild-type ATTR-CM) first-, second-, or third-degree heart block.
- Wild-type ATTR-CM is associated with aortic stenosis, especially paradoxical low-flow, low-gradient aortic stenosis.
- **Carpal tunnel syndrome (especially bilateral disease), lumbar spinal stenosis, and biceps tendon rupture can be highly suggestive of ATTR.**[9,11,12]
- Sensorimotor peripheral neuropathy, autonomic dysfunction, and orthostatic hypotension are seen in hereditary ATTR with neurologic involvement.
- Gastrointestinal symptoms (unintentional weight loss, early satiety, nausea, diarrhea, constipation) are seen primarily in hereditary ATTR.

Physical Examination
- Cardiac examination findings of cardiac amyloidosis are consistent with restrictive cardiomyopathy and include peripheral edema, elevated jugular venous pressure, hepatojugular reflux, and rales.
- Findings of right-sided heart failure (ascites, peripheral edema) are particularly prominent in patients with AL-CM, especially in those with significant proteinuria.
- Orthostatic hypotension is indicative of autonomic dysfunction.
- Neurologic examination may demonstrate findings of symmetric sensorimotor polyneuropathy, carpal tunnel syndrome, or spinal stenosis.
- Periorbital purpura ("raccoon eyes") and macroglossia are seen in a minority of patients but are pathognomonic for AL.

Initial Diagnostic Testing
Electrocardiography
- **Individual electrocardiographic findings have limited diagnostic accuracy for cardiac amyloidosis** (Fig. 22-1A and Table 22-2).
- A hallmark finding of cardiac amyloidosis is low-voltage QRS amplitude, especially in the limb leads (≤5 mm). This is seen in only 30% to 50% of patients with cardiac amyloidosis, with 49% sensitivity and 91% specificity in patients with cardiac biopsy-proven disease.[13-15]
- Pseudoinfarct pattern (Q waves in the early precordial leads mimicking a prior anteroseptal myocardial infarction) is another hallmark finding of cardiac amyloidosis, though it is present in only 25% to 50% of patients.[14-16]
- Relative low voltage on electrocardiography (S wave in V1 + R wave in V5 or V6 ≤ 15 mm) in the setting of left ventricular hypertrophy on echocardiography is another classic finding, though it appears to have poor specificity for cardiac amyloidosis.[14]
- Other electrocardiographic findings of cardiac amyloidosis include:
  - Intraventricular conduction delay, seen in 20% to 50% of patients.[13,16]
  - First-, second-, or third-degree atrioventricular block, seen in 15% to 40% of patients.[13,16]
  - Atrial fibrillation and atrial flutter, seen in 24% of patients.[14,16]

Transthoracic Echocardiography
- **Hallmark findings of cardiac amyloidosis on transthoracic echocardiography (TTE) include increased left and right ventricular wall thickness, diastolic**

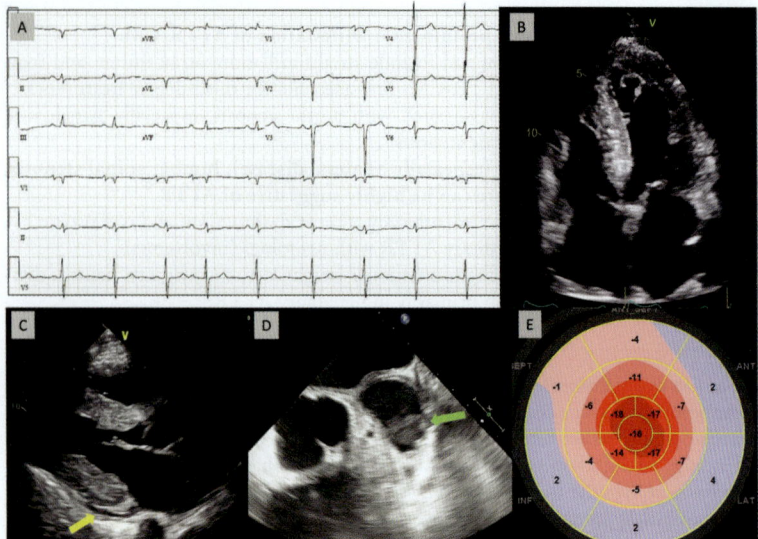

Figure 22-1. Electrocardiographic findings in cardiac amyloidosis. (A) Electrocardiography demonstrates pseudoinfarct pattern (Q waves in V1-V2), poor R wave progression, and low QRS voltage in the limb leads. (B) Apical four-chamber view displays left ventricular (LV) hypertrophy, biatrial enlargement, and thickened interventricular septum. (C) Parasternal long-axis view shows left atrial enlargement and LV septal thickening. (D) Left atrial appendage thrombus on transesophageal echocardiography. (E) Relative apical sparing of LV longitudinal strain. (From Zhang KW, Zhang R, Deych E, Stockerl-Goldstein KE, Gorcsan J, Lenihan DJ. A multi-modal diagnostic model improves detection of cardiac amyloidosis among patients with diagnostic confirmation by cardiac biopsy. *Am Heart J.* 2021;232:137-145; Boldrini M, Cappelli F, Chacko L, et al. Multiparametric echocardiography scores for the diagnosis of cardiac amyloidosis. *JACC Cardiovasc Imaging.* 2020;13(4).)

dysfunction, biatrial enlargement, and a small pericardial effusion (Fig. 22-1B-C).
- Left ventricular ejection fraction (LVEF) is typically preserved ($\geq$ 50%), though mild or even severe reductions in LVEF may be seen in patients with advanced disease.
- Increased relative left ventricular wall thickness (>0.6), increased left atrial pressure by E/e′ (>11), and reduced tricuspid annular plane systolic excursion (TAPSE; $\leq$19 mm) are suggestive of cardiac amyloidosis among patients with increased left ventricular wall thickness.[17]
- Intracardiac thrombus (such as left atrial appendage thrombus) is more common in patients with cardiac amyloidosis, including those on systemic anticoagulation (Fig. 22-1D).[18]
- Speckle tracking strain analysis can be helpful to assess for cardiac amyloidosis.
  - Global longitudinal strain (GLS) is usually severely abnormal in patients with cardiac amyloidosis (>−13%; normal $\leq$−19%).[14,17]

TABLE 22-1 Clinical Manifestations of Light Chain and Transthyretin Amyloidosis

Type of amyloid	Cardiovascular	Neurologic	Gastrointestinal	Renal	Other
Wild-type ATTR	**Left-sided heart failure** **Atrial fibrillation/flutter** Heart block Calcific aortic stenosis	**Carpal tunnel syndrome** Lumbar spinal stenosis	Rare	Renal impairment	Biceps tendon rupture
Hereditary ATTR[a]	**Left-sided heart failure** **Atrial fibrillation/flutter**	Carpal tunnel syndrome Lumbar spinal stenosis Peripheral neuropathy **Autonomic dysfunction**	Dysmotility	Renal impairment	Biceps tendon rupture
AL	**Biventricular heart failure** **Atrial fibrillation/flutter**	Peripheral neuropathy **Autonomic dysfunction**	Dysmotility Hepatic dysfunction	**Nephrotic syndrome** Renal impairment	Macroglossia Periorbital purpura

Note: Highly prominent clinical signs and symptoms are bolded.

ATTR, transthyretin amyloidosis; AL, light chain amyloidosis.

[a]Varying mutations leading to hereditary ATTR present with unique phenotypes that may be cardiac or neurologic predominant. Those presented here pertain to the most common variant in the United States, Val122Ile.

Zhang KW, Vallabhaneni S, Alvarez-Cardona JA, Krone RJ, Mitchell JD, Lenihan DJ. Cardiac amyloidosis for the primary care provider: A practical review to promote earlier recognition of disease. *Am J Med.* 2021;134:587-595.

- Relative apical sparing of left ventricular longitudinal strain (LS) is also suggestive of cardiac amyloidosis (Fig. 22-1E). This is thought to reflect preferential deposition of amyloid fibrils in the mid- and basal segments of the heart.
  a. The apical sparing ratio of LS is calculated as (average LS of apical segments)/(average LS of mid segments + average LS of basal segments), with a cut-off of 1.0 for cardiac amyloidosis.[19]
  b. Apical sparing of LS has 60% to 70% sensitivity and 70% to 80% specificity for cardiac amyloidosis.[14,17]
- Other suggestive strain findings for cardiac amyloidosis include increased LVEF to GLS ratio (>3.8) and increased ratio of apical septal LS to basal septal LS (>3.1).[17]

Cardiac Biomarkers
- Mild elevation in serum troponin levels on multiple occasions is commonly seen in patients with cardiac amyloidosis.
- Brain natriuretic peptide (BNP) levels are often markedly elevated. In patients with established AL, N-terminal (NT)-proBNP is highly sensitive for cardiac involvement.[20]
- Other novel biomarkers, including hepatocyte growth factor, may help to differentiate cardiac amyloidosis from other types of heart failure.[21]

Establishing the Diagnosis of Cardiac Amyloidosis

- Once cardiac amyloidosis is suspected, definitive diagnostic testing should be pursued (Fig. 22-2).
- **Endomyocardial biopsy with mass spectrometry is the gold standard for diagnosis of cardiac amyloidosis.**
- ^{99m}Technetium (Tc)-labeled bone scintigraphy has been validated for noninvasive diagnosis of ATTR-CM with 91% sensitivity and 100% specificity in the absence of a monoclonal protein.[22]
- Noncardiac biopsy with mass spectrometry in combination with cardiac magnetic resonance imaging (CMR) can be used for diagnosis of AL-CM in many cases.

^{99m}Technetium-Labeled Bone Scintigraphy
- Traditionally used as bone tracers, ^{99m}Tc-labeled bisphosphonates also localize to cardiac transthyretin amyloid deposits by an unknown mechanism.
- ^{99m}Tc-labeled pyrophosphate (PYP) is most commonly used in the United States. ^{99m}Tc-labeled 3,3-diphosphono-1,2-propanodicarboxylic acid (DPD) and ^{99m}Tc-labeled hydroxymethylene diphosphonate (HDMP) are also validated tracers for the diagnosis of ATTR-CM.
- **Scans are scored based on a semiquantitative grading scale: grade 3 = cardiac uptake greater than bone; grade 2 = cardiac uptake equal to bone; grade 1 = cardiac uptake less than bone; grade 0 = no cardiac uptake** (Fig. 22.3A-C).
- **A study is considered positive for ATTR-CM in the setting of grade 2 or 3 uptake (91% sensitivity, 87% specificity).**[22]
- **Single-photon emission computed tomography (SPECT) imaging should be used to confirm intramyocardial tracer uptake and not blood pool uptake** (Fig. 22-3D).

TABLE 22-2 Diagnostic Testing in Cardiac Amyloidosis

Lab Testing	ECG Prevalence	Echocardiography Sensitivity, Specificity[a]	Cardiac MRI
Elevated NT-proBNP	Poor R wave progression 60%-70%	Increased ejection fraction to longitudinal strain ratio 62%, 65%	Diffuse sub-endocardial LGE
Persistent mild troponin elevation without ischemic symptoms	Pseudoinfarct pattern 18%-39%	Relative apical sparing on longitudinal strain 71%, 73%	Prolonged T1 relaxation times
Abnormal free light chain levels (AL)	Atrioventricular block 13%-41%	Diastolic dysfunction with increased E/A ratio 74%, 75%	Increased extracellular volume
Monoclonal protein on SPEP or UPEP (AL)	Low QRS voltage 18%-60%	RV dysfunction with decreased TAPSE 67%, 64%	LV hypertrophy

ECG, electrocardiogram; NT-proBNP, N-terminal pro brain natriuretic peptide; AL, light chain amyloidosis; LGE, late gadolinium enhancement; SPEP, serum protein electrophoresis; UPEP, urine protein electrophoresis; RV, right ventricle; TAPSE, tricuspid annular plane systolic excursion; LV, left ventricle.

[a]Reported sensitivity and specificity are for patients identified as having increased septal wall thickness >12 mm on echocardiogram.

From Cyrille NB, Goldsmith J, Alvarez J, Maurer MS. Prevalence and prognostic significance of low QRS voltage among the three main types of cardiac amyloidosis. *Am J Cardiol.* 2014;114(7):1089-1093. doi:10.1016/j.amjcard.2014.07.026; Zhang KW, Zhang R, Deych E, Stockerl-Goldstein KE, Gorcsan J, Lenihan DJ. A multi-modal diagnostic model improves detection of cardiac amyloidosis among patients with diagnostic confirmation by cardiac biopsy. *Am Heart J.* 2021;232: 137-145. doi:10.1016/j.ahj.2020.11.006; Murtagh B, Hammill SC, Gertz MA, Kyle RA, Tajik AJ, Grogan M. Electrocardiographic findings in primary systemic amyloidosis and biopsy-proven cardiac involvement. *Am J Cardiol.* 2005;95(4): 535-537. doi:10.1016/j.amjcard.2004.10.028; Cappelli F, Vignini E, Martone R, et al. Baseline ECG features and arrhythmic profile in transthyretin versus light chain cardiac amyloidosis. *Circ Heart Fail.* 2020;13(3):e006619. doi:10.1161/CIRCHEARTFAILURE.119.006619; Boldrini M, Cappelli F, Chacko L, et al. Multiparametric echocardiography scores for the diagnosis of cardiac amyloidosis. *JACC Cardiovasc Imaging.* 2020;13(4):909-920. doi:10.1016/j.jcmg.2019.10.011

- As a quantitative measure, a heart-to-contralateral lung ratio of tracer uptake >1.5 is consistent with the diagnosis of ATTR-CM.[22]
- **Because the majority of false-positive scans are due to AL-CM, AL must be excluded prior to interpreting the 99mTc scan.**

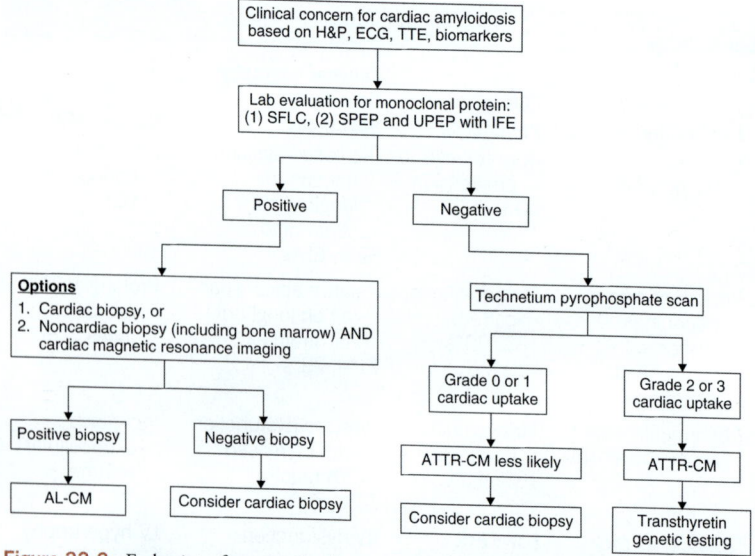

Figure 22-2. Evaluation of suspected cardiac amyloidosis. AL-CM, light chain cardiac amyloidosis; ATTR, transthyretin cardiac amyloidosis; H&P, history and physical examination; IFE, immunofixation; SFLC, serum free light chain; SPEP, serum protein electrophoresis; TTE, transthoracic echocardiogram; UPEP, urine protein electrophoresis. (From Zhang KW, Zhang R, Deych E, Stockerl-Goldstein KE, Gorcsan J, Lenihan DJ. A multi-modal diagnostic model improves detection of cardiac amyloidosis among patients with diagnostic confirmation by cardiac biopsy. *Am Heart J.* 2021;232:137-145.)

- AL can be excluded with normal findings on the following three lab tests:
  1. Serum free light chain assay
  2. Serum protein electrophoresis with immunofixation
  3. Urine protein electrophoresis with immunofixation
- Abnormal findings may be suggestive of renal impairment or a monoclonal gammopathy (including AL) and require hematology consultation in most cases.
- Other causes of false-positive ^{99m}Tc scans include hydroxychloroquine cardiotoxicity, metastatic myocardial calcification, and myocardial infarction.

Cardiac Magnetic Resonance Imaging
- Diffuse, subendocardial late gadolinium enhancement (LGE) is highly specific for cardiac amyloidosis (Fig. 22-4) (86% sensitivity), though other nonvascular patterns of LGE can also be seen.[23]
- Prolonged native T1 relaxation times may identify cardiac amyloidosis without need for gadolinium contrast.[24]
- Increased extracellular volume is also characteristic of cardiac amyloidosis and may improve diagnostic accuracy of CMR.[25]
- When possible, tissue biopsy should be pursued in conjunction with CMR to confirm the diagnosis of amyloidosis and determine the amyloid fibril type.
- Endomyocardial biopsy
  - Endomyocardial biopsy with mass spectrometry is the diagnostic gold standard for cardiac amyloidosis and is safely performed at experienced centers.

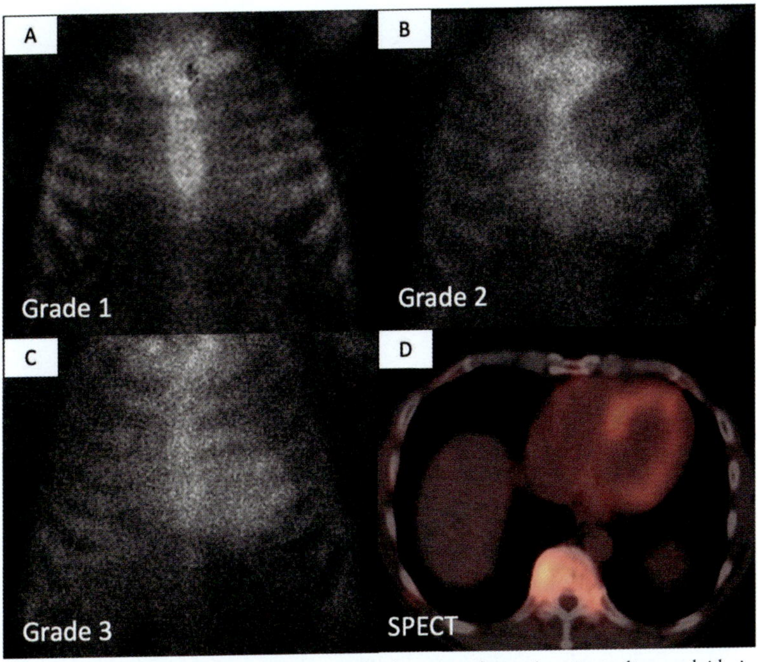

Figure 22-3. Tc^{99} Pyrophosphate scan in the diagnosis of transthyretin cardiac amyloidosis. Planar (A-C) and single-photon emission computed tomography (SPECT) images (D) from technetium-99 pyrophosphate scan in patients with grade 1-3 uptake. SPECT imaging is critical to ensure tracer uptake within the myocardium, and thereby rule out a false-positive result from blood pooling within the left ventricular cavity.

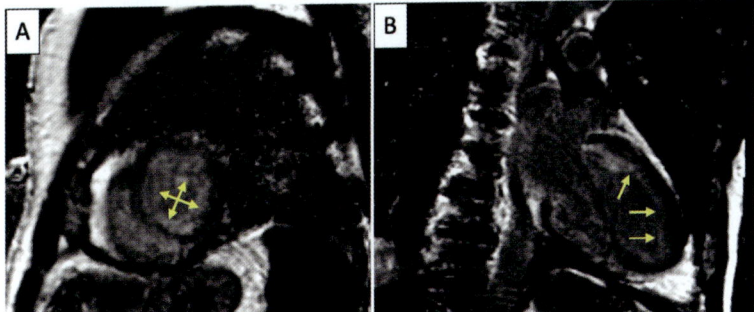

Figure 22-4. Cardiac Magnetic Resonance Imaging (MRI) findings in cardiac amyloidosis. Cardiac MRI images with arrows identifying diffuse subendocardial late gadolinium enhancement on (A) short axis and (B) two chamber views.

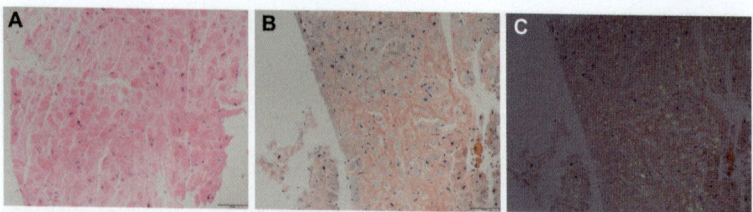

Figure 22-5. Endomyocardial biopsy findings in cardiac amyloidosis. Light microscopy slides of endomyocardial biopsy in a patient with cardiac amyloidosis demonstrate extracellular amyloid deposition (yellow arrows) with (A) Hematoxylin and eosin staining at 20×, (B) congo red staining at 20×, and (C) congo red staining under polarized light.

- Histopathologic examination classically reveals apple-green birefringence with Congo red staining under polarized light microscopy (Fig. 22-5).
- Right heart catheterization at the time of biopsy may help to guide heart failure management.
- Noncardiac biopsy
  - **To maximize diagnostic yield, biopsy of a clinically involved organ should be pursued.**
  - Diagnostic sensitivity of fat pad biopsy is higher for AL (80%) than hereditary ATTR (55%) or wild-type ATTR (15%).[26,27]
  - In patients with suspected cardiac amyloidosis, a bone marrow biopsy showing a plasma cell neoplasm without amyloid deposition may represent AL *or* a monoclonal gammopathy with concurrent ATTR. Hematology/Oncology consultation is recommended.
- Transthyretin genotyping is necessary for all patients with ATTR to evaluate for the presence of hereditary variants.

REFERENCES

1. Zhang KW, Stockerl-Goldstein KE, Lenihan DJ. Emerging therapeutics for the treatment of light chain and transthyretin amyloidosis. *JACC Basic Transl Sci.* 2019;4(3):438-448. doi:10.1016/j.jacbts.2019.02.002
2. Bishop E, Brown EE, Fajardo J, Barouch LA, Judge DP, Halushka MK. Seven factors predict a delayed diagnosis of cardiac amyloidosis. *Amyloid.* 2018;25(3):174-179. doi:10.1080/13506129.2018.1498782
3. Quock TP, Yan T, Chang E, Guthrie S, Broder MS. Epidemiology of AL amyloidosis: a real-world study using US claims data. *Blood Adv.* 2018;2(10):1046-1053. doi:10.1182/bloodadvances.2018016402
4. Lee Chuy K, Drill E, Yang JC, et al. Incremental value of global longitudinal strain for predicting survival in patients with advanced AL amyloidosis. *JACC CardioOncol.* 2020;2(2):223-231. doi:10.1016/j.jaccao.2020.05.012
5. Kyle RA, Larson DR, Therneau TM, et al. Long-term follow-up of monoclonal gammopathy of undetermined significance. *N Engl J Med.* 2018;378(3):241-249. doi:10.1056/nejmoa1709974
6. Maurer MS, Hanna M, Grogan M, et al. Genotype and phenotype of transthyretin cardiac amyloidosis: THAOS (Transthyretin Amyloid Outcome Survey). *J Am Coll Cardiol.* 2016;68(2):161-172. doi:10.1016/j.jacc.2016.03.596

7. González-López E, Gallego-Delgado M, Guzzo-Merello G, et al. Wild-type transthyretin amyloidosis as a cause of heart failure with preserved ejection fraction. *Eur Heart J.* 2015;36(38):2585-2594. doi:10.1093/eurheartj/ehv338
8. Scully PR, Patel KP, Treibel TA, et al. Prevalence and outcome of dual aortic stenosis and cardiac amyloid pathology in patients referred for transcatheter aortic valve implantation. *Eur Heart J.* 2020;41(29):2759-2767. doi: 10.1093/eurheartj/ehaa170
9. Milandri A, Farioli A, Gagliardi C, et al. Carpal tunnel syndrome in cardiac amyloidosis: implications for early diagnosis and prognostic role across the spectrum of aetiologies. *Eur J Heart Fail.* 2020;22(3):507-515. doi:10.1002/ejhf.1742
10. Sperry BW, Reyes BA, Ikram A, et al. Tenosynovial and cardiac amyloidosis in patients undergoing carpal tunnel release. *J Am Coll Cardiol.* 2018;72(17):2040-2050. doi:10.1016/j.jacc.2018.07.092
11. Geller HI, Singh A, Alexander KM, Mirto TM, Falk RH. Association between ruptured distal biceps tendon and wild-type transthyretin cardiac amyloidosis. *JAMA.* 2017;318(10):962-963. doi:10.1001/jama.2017.9236
12. Westermark P, Westermark GT, Suhr OB, Berg S. Transthyretin-derived amyloidosis: Probably a common cause of lumbar spinal stenosis. *Ups J Med Sci.* 2014;119(3):223-228. doi:10.3109/03009734.2014.895786
13. Cyrille NB, Goldsmith J, Alvarez J, Maurer MS. Prevalence and prognostic significance of low QRS voltage among the three main types of cardiac amyloidosis. *Am J Cardiol.* 2014;114(7):1089-1093. doi:10.1016/j.amjcard.2014.07.026
14. Zhang KW, Zhang R, Deych E, Stockerl-Goldstein KE, Gorcsan J, Lenihan DJ. A multimodal diagnostic model improves detection of cardiac amyloidosis among patients with diagnostic confirmation by cardiac biopsy. *Am Heart J.* 2021;232:137-145. doi:10.1016/j.ahj.2020.11.006
15. Murtagh B, Hammill SC, Gertz MA, Kyle RA, Tajik AJ, Grogan M. Electrocardiographic findings in primary systemic amyloidosis and biopsy-proven cardiac involvement. *Am J Cardiol.* 2005;95(4):535-537. doi:10.1016/j.amjcard.2004.10.028
16. Cappelli F, Vignini E, Martone R, et al. Baseline ECG features and arrhythmic profile in transthyretin versus light chain cardiac amyloidosis. *Circ Heart Fail.* 2020;13(3):e006619. doi:10.1161/CIRCHEARTFAILURE.119.006619
17. Boldrini M, Cappelli F, Chacko L, et al. Multiparametric echocardiography scores for the diagnosis of cardiac amyloidosis. *JACC Cardiovasc Imaging.* 2020;13(4):909-920. doi:10.1016/j.jcmg.2019.10.011
18. Martinez-Naharro A, Gonzalez-Lopez E, Corovic A, et al. High prevalence of intracardiac thrombi in cardiac amyloidosis. *J Am Coll Cardiol.* 2019;73(13):1733-1734. doi:10.1016/j.jacc.2019.01.035
19. Phelan D, Collier P, Thavendiranathan P, et al. Relative apical sparing of longitudinal strain using two-dimensional speckle-tracking echocardiography is both sensitive and specific for the diagnosis of cardiac amyloidosis. *Heart.* 2012;98(19):1442-1448. doi:10.1136/heartjnl-2012-302353
20. Palladini G, Campana C, Klersy C, et al. Serum N-terminal pro-brain natriuretic peptide is a sensitive marker of myocardial dysfunction in AL amyloidosis. *Circulation.* 2003;107(19):2440-2445. doi:10.1161/01.CIR.0000068314.02595.B2
21. Zhang KW, Miao J, Mitchell JD, et al. Plasma hepatocyte growth factor for diagnosis and prognosis in light chain and transthyretin cardiac amyloidosis. *JACC CardioOncol.* 2020;2(1):56-66. doi:10.1016/j.jaccao.2020.01.006
22. Gillmore JD, Maurer MS, Falk RH, et al. Nonbiopsy diagnosis of cardiac transthyretin amyloidosis. *Circulation.* 2016;133(24):2404-2412. doi:10.1161/CIRCULATIONAHA.116.021612
23. Maceira AM, Joshi J, Prasad SK, et al. Cardiovascular magnetic resonance in cardiac amyloidosis. *Circulation.* 2005;111(2):186-193. doi:10.1161/01.CIR.0000152819.97857.9D
24. Baggiano A, Boldrini M, Martinez-Naharro A, et al. Noncontrast magnetic resonance for the diagnosis of cardiac amyloidosis. *JACC Cardiovasc Imaging.* 2020;13(1, Part 1):69-80. doi:https://doi.org/10.1016/j.jcmg.2019.03.026

25. Banypersad SM, Sado DM, Flett AS, et al. Quantification of myocardial extracellular volume fraction in systemic AL amyloidosis: an equilibrium contrast cardiovascular magnetic resonance study. *Circ Cardiovasc Imaging.* 2013;6(1):34-39. doi:10.1161/CIRCIMAGING.112.978627
26. Quarta CC, Gonzalez-Lopez E, Gilbertson JA, et al. Diagnostic sensitivity of abdominal fat aspiration in cardiac amyloidosis. *Eur Heart J.* 2017;38(24):1905-1908. doi:10.1093/eurheartj/ehx047
27. Fine NM, Arruda-Olson AM, Dispenzieri A, et al. Yield of noncardiac biopsy for the diagnosis of transthyretin cardiac amyloidosis. *Am J Cardiol.* 2014;113(10):1723-1727. doi:10.1016/j.amjcard.2014.02.030

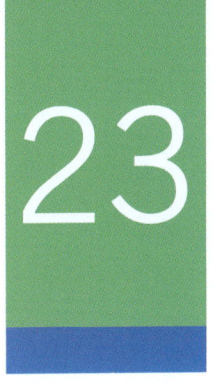

23 Light Chain Amyloidosis: Latest Treatment Strategies

Scott R. Goldsmith and Keith E. Stockerl-Goldstein

GENERAL PRINCIPLES

- Most patients with light chain amyloidosis (AL) have systemic involvement (eg, renal, cardiac, hepatic) at the time of diagnosis. Survival benefits have been demonstrated with early systemic therapy, including both transplant and nontransplant modalities.
- Patients with noncardiac, organ-specific light chain amyloid deposition should undergo a complete workup to rule out systemic disease. These patients are either monitored clinically or treated with local therapy depending on organ involvement and symptoms.
- Treatment strategies hinge on patient- and disease-related factors that determine eligibility for stem cell transplantation.
- A thorough evaluation of the extent and severity of organ involvement is integral to determining treatment strategy and organ response (Table 23-1).
- Current therapeutic strategies target the amyloidogenic plasma cell clone, whereas investigational therapies target the amyloidogenic light chains and amyloid fibrils themselves.
- Treatment and monitoring paradigms are evolving rapidly.
- Clinical trial enrollment is strongly encouraged.
- **Management should be guided by a multidisciplinary team with expertise in the complexities of AL.**

STAGING

- As cardiac involvement is highly prognostic of outcomes, all AL staging systems to date have relied heavily on cardiac biomarkers.
- **The original Mayo classification system utilizes cardiac troponin T (cTnT) or cardiac troponin I (cTnI) and N-terminal pro-B-type natriuretic peptide (NT-proBNP) levels to designate three stages of disease (I-III) with progressively worsening overall mortality.**[1] **Patients receive 1 point each for cTnT ≥ 0.025 ng/mL and NT-proBNP ≥ 1800 pg/mL.**
- **A 2012 revision of the original Mayo system added an additional parameter, difference between involved and uninvolved free light chains (dFLCs) ≥ 18 mg/dL, which improved risk stratification** (Table 23-2).[2] **This system is commonly used clinically.**
- The European modification of the original Mayo system does not incorporate dFLC, but subdivides stage III into IIIA and IIIB for patients with NT-proBNP

TABLE 23-1 Organ-Specific Criteria for Involvement With Light Chain Amyloidosis, Response to Therapy, and Disease Progression

Organ	Involvement criteria	Response criteria	Response criteria
Heart	Biopsy verification with clinical or lab evidence of cardiac dysfunction OR Noncardiac biopsy verification AND mean wall thickness on echo >12 mm OR elevated NT-proBNP in the absence of renal failure or atrial fibrillation	Mean IVS thickness decreases by 2 mm, 20% improvement of EF, and ≥2 NYHA class decrease in subjects with baseline NYHA class III or IV OR NT-proBNP reduction >30% and ≥300 ng/L in patients with baseline NT-proBNP ≥650 ng/L (must have eGFR ≥45 mL/min/1.73 m²)	>30% increase in NT-proBNP and >300 ng/L OR ≥33% increase in cTn OR ≥10% decrease in EF
Kidney	Biopsy verification with clinical or lab evidence of renal dysfunction OR Nonrenal biopsy verification AND 24-hour UPro >0.5 g/day (other causes excluded)	50% decrease in 24-hour UPro without reduction of eGFR by ≥25% or an increase in sCr ≥0.5 mg/dL	50% increase in 24-hour UPro to >1 g/day OR 25% increase of sCr OR 25% decrease of CrCl
Liver	Biopsy verification with clinical or lab evidence of hepatic dysfunction OR Non-hepatic biopsy verification AND hepatomegaly >15 cm (not cardiac-related) OR alk-phos >1.5 ULN	50% decrease in abnormal alk-phos OR 2 cm decrease in hepatomegaly	50% increase in alk-phos above the lowest value

Lung	Biopsy verification with respiratory symptoms and interstitial pulmonary infiltrate	N/A
Nerve	Clinical manifestation of peripheral neuropathy (ie, symmetrical sensorimotor neuropathy) or autonomic neuropathy (ie, delayed gastric emptying, orthostatic hypotension, urinary dysfunction)	N/A
Soft Tissue	Macroglossia, skin deposits, muscular deposits, lymphadenopathy	N/A

alk-phos, alkaline phosphatase; CrCl, creatinine clearance; cTn, cardiac troponin; EF, ejection fraction; eGFR, estimated glomerular filtration rate; IVS, intraventricular septum; NT-proBNP, N-terminal pro-B-type natriuretic peptide; NYHA, New York Heart Association; sCr, serum creatinine; ULN, upper limit of normal; UPro, urinary protein.

Adapted from Gertz MA, Comenzo R, Falk RH, et al. Definition of organ involvement and treatment response in immunoglobulin light chain amyloidosis (AL): a consensus opinion from the 10th International Symposium on Amyloid and Amyloidosis, Tours, France, 18-22 April 2004. *Am J Hematol.* 2005;79(4):319-328. Merlini G, Seldin DC, Gertz MA. Amyloidosis: pathogenesis and new therapeutic options. *J Clin Oncol.* 2011;29(14):1924-1933; Comenzo RL, Reece D, Palladini G, et al. Consensus guidelines for the conduct and reporting of clinical trials in systemic light-chain amyloidosis. *Leukemia.* 2012;26(11):2317-2325. doi:10.1038/leu.2012.100.

TABLE 23-2 Revised Prognostic Staging System (2012 Mayo System) for Light Chain Amyloidosis

Stage	Points	Median OS (months)
I	0	94.1
II	1	40.3
III	2	14
IV	3	5.8

Patients receive 1 point for each of the following: dFLC ≥ 18 mg/dL; cTnT[a] ≥ 0.025 ng/mL; NT-proBNP ≥ 1800 pg/mL

cTnT, cardiac troponin T; dFLC, difference in involved and uninvolved free light chain; NT-proBNP, N-terminal pro-B-type natriuretic peptide; OS, overall survival.

[a]High-sensitivity cTnT, with a cutoff value of 40 pg/mL, has been recently validated as a substitute for the fourth-generation cTnT for staging purpose, Kumar SK, Gertz MA, Dispenzieri A. Validation of Mayo Clinic staging system for light chain amyloidosis with high-sensitivity troponin. *J Clin Oncol.* 2019;37(2):171-173.

Staging system and survival data adapted from Kumar S, Dispenzieri A, Lacy MQ, et al. Revised prognostic staging system for light chain amyloidosis incorporating cardiac biomarkers and serum free light chain measurements. *J Clin Oncol.* 2012;30(9):989-995.

1800-8500 pg/mL or >8500 pg/mL, respectively. This system is often employed in clinical trials.[3]
- The high-sensitivity cTnT (hs-cTnT) assay has also been validated in lieu of the fourth-generation cTnT assay (using a cutoff of ≥40 pg/mL) and provides similar prognostic information.[4,5]

TREATMENT

Initial Therapy

- Clinical trials are preferred if available.
- Patients without concomitant multiple myeloma (MM) and with bone marrow plasma cell (BMPC) burden <10% can proceed to autologous stem cell transplantation (ASCT) directly, assuming they are eligible for transplant (see *Determining Transplant Eligibility*).
- Although ASCT for those eligible is standard at many centers, some centers defer transplant and employ upfront novel regimens with high response rates.
- **Only about 20% of AL patients are eligible for ASCT at diagnosis; therefore, the majority are treated with bortezomib-based combination chemotherapy. Transplant-eligible patients with concomitant MM or higher BMPCs at diagnosis generally undergo two to four cycles of cytoreduction with bortezomib-based therapy prior to ASCT.**
- Unlike in MM without amyloidosis, immunomodulatory drugs (IMiDs) are not frequently used for frontline therapy because of poor patient tolerance. Additionally, these agents have been associated with increases in cardiac biomarkers, which may complicate assessment of treatment response.[5]
- **Cyclophosphamide, bortezomib, and dexamethasone (CyBorD)** is the most commonly used frontline regimen.
  - Hematologic response is seen in 60% to 70% of patients and cardiac response in about 33% of patients at 12 months.[6]

- Overall survival among responders is comparable to that seen after ASCT.
- Notable toxicities are lethargy, fluid overload, infection, sensory neuropathy, and gastrointestinal upset.
- Patients should receive herpesvirus prophylaxis while on bortezomib.
- **Daratumumab (Dara) plus CyBorD is a novel combination being evaluated as frontline therapy in the phase 3 ANDROMEDA study and will likely represent a new standard of care.**
  - Daratumumab is a monoclonal antibody targeting CD38-expressing plasma cells.
  - Primary analysis of ANDROMEDA demonstrated a significantly higher hematologic overall response rate (92% vs. 77%), complete response (53% vs. 18%), and very good partial response (VGPR; 79% vs. 49%), as well as cardiac response (42% vs. 22%) for Dara-CyBorD compared to the CyBorD control arm.[7]
  - Toxicities were comparable to CyBorD without observed synergistic toxicities. Cardiac failure was rarely reported in both study arms.
  - Longer follow-up duration is needed to determine potential improvements in progression and survival outcomes on Dara-CyBorD as compared to CyBorD.
- **Bortezomib, melphalan, and dexamethasone (BMD)** can be used for transplant-ineligible patients, although it has not been compared directly to CyBorD. BMD yielded a superior hematologic response and better overall survival compared to melphalan and dexamethasone, although with increased neuropathy, gastrointestinal toxicity, and fluid retention.[8] Herpesvirus prophylaxis is required.
- **Melphalan and dexamethasone** is a regimen for patients ineligible for ASCT who cannot receive bortezomib for reasons such as preexisting neuropathy.

Autologous Stem Cell Transplantation
- High-dose therapy (HDT) with myeloablative doses of melphalan followed by ASCT rescue is a key component of therapy in carefully selected patients with AL.
- In such patients, HDT with ASCT has been associated with deeper hematologic responses and survival benefits.
- HDT aims to eliminate the amyloidogenic plasma cell clone, thereby preventing light chain amyloid production.
- Traditionally, transplant-eligible AL patients without concomitant MM and with <10% BMPCs would proceed to ASCT without induction therapy, whereas those with concomitant MM, ≥10% BMPCs, or anticipated delays to transplant would receive induction therapy to control or reduce the burden of disease. The efficacy of novel agents, including proteasome inhibitors and monoclonal antibodies, may in the future support their routine use in all AL patients as pretransplant induction therapy or supplant the need for ASCT altogether.
- **Patients with AL are at significantly higher risk of morbidity and mortality with ASCT as compared to patients with MM because of unique complications during stem cell mobilization, including arrhythmias, sepsis, and gastrointestinal hemorrhage. Therefore, in addition to meticulous patient selection, management by a multidisciplinary team at an institution with experience performing ASCT for AL is necessary.**

Determining Transplant Eligibility
- Attention to and refinement of patient eligibility criteria over the past three decades has resulted in a 40% reduction in early post-ASCT mortality.[9]
- In retrospective studies and clinical trials, increased risk for transplant-related mortality is associated with age, >2 organs significantly involved, advanced cardiac

disease (symptomatic congestive heart failure [CHF], arrhythmias, baseline hypotension), and renal dysfunction.
- **Consensus guidelines, such as the mSMART criteria, have been developed in order to standardize the approach to patient selection for ASCT** (Table 23-3). **However, transplant criteria are usually center specific.**
- Cardiopulmonary exercise testing in patients with cardiac involvement is both prognostic for survival and predictive of tolerance of ASCT.[10,11] Therefore, it is recommended for all AL patients being considered for ASCT.
- Pre-ASCT cardiac or renal transplantation may make a previously transplant-ineligible patient a suitable candidate for ASCT.
- Patients with AL may have an acquired factor X deficiency because of adsorption of the coagulation factor to the light chain amyloid fibrils. This can lead to a severe coagulopathy and is associated with exceedingly high transplant-related mortality if unrecognized.

Transplantation and Risk-Adapted Approach
- Peripheral blood stem cells are collected by leukapheresis after mobilization with granulocyte colony-stimulating factor (filgrastim) and occasionally plerixafor.
  - Life-threatening complications during stem cell mobilization, such as spontaneous splenic rupture and arrhythmias, occur more frequently in patients with AL as compared to others undergoing mobilization. Vigilant monitoring and possibly inpatient admission during the mobilization and collection process are warranted.
- A minimum collection of 2.0×10^6 CD34$^+$ cells/kg of body weight is usually necessary.
- **Risk-adapted approaches to melphalan dosing have incorporated factors such as patient age, left ventricular ejection fraction, presence and severity of cardiac**

TABLE 23-3　mSMART Eligibility Criteria for Autologous Stem Cell Transplantation

Variable	Parameter
"Physiologic" age	≤70 years
ECOG performance status	≤2
Systolic blood pressure	≥90 (optimally ≥100)
Cardiac troponin T	≤0.06 ng/mL (hs-TnT <75 ng/mL)
Creatinine clearance	≥30 mL/min (unless on chronic dialysis)
NYHA functional class	I or II

Patients should meet all of the above eligibility criteria in order to be eligible for high-dose therapy with autologous stem cell transplantation. "Physiologic" age requires careful clinical evaluation.

ECOG, Eastern Cooperative Oncology Group; hs-TnT, high-sensitivity troponin T; NYHA, New York Heart Association.

Adapted from mSMART Guidelines for Treatment, v9 Oct 2020. https://www.msmart.org/treatment-guidlines

involvement, yield of stem cells from collection, number of organs involved, and renal dysfunction.
- Based on these factors, patients might receive full-dose (200 mg/m^2), intermediate-dose (140 mg/m^2), or low-dose (100 mg/m^2) melphalan.
- Studies have demonstrated that patients who receive full-dose melphalan have significantly better hematologic response and survival compared to attenuated dosing, even after adjusting for confounding covariates. Therefore, pursuing a nontransplant strategy may be favored over intermediate- or low-dose melphalan if full dose is likely to be prohibitively toxic. Patients with a creatinine clearance (CrCl) <30 mL/min or on chronic dialysis should receive 140 mg/m^2.
- Patients usually remain hospitalized until durable engraftment occurs, with reliable reconstitution of neutrophils (>500/μL) and platelets (>20,000/μL).
  - The hospitalization course typically includes transfusion support, cardiac monitoring, and management of infections, bleeding, and gastrointestinal complications.
  - **Careful management of fluid status is essential in patients with AL cardiomyopathy and is best managed in consultation with cardio-oncology.**

Cardiac Transplantation with Subsequent Autologous Stem Cell Transplantation
- **In patients who are ineligible for ASCT because of severe restrictive cardiomyopathy, heart transplantation (HT) in carefully selected patients with minimal involvement of other organs may be feasible with the intent of proceeding to ASCT within a reasonable time frame.**[12]
- Several small series have demonstrated the feasibility of this approach with outcomes comparable to patients who receive HT for non-amyloid causes; subsequent ASCT is considered necessary to halt the production of amyloidogenic light chains.
- In general, HT is reserved for AL patients without MM and with low BMPCs who are expected to have longer progression-free intervals after ASCT.
- Careful pre-HT evaluation as to the extent of systemic involvement is paramount and may be aided by techniques such as iodine-123 (^{123}I)-labeled serum amyloid P (SAP) component scintigraphy.[13]
- Optimal timing of post-HT ASCT remains unknown, as the desire to minimize further accumulation of amyloid by earlier ASCT is counterbalanced by the need for stronger immunosuppression in the early post-HT period, which elevates the risk of peri-ASCT infection. In general, a delay of 6 to 8 months post-HT is common.[14]
- Adjustment of HT immunosuppression prior to mobilization and collection is often necessary as certain medications (eg, azathioprine) may affect stem cell quality and yield.
- Disease relapse and systemic amyloid accumulation, including within the transplanted heart, is an important cause of posttransplant morbidity and mortality, highlighting the need for continued monitoring, treatment, and innovation.

Therapy for Relapsed/Refractory Disease
- **As comparative prospective trials for relapsed/refractory AL have not been conducted, treatment is chosen based on prior therapies, physician preference, toxicities, and specific organ involvement.**
- Clinical trials are preferred.
- Repeating the initial therapy is a reasonable approach if it was previously effective, especially if there is a long interval between initial completion and relapse; trials of the above-listed frontline regimens are reasonable.

- IMiDs (eg, lenalidomide, pomalidomide) may lead to disease response but can also be associated with elevations in cardiac biomarkers that may complicate assessment of cardiac response to therapy. Prescribed doses should be lower than those used in MM patients, and caution should be exercised in patients with significant cardiac and renal involvement. Because of the association of IMiDs with thrombosis, thromboprophylaxis is needed.
- Selected therapies for relapsed/refractory disease, response rates, and notable toxicities are summarized in Table 23-4.

Amyloid Fibril-Targeting Therapy
Adjuvant Doxycycline
- Based on *in vitro* and *in vivo* models, doxycycline has been posited to inhibit amyloid fibril formation or decrease the toxic effects of the amyloidogenic light chains on cardiac tissue.
- A retrospective study examining the impact of post-ASCT antibiotic prophylaxis demonstrated that those receiving doxycycline had improved overall survival compared to those receiving penicillins.[15]

TABLE 23-4 Therapy Options for Relapsed/Refractory Light Chain Amyloidosis[a]

Therapy	Response	Toxicities
Daratumumab[20,21] (subcutaneous may be preferred because of risk of volume overload from intravenous formulation)	60%-80% hematologic 30%-50% cardiac	CHF (14% Gr 3/4 in one trial), AFib (18% Gr 3/4 in one trial), orthostatic hypotension, respiratory infections (upper and lower), infusion reactions
Lenalidomide[22,23] ± dex ± cyclophosphamide	60%-70% hematologic 5%-20% cardiac	Rising cardiac biomarkers, thrombotic events, fatigue, edema, respiratory infections, rash
Pomalidomide[24] ± dex	50%-70% hematologic 15% cardiac	Arrhythmias, CHF (rare), dyspnea, myelosuppression, neuropathy
Bortezomib[25] ± dex ± melphalan	70%-80% hematologic 13% cardiac	Neuropathy, gastrointestinal disorders CHF and arrythmias reported, but rare
Ixazomib[26] ± dex	50% hematologic 18% cardiac	Cardiac arrhythmias, CHF, rash, gastrointestinal disorders, pneumonia, edema

AFib, atrial fibrillation; CHF, congestive heart failure; dex, dexamethasone; Gr, grade.
[a]Frontline regimens that were effective with long intervals between discontinuation and relapse may be retried.

- Safety, tolerability, and preliminary efficacy of doxycycline added to chemotherapy or after ASCT have been suggested based on small retrospective case-control studies and small prospective single-arm trials comparing outcomes with historical controls; survival benefits have been suggested.[16] A recent randomized control trial of 140 patients did not demonstrate a significant benefit in hematologic or cardiac PFS in which doxycycline was added to CyBorD compared to placebo.[17]
- **Although larger randomized controlled trials are needed, some guidelines and experts suggest adjuvant doxycycline based on the low risk and possible benefit in patients with AL cardiomyopathy.**

Investigational Agents
- GSK2315698 is a monoclonal antibody targeting the SAP component of amyloid deposits that induced phagocytic clearance of amyloid deposits *in vivo*. A phase 2 trial of GSK2315698 in cardiac amyloidosis was terminated prematurely because of an adverse risk/benefit profile.
- CAEL-101 is a light chain–reactive monoclonal antibody that was safe and tolerable in phase 1 and 2 studies with promising efficacy based on organ response.[18] It is currently being investigated in two placebo-controlled phase 3 trials in combination with CyBorD.

ASSESSMENT OF TREATMENT RESPONSE

- Consensus guidelines for hematologic response (Table 23-5) and organ response (Table 23-1) are shown.

TABLE 23-5 Consensus Hematologic Response Criteria for Light Chain Amyloidosis

Response	Criteria
Complete response (CR)	Negative serum and urine IFE, normal FLC ratio
Very good partial response (VGPR)	dFLC[a] <4 mg/dL
Partial response (PR)	dFLC[a] decrease by >50%
No response (NR)	Less than PR
Progression	From CR: Any detectable M-protein or abnormal FLC ratio (FLC must double) From PR: 50% increase in serum M-protein to >0.5 g/dL OR 50% increase in urine M-protein to >200 mg/day FLC increase of 50% to >10 mg/dL

dFLC, difference between involved and uninvolved free light chains; FLC, free light chain; IFE, immunofixation.

[a]Change in dFLC is not applicable for patients with pretreatment dFLC <5 mg/dL; posttreatment dFLC <1 mg/dL has been associated with a survival benefit in such patients.

Adapted from Comenzo RL, Reece D, Palladini G, et al. Consensus guidelines for the conduct and reporting of clinical trials in systemic light-chain amyloidosis. *Leukemia.* 2012;26(11):2317-2325. doi:10.1038/leu.2012.100 and Palladini G, Dispenzieri A, Gertz MA, et al. New criteria for response to treatment in immunoglobulin light chain amyloidosis based on free light chain measurement and cardiac biomarkers: impact on survival outcomes. *J Clin Oncol.* 2012;30(36):4541-4549. doi:10.1200/JCO.2011.37.7614

- Criteria for hematologic response are evolving. Some investigators have demonstrated that normalization of the FLC ratio is not associated with improved organ response, progression-free survival, or overall survival, but that dFLC <1 mg/dL or decline of the absolute value of the involved FLC (iFLC) ≤2 mg/dL may be better prognostic discriminators.[6,19]
- The goal of treatment with chemotherapy or ASCT is to attain a hematologic VGPR or better to prevent further amyloid deposition.
- **Organ responses are seen less frequently than hematologic responses and may not be apparent for 6 months or more after achievement of a hematologic response.**
- Treatment changes should be considered for patients who do not achieve at least a partial response after two cycles of therapy or do not achieve at least a VGPR after four to six cycles of therapy.

REFERENCES

1. Dispenzieri A, Gertz MA, Kyle RA, et al. Serum cardiac troponins and N-terminal pro-brain natriuretic peptide: a staging system for primary systemic amyloidosis. *J Clin Oncol.* 2004;22(18):3751-3757.
2. Kumar S, Dispenzieri A, Lacy MQ, et al. Revised prognostic staging system for light chain amyloidosis incorporating cardiac biomarkers and serum free light chain measurements. *J Clin Oncol.* 2012;30(9):989-995.
3. Dittrich T, Kimmich C, Hegenbart U, Schönland SO. Prognosis and staging of AL amyloidosis. *Acta Haematol.* 2020;143(4):388-400.
4. Kumar SK, Gertz MA, Dispenzieri A. Validation of Mayo Clinic staging system for light chain amyloidosis with high-sensitivity troponin. *J Clin Oncol.* 2019;37(2):171-173.
5. Jelinek T, Kufova Z, Hajek R. Immunomodulatory drugs in AL amyloidosis. *Crit Rev Oncol Hematol.* 2016;99:249-260.
6. Manwani R, Cohen O, Sharpley F, et al. A prospective observational study of 915 patients with systemic AL amyloidosis treated with upfront bortezomib. *Blood.* 2019;134(25):2271-2280.
7. Kastritis E, Palladini G, Minnema MC, et al; ANDROMEDA Trial Investigators. Daratumumab-based treatment for immunoglobulin light-chain amyloidosis. *N Engl J Med.* 2021;385(1):46-58. doi:10.1056/NEJMoa2028631.
8. Kastritis E, Leleu X, Arnulf B, et al. Bortezomib, melphalan, and dexamethasone for light-chain amyloidosis. *J Clin Oncol.* 2020;38(28):3252-3260.
9. Comenzo RL, Gertz MA. Autologous stem cell transplantation for primary systemic amyloidosis. *Blood.* 2002;99(12):4276-4282.
10. White PS, Phull P, Brauneis D, et al. High-dose melphalan and stem cell transplantation in AL amyloidosis with elevated cardiac biomarkers. *Bone Marrow Transplant.* 2018;53(12):1593-1595.
11. Nicol M, Deney A, Lairez O, et al. Prognostic value of cardiopulmonary exercise testing in cardiac amyloidosis. *Eur J Heart Fail.* 2021;23(2):231-239.
12. Mehra MR, Canter CE, Hannan MM, et al. The 2016 International Society for Heart Lung Transplantation listing criteria for heart transplantation: a 10-year update. *J Heart Lung Transplant.* 2016;35(1):1-23.
13. Gillmore JD, Goodman HJ, Lachmann HJ, et al. Sequential heart and autologous stem cell transplantation for systemic AL amyloidosis. *Blood.* 2006;107(3):1227-1229.
14. Davis MK, Kale P, Liedtke M, et al. Outcomes after heart transplantation for amyloid cardiomyopathy in the modern era. *Am. J. Transplant* 2015;15(3):650-658.
15. Kumar SK, Dispenzieri A, Lacy MQ, et al. Doxycycline used as post transplant antibacterial prophylaxis improves survival in patients with light chain amyloidosis undergoing autologous stem cell transplantation. *Blood.* 2012;120(21):3138.

16. D'Souza A, Szabo A, Flynn KE, et al. Adjuvant doxycycline to enhance anti-amyloid effects: Results from the dual phase 2 trial. *EClinicalMedicine*. 2020;23:100361.
17. Shen KN, Fu WJ, Wu Y, et al. Doxycycline combined with bortezomib-cyclophosphamide-dexamethasone chemotherapy for newly diagnosed cardiac light-chain amyloidosis: a multicenter randomized controlled trial. *Circulation. 2021*. doi:10.1161/CIRCULATIONAHA.121.055953. Epub ahead of print.
18. Valent J, Silowsky J, Kurman MR, et al. Cael-101 Is well-tolerated in AL amyloidosis patients receiving concomitant cyclophosphamide-bortezomib-dexamethasone (CyborD): a phase 2 dose-finding study (NCT04304144). *Blood*. 2020;136(suppl 1):26-27.
19. Muchtar E, Dispenzieri A, Leung N, et al. Optimizing deep response assessment for AL amyloidosis using involved free light chain level at end of therapy: failure of the serum free light chain ratio. *Leukemia*. 2019;33(2):527-531.
20. Roussel M, Merlini G, Chevret S, et al. A prospective phase 2 trial of daratumumab in patients with previously treated systemic light-chain amyloidosis. *Blood*. 2020;135(18):1531-1540.
21. Sanchorawala V, Sarosiek S, Schulman A, et al. Safety, tolerability, and response rates of daratumumab in relapsed AL amyloidosis: results of a phase 2 study. *Blood*. 2020;135(18):1541-1547.
22. Sanchorawala V, Wright DG, Rosenzweig M, et al. Lenalidomide and dexamethasone in the treatment of AL amyloidosis: results of a phase 2 trial. *Blood*. 2006;109(2):492-496.
23. Sanchorawala V, Finn KT, Fennessey S, et al. Durable hematologic complete responses can be achieved with lenalidomide in AL amyloidosis. *Blood*. 2010;116(11):1990-1991.
24. Dispenzieri A, Buadi F, Laumann K, et al. Activity of pomalidomide in patients with immunoglobulin light-chain amyloidosis. *Blood*. 2012;119(23):5397-5404.
25. Reece DE, Hegenbart U, Sanchorawala V, et al. Long-term follow-up from a phase 1/2 study of single-agent bortezomib in relapsed systemic AL amyloidosis. *Blood*. 2014;124(16):2498-2506.
26. Dispenzieri A, Kastritis E, Wechalekar AD, et al. Primary results from the phase 3 Tourmaline-AL1 trial of ixazomib-dexamethasone versus physician's choice of therapy in patients (pts) with relapsed/refractory primary systemic AL amyloidosis (RRAL). *Blood*. 2019;134(Suppl_1):139. doi:10.1182/blood-2019-124409.

24 Cardiac Amyloidosis: Latest Treatment Strategies for Transthyretin Amyloidosis

Mario Rodriguez Rivera and Justin M. Vader

GENERAL PRINCIPLES

- Transthyretin cardiac amyloidosis (ATTR-CM) is a form of restrictive cardiomyopathy resulting from the deposition of misfolded transthyretin protein as amyloid fibrils in myocardium.[1]
- Transthyretin-directed therapy with either transthyretin stabilizers or transthyretin synthesis inhibitors prevents additional transthyretin amyloid fibril deposition.
- Fluid overload, arrhythmias, and orthostatic hypotension (OH) are additional components of ATTR-CM management.
- In carefully selected patients with end-stage heart failure because of ATTR-CM, heart transplantation is an effective treatment option.
- A multidisciplinary care team is frequently necessary for the care of patients with ATTR-CM and may include general cardiologists, cardio-oncologists, electrophysiologists, neurologists, and advanced heart failure specialists.

BACKGROUND

- Transthyretin, also called prealbumin, is a ubiquitous protein synthesized predominantly in the liver and choroid plexus that circulates in the blood and cerebrospinal fluid, transporting thyroxine and retinol.[2]
- Transthyretin circulates predominantly as a homotetramer, rich in beta-pleated sheets that interact to stabilize the structure. Disruptions of the homotetrameric protein structure lead to dissociation into protein monomers that misfold and aggregate in tissue as amyloid fibrils, resulting in transthyretin amyloidosis (ATTR).[1]
- **ATTR can occur in older individuals as the result of the deposition of genetically normal or "wild-type" transthyretin amyloid fibrils (wild-type ATTR).**
- **ATTR can also occur in an accelerated hereditary form (hereditary ATTR) with a predilection for cardiac and neuronal involvement.** Several known genetic mutations in the transthyretin gene are associated with hereditary ATTR (see Chapter 22, Cardiac Amyloidosis: General Diagnostic Approach).[2]
- Overall survival with ATTR is largely determined by cardiac involvement with disease, with a median survival of 2 to 4 years after diagnosis of ATTR-CM when left untreated.[2]

STAGING AND PROGNOSIS OF TRANSTHYRETIN CARDIAC AMYLOIDOSIS

- The main determinant of survival and prognosis in ATTR is cardiac involvement.[3]
- Current staging systems for ATTR-CM utilize serum cardiac biomarkers and/or glomerular filtration rate (GFR) and include the Mayo Clinic staging system and the UK National Amyloidosis Center staging system (Table 24-1).[4-6]

TRANSTHYRETIN-DIRECTED THERAPY

- Selection of transthyretin-directed therapy is based on the presence of cardiomyopathy and/or polyneuropathy, as well as the distinction between wild-type and hereditary ATTR (Table 24-2).

Transthyretin Stabilizers
Tafamidis
- Tafamidis is an orally bioavailable small molecule that exhibits potent and selective transthyretin binding, leading to transthyretin tetramer stabilization and reduction in transthyretin amyloid fibril formation.[2,7]

TABLE 24-1 Prognosis and Staging Systems for Transthyretin Cardiac Amyloidosis

	Patient population	Biomarker levels	Median survival by stage		
			Stage I (both normal)	Stage II (one abnormal)	Stage III (both abnormal)
Mayo Clinic[a] Staging System	wtATTR	NT-proBNP <3000 pg/mL	66 months	40 months	20 months
		Troponin <0.05 ng/mL			
UK Staging System[b]	wtATTR, hATTR	NT-proBNP <3000 pg/mL	69 months	46.7 months	24.1 months
		eGFR <45mL/min			

eGFR, estimated glomerular filtration rate; hATTR, hereditary transthyretin amyloidosis; NT-proBNP, N-terminal pro-brain natriuretic peptide; wtATTR, wild-type transthyretin amyloidosis.
[a]Grogan M, Scott C, Kyle R, et al. Natural history of wild-type transthyretin cardiac amyloidosis and risk stratification using a novel staging system. *J Am Coll Cardiol*. 2016;6:1014-1020.
[b]Gillmore JD, Damy T, Fontana M, et al. A new staging system for cardiac transthyretin amyloidosis. *Eur Heart J*. 2018;3:2799-2806.

- In the ATTR-ACT trial of 441 patients with either wild-type or hereditary ATTR-CM, tafamidis reduced all-cause mortality (hazard ratio [HR] 0.70, 95% confidence interval [CI] 0.51-0.96) and cardiovascular hospitalization (HR 0.68, 95% CI 0.56-0.81) as compared to placebo.[8]
  - Tafamidis was also associated with lower rates of decline in 6-minute walk distance and quality of life.
  - Patients with New York Heart Association (NYHA) class IV symptoms, severe aortic stenosis, and impaired renal function (GFR <25 mL·min^{-1}·1.73 m^{-2} body surface area) were excluded.
- **Tafamidis is approved by the U.S. Food and Drug Administration (FDA) for treatment of ATTR-CM. The benefits of tafamidis in patients with NYHA class IV symptoms and/or advanced renal dysfunction (GFR <25 mL·min^{-1}·1.73 m^{-2}) are uncertain.**
- Currently, tafamidis represents the standard of care for patients with wild-type ATTR-CM or hereditary ATTR-CM without polyneuropathy.

Diflunisal
- The nonsteroidal anti-inflammatory drug (NSAID) diflunisal was the first transthyretin stabilizer recognized. Diflunisal binds with higher affinity to the central hormone-binding funnel than thyroxine, thus stabilizing the transthyretin tetramer.[7,9] *In vitro* studies showed that diflunisal 250 mg twice daily slows transthyretin amyloid fibril aggregation.
- A phase III trial in patients with hereditary ATTR with polyneuropathy showed that diflunisal reduced the rate of disease progression and improved quality of life. No large randomized controlled trials have evaluated diflunisal in ATTR-CM, with only small retrospective data suggesting efficacy and tolerability.[2]
- **As an NSAID, concerns for thrombocytopenia, kidney dysfunction, and gastrointestinal bleeding accompany the use of diflunisal.**
- In clinical practice, use of diflunisal may be considered in carefully selected patients with normal renal function and stable volume status when tafamidis is not available.

Transthyretin Synthesis Inhibitors
- **Patisiran and inotersen are approved by the FDA for treatment of hereditary ATTR with polyneuropathy.** Phase III studies of patisiran (NCT03997383) and a newer formulation of inotersen (NCT04136171) in ATTR-CM are ongoing.

Patisiran
- Patisiran is a double-stranded small interfering RNA that targets the 3'-untranslated region of the transthyretin gene, interrupting cellular RNA transcription and leading to an overall reduction in transthyretin protein synthesis.[2]
- In the APOLLO trial of patients with hereditary ATTR with polyneuropathy, patisiran improved neuropathy impairment scores and quality of life in the overall cohort and in the 56% of subjects with cardiac involvement. **Patients with NYHA class III and IV symptoms were excluded from the trial.**[10]
- Patisiran also reduced N-terminal pro-brain natriuretic peptide (NT-proBNP) levels, reduced left ventricular (LV) wall thickness, and mitigated worsening of global longitudinal strain, suggesting cardiac benefit.[10]

TABLE 24-2 Therapeutic Options for Transthyretin Amyloidosis With Cardiac and/or Neurologic Involvement

Drug name	FDA approval and indication	Dose, route, and frequency	Clinical trial key exclusion criteria	Side effects and monitoring
Transthyretin stabilizers				
Diflunisal	Approved as NSAID (off-label use in ATTR)	250 mg oral, twice daily	NYHA class IV, eGFR <30 mL/min, anticoagulation	Bleeding, renal dysfunction
Tafamidis	Approved for wild-type and hereditary ATTR-CM	61 or 80 mg oral, daily	NYHA class IV, eGFR <25 mL/min, 6MWT <100m	GI symptoms
Transthyretin synthesis inhibitors				
Patisiran	Approved for hereditary ATTR with neuropathy	0.3 mg/kg intravenous, every 3 weeks (premedication with steroids, H1/H2 blockers)	NYHA class III-IV, liver transplant	Vitamin A deficiency, infusion-related reactions
Inotersen	Approved for hereditary ATTR with neuropathy	284 mg subcutaneous, weekly	Platelets <125×10^9/L, creatinine clearance <60 mL·min^{-1}·1.73 m^{-2}, NYHA class III-IV, liver transplant	Vitamin A deficiency, infusion-related reactions, thrombocytopenia, glomerulonephritis

6MWT: 6-minute walk test; ATTR, transthyretin amyloidosis; ATTR-CM, transthyretin amyloid cardiomyopathy; eGFR, estimated glomerular filtration rate; FDA, Food and Drug Administration; GI, gastrointestinal; NSAID, nonsteroidal anti-inflammatory drug; NYHA, New York Heart Association.

- The ongoing APOLLO-B trial (NCT03997383) will determine the efficacy of patisiran for treatment of ATTR-CM.
- Patisiran is currently a first-line treatment option for patients with hereditary ATTR with polyneuropathy.

Inotersen

- Inotersen is a second-generation antisense oligonucleotide (ASO) that binds to the 3′-untranslated region of transthyretin messenger RNA (mRNA), forming an RNA-DNA hybrid that triggers mRNA degradation and reduces transthyretin protein synthesis.[1,2]
- In the NEURO-TTR trial of patients with hereditary ATTR with polyneuropathy, inotersen significantly improved neuropathy impairment scores and quality of life in the overall cohort and in the 63% of subjects with cardiomyopathy. **Patients with NYHA class III and IV symptoms were excluded from the trial.**[11]
- There were no significant differences in LV ejection fraction, global longitudinal strain, LV wall thickness, LV mass, or lateral E/e′ ratio after 15 months of inotersen therapy as compared to placebo therapy.
- **Thrombocytopenia and glomerulonephritis are important safety concerns for inotersen.** Inotersen is contraindicated in patients with platelets <100,000/mm^3 and weekly platelet monitoring is recommended. Inotersen should not be given to patients who develop a urine protein: creatinine >1000 mg/g or estimated GFR <45 mL/min/1.73 m^2. Because of these concerns, inotersen is currently available only through a restricted distribution program under a Risk Evaluation and Mitigation Strategy (REMS). The safety of inotersen in patients with a prior liver transplant for hereditary ATTR is not established.
- The ongoing CARDIO-TTRansform trial (NCT04136171) will determine the efficacy of a newer formulation of inotersen for treatment of ATTR-CM.
- Inotersen is currently a first-line treatment option for patients with hereditary ATTR with polyneuropathy.

MANAGEMENT OF SYMPTOMATIC HEART FAILURE

- ATTR-CM results in restrictive cardiac physiology with elevated cardiac filling pressures and a fixed and reduced stroke volume. As the disease progresses, patients may also develop a reduced LV ejection fraction.
- **Loop diuretics are the mainstay of decongestive therapy for management of volume overload in ATTR-CM.** In patients with high loop diuretic dosing requirements, thiazide or thiazide-like diuretics may be added to overcome diuretic resistance. Caution is required regarding renal dysfunction from excessive preload reduction.
- **Traditional guideline-directed medical therapy for heart failure (beta-blockers, renin-angiotensin-aldosterone-system inhibitors, and angiotensin receptor-neprilysin inhibitors) is not routinely recommended in patients with ATTR-CM.**
  - Vasodilating therapies are generally poorly tolerated because of hypotension.[12]
  - Heart rate–lowering agents, such as beta-blockers, may not be tolerated because of a dependence on elevated heart rate to maintain cardiac output in the setting of a fixed and reduced LV stroke volume.[12]
  - Mineralocorticoid receptor antagonists have been demonstrated to reduce heart failure hospitalizations in patients with heart failure with preserved ejection

fraction and may be with a reasonable choice in normotensive or hypertensive ATTR-CM patients with fluid retention.[13]
- The benefit of any of these therapies in patients with ATTR-CM is unknown as these patients were routinely excluded from heart failure clinical trials.
- Patients who progress to NYHA class IV or end-stage heart failure should be referred for evaluation for advanced heart failure therapies. The I NEED HELP acronym is an easy reminder of the clinical criteria for advanced heart failure therapy referral (Table 24-3).[14]

ADVANCED HEART FAILURE THERAPIES

- **In carefully selected patients with ATTR-CM, cardiac transplantation is an effective treatment option with outcomes that are similar to patients with non-amyloid causes of heart failure.**[15-17]
- In addition to the standard cardiac transplantation evaluation process, a thorough diagnostic evaluation is required to (a) confirm the amyloid fibril type, preferably using endomyocardial biopsy with mass spectrometry, and (b) to determine the extent of extracardiac involvement with amyloidosis.

TABLE 24-3 I NEED HELP—Indicators for Advanced Heart Failure Referral

Inotropes	Previous or ongoing inotrope requirement
NYHA class/**N**atriuretic peptides	Persistent NYHA Class III, IV symptoms and/or persistently high BNP or NT-proBNP
End-organ dysfunction	Worsening renal or liver dysfunction in the setting of heart failure
Ejection fraction	Very low left ventricular ejection fraction <20%
Defibrillator shocks	Recurrent appropriate defibrillator shocks
Hospitalizations	>1 hospitalization for heart failure in the last 6-12 months
Edema/**E**scalating diuretics	Persisting fluid overload and/or increasing diuretic requirement
Low blood pressure	Consistently low systolic BP <90-100 mm Hg
Prognostic medication	Inability to uptitrate (or need to cease/decrease) ACEI, β-blocker, ARNIs, or MRAs

ACEI, angiotensin-converting enzyme inhibitor; ARNI, angiotensin receptor-neprilysin inhibitor; BNP, brain natriuretic peptide; BP, blood pressure; MRA, mineralocorticoid receptor antagonist; NT-proBNP, N-terminal pro-brain natriuretic peptide; NYHA, New York Heart Association.

From Baumwol J. "I Need Help"—a mnemonic to aid timely referral in advanced heart failure. *J Heart Lung Transpl.* 2017;36:593-594.

- In patients with hereditary ATTR-CM, combined heart-liver transplant should be considered to restore normal transthyretin production, prevent the progression of neuropathy, and prevent recurrence of amyloidosis in the transplanted heart.
- The United Network for Organ Sharing (UNOS) heart transplant allocation system provides modified listing criteria for patients with restrictive cardiomyopathy such as ATTR-CM.
- LV assist device therapy for patients with ATTR-CM is uncommon because of small LV cavity size, which impairs device inflow, and frequent coexisting right ventricular dysfunction. **Outcomes with durable mechanical circulatory support appear to be worse in patients with cardiac amyloidosis as compared to those with non-amyloid cardiomyopathies.**[18] There are limited data to support total artificial heart as a bridge to heart transplantation in cardiac amyloidosis patients without significant extracardiac disease.[15]

MANAGEMENT OF ORTHOSTATIC HYPOTENSION

- OH is present in nearly 60% of patients with hereditary ATTR. The development of normal or low blood pressure in previously hypertensive patients should prompt consideration of amyloidosis.[19]
- Neuronal mechanisms of OH because of transthyretin amyloid infiltration include impaired norepinephrine release from sympathetic neurons, reduced circulating norepinephrine levels, and reduced sympathetic cardiac innervation.[20,21]
- Cardiac mechanisms of OH include reduced LV stroke volume because of reduced LV chamber volume and reduced heart rate because of infiltration of the sinoatrial node or cardiac conduction system.[22,23]
- **The goal of OH treatment is not to restore normal standing blood pressure, but to improve quality of life and reduce morbidity and mortality associated with OH.**[22]
- **Treatment approach includes avoiding aggravating factors, nonpharmacologic and pharmacologic measures** (Table 24-4).

Aggravating Factors
- Aggravating factors include the use of vasodilators (which reduce peripheral resistance) and diuretics (which reduce ventricular preload) as well as medications that inhibit norepinephrine reuptake (as in certain antidepressants).
- Iron deficiency anemia can worsen OH and should be treated if present.[22]

Nonpharmacologic Management
- Intravascular volume depletion should be avoided and patients should be counseled on the diuretic effect of caffeinated and alcoholic beverages. Fluid intake should be around 2 L/day as congestion signs and symptoms allow. In patients without significant edema, liberalized dietary salt intake or even salt tablets may be considered.[22]
- Exercise is encouraged, beginning in the supine position if possible. Progress toward a supine or sitting position should be pursued.
- Small frequent meals may reduce postprandial hypotension, whereas large carbohydrate-rich meals may exacerbate postprandial hypotension.
- Compression stockings are recommended, but may not be tolerated in the setting of painful neuropathy.

TABLE 24-4	Pharmacologic Options for Orthostatic Hypotension		
	Mechanism of action	**Dose, route, and frequency**	**Side effects**
Fludrocortisone	Increase sodium and water retention	0.1-0.2 mg/day oral	Edema and hypokalemia
	Enhance pressor responsiveness		
Midodrine	α-1 adrenoreceptor agonist	2.5-10 mg 3 times/day oral	Supine hypertension, piloerection, urinary retention
Droxidopa	α,β-adrenoreceptor agonist	100-600 mg 3 times/day oral	Supine hypertension
	(metabolized to norepinephrine)		

Pharmacologic Management

- Fludrocortisone is a synthetic mineralocorticoid hormone that increases blood pressure through renal sodium retention and enhanced sensitization to catecholamines. Use of this agent is discouraged in ATTR because of increased risk of volume retention and end-organ damage from supine hypertension. When used, monitoring for supine hypertension, fluid retention, and hypokalemia is recommended.[22]
- **Sympathomimetic agents are preferred over fludrocortisone.**
  - Midodrine is an α-1 adrenergic stimulant that is FDA-approved for treatment of neurogenic OH.
    - Midodrine raises blood pressure by increasing arterial vasoconstriction, and possible side effects include supine hypertension and urinary retention.
    - Midodrine should be started at 2.5 to 5 mg 3 times daily and titrated to a maximum daily dose of 15 mg with the last dose given ≥3 hours before bedtime to avoid supine hypertension.[22]
  - Droxidopa (L-dihydroxyphenylserine) is a synthetic amino acid that is FDA-approved for the treatment of symptomatic neurogenic OH associated with Parkinson disease, multiple system atrophy, pure autonomic failure, and nondiabetic autonomic neuropathy (including ATTR).
    - Droxidopa is metabolized to norepinephrine and raises upright systolic blood pressure. Supine hypertension may be reduced on droxidopa compared to midodrine.
    - Droxidopa should be started at 100 mg 3 times daily and titrated in increments of 100 mg 3 times daily every 24 to 48 hours to symptomatic response (maximum dose of 1800 mg/day).

- The last dose should be given ≥3 hours before bedtime to avoid supine hypertension.
- Ambulatory blood pressure monitoring may be used to tailor the dose.[22,23]

MANAGEMENT OF RHYTHM DISTURBANCES

- Amyloid fibrils may infiltrate the conduction system, resulting in conduction block, ventricular arrhythmias, and atrial arrhythmias.[1]
- Atrial dysfunction is common in patients with cardiac amyloidosis. Amyloid fibrils infiltrate the atrial myocardium, resulting in contractile dysfunction. Chronically elevated ventricular filling pressures exacerbate atrial dilatation, promoting atrial arrhythmias.
- Atrial fibrillation (AF) is the most common supraventricular arrhythmia in patients with cardiac amyloidosis and is associated with a high prevalence of atrial thrombus. Atrial thrombi are common even in patients with cardiac amyloidosis in sinus rhythm.[24,25]
- **Patients with cardiac amyloidosis and AF should be anticoagulated with warfarin or a direct oral anticoagulant irrespective of CHADS2-VASC score.** Anticoagulation may be reasonable in cardiac amyloidosis patients *without* known AF who have severe LV diastolic dysfunction and low atrial appendage emptying velocities.[1,24,25]
- Several pharmacologic considerations apply regarding treatment of AF in patients with cardiac amyloidosis:
  - **Amiodarone is the drug of choice both for rate and rhythm control in patients with AF.**[1]
  - Rate control using β-blockers and nondihydropyridine calcium channel blockers may be complicated by the negative inotropic properties of these drugs.
  - Digoxin binds avidly to amyloid fibrils *in vitro*, theoretically increasing the risk for toxicity in cardiac amyloidosis. Therefore, digoxin should be used with caution and only at low doses.[12]
  - Cardioversion and catheter-based ablation of AF may be considered in select cases.
- Syncope may result from arrhythmia or hypotension. Evaluation of syncope should include ambulatory cardiac arrhythmia monitoring. Pacemakers are indicated in accordance with bradycardia and cardiac implantable electronic device guidelines.[1]
- Ventricular arrhythmias are less common than atrial arrhythmias and occur in 17% of patients. Implantable cardioverter defibrillators (ICDs) are recommended for secondary prevention of cardiac death in cases of resuscitated sudden cardiac death when expected survival is >1 year. However, the most common mechanism of death in patients with cardiac amyloidosis is electromechanical dissociation.[1,26,27]
- Use of ICDs for primary prevention of sudden cardiac death in patients with ATTR-CM is not well established. Heart Rhythm Society guidelines assign a class IIb indication for ICD placement in patients with light chain cardiac amyloidosis and nonsustained ventricular tachycardia with expected survival >1 year. **Routine use of primary prevention ICD in patients with cardiac amyloidosis is otherwise not recommended.**[26]

REFERENCES

1. Kittelson M, Maurer M, Ambardekar A, et al. Cardiac amyloidosis: evolving diagnosis and management: a scientific statement from the American Heart Association. *Circulation*. 2020;142:e7-e22.
2. Zhang K, Stockerl-Goldstein K, Lenihan D. Emerging therapeutics for the treatment of light chain and transthyretin amyloidosis. *J Am Coll Cardiol Basic Transl Sci*. 2019;4:438-448.
3. Ruberg F, Grogan M, Hanna M, et al Transthyretin amyloid cardiomyopathy. *J Am Coll Cardiol*. 2019;73:2872-2891.
4. Grogan M, Scott C, Kyle R, et al. Natural history of wild-type transthyretin cardiac amyloidosis and risk stratification using a novel staging system. *J Am Coll Cardiol*. 2016;6:1014-1020.
5. Gillmore JD, Damy T, Fontana M, et al. A new staging system for cardiac transthyretin amyloidosis. *Eur Heart J*. 2018;3:2799-2806.
6. Cappelli F, Martone R, Gabriele M, et al. Biomarkers and prediction of prognosis in transthyretin-related cardiac amyloidosis: direct comparison of two staging systems. *Canadian J Cardiol*. 2020;36:424-431.
7. Peterson SA, Klabunde T, Lashuel HA, et al. Inhibiting transthyretin conformational changes that lead to amyloid fibril formation. *Proc Natl Acad Sci USA*. 1998;95:12956-12960.
8. Maurer MS, Schwartz JH, Gundapaneni B, et al. Tafamidis treatment for patients with transthyretin amyloid cardiomyopathy. *N Engl J Med*. 2018;379:1007-1016.
9. Sekijima Y, Dendle MA, Kelly JW. Orally administered diflunisal stabilizes transthyretin against dissociation required for amyloidogenesis. *Amyloid*. 2006;1:236-249.
10. Adams D, Gonzalez Duarte A, Riordan W, et al. Patisiran, an RNAi therapeutic, for hereditary transthyretin amyloidosis. *N Engl J Med*. 2018;379:11-21.
11. Benson M, Waddington-Cruz M, Berk J, et al. Inotersen treatment for patients with hereditary transthyretin amyloidosis. *N Engl J Med*. 2018;379:22-31.
12. Step J, Bhimaraj A, Cordero-Reyes A, et al. Heart transplantation and end-stage cardiac amyloidosis: a review and approach to evaluation and management. *Methodist Debakey Cardiovasc J*. 2012;8(3):8-16.
13. Pitt B, Pfeffer M, Assman S, et al. Spironolactone for heart failure with preserved ejection fraction. *N Engl J Med*. 2014;370:1383-1392.
14. Baumwol J. "I Need Help"—a mnemonic to aid timely referral in advanced heart failure. *J Heart Lung Transpl*. 2017;36:593-594.
15. Kittleson M, Cole R, Patel J, et al. Mechanical circulatory support for cardiac amyloidosis. *Clin Transplant*. 2019;33:e13663.
16. Chen Q, Moriguchi J, Levine R, et al. Outcomes of heart transplantation in cardiac amyloidosis patients: a single center experience. *Transplant Proc*. 2021;53:329-334.
17. Barret C, Alexander A, Zhou H, et al. Outcomes in patients with cardiac amyloidosis undergoing heart transplantation. *JACC Heart Fail*. 2020;8:461-468.
18. Michelis K, Zhong L, Tang W, et al. Durable mechanical circulatory support in patients with amyloid cardiomyopathy; insights from INTERMACS. *Circ Heart Fail*. 2020;13:e007931.
19. Gonzalez-Duarte A, Mundayat R, Shapiro B. Assessing the onset and characteristics of orthostatic hypotension in patients with transthyretin amyloidosis from the transthyretin amyloidosis outcomes survey (THAOS). *J Neurol Sci*. 2017;381:914-915.
20. Kaufman H, Kaufman L, Palma J. Baroreflex dysfunction. *N Engl J Med*. 2020;382:163-178
21. Tanaka M, Hongo M, Kinoshita U, et al. Iodine-123 metaiodobenzylguanidine scintigraphic assessment of myocardial sympathetic innervation in patients with familial amyloid polyneuropathy. *J Am Coll Cardiol*. 1998;29(1):168-174
22. Palma J, Gonzalez A, Kaufman H. Orthostatic hypotension in hereditary transthyretin amyloidosis: epidemiology, diagnosis and management. *Clin Auton Res*. 2019;29(suppl 1):S33-S44.
23. Chen J, Han Y, Tang J, et al. Standing and supine blood pressure outcomes associated with droxidopa and midodrine in patients with neurogenic orthostatic hypotension: a bayesian meta-analysis and mixed treatment comparison of randomized trials. *Ann Pharmacother*. 2018;52(12):1182-1194.

24. Feng D, Edwards WD, Oh JK, et al. Intracardiac thrombosis and embolism in patients with cardiac amyloidosis. *Circulation.* 2007;116:2420-2426.
25. El-Am E, Dispenzieri A, Melduni R, et al. Direct current cardioversion of atrial arrhythmias in adults with cardiac amyloidosis. *J Am Coll Cardiol.* 2019;73:589-597.
26. Towbin JA, McKenna WJ, Abrams DJ, et al. 2019 HRS expert consensus statement on evaluation, risk stratification, and management of arrhythmogenic cardiomyopathy: executive summary. *Heart Rhythm.* 2019;16:e373-e407.
27. Hörnsten R, Wiklund U, Olofsson B-O, Jensen SM, Suhr OB. Liver transplantation does not prevent the development of life-threatening arrhythmia in familial amyloidotic polyneuropathy, Portuguese-type (ATTR Val30Met) patients. *Transplantation.* 2004;78:112-116.

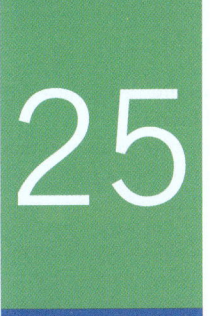

Cancer Survivors and Advanced Heart Failure Therapies

Benjamin J. Kopecky, Ankit Bhatia, and Jose A. Alvarez-Cardona

GENERAL PRINCIPLES

Definition

- **Advanced heart failure (AHF)** is variably defined by the multiple medical societies (American College of Cardiology [ACC]/American Heart Association [AHA], European Society of Cardiology, INTERMACS, Heart Failure Society of America) but generally is identified as progressive or persistent symptoms of heart failure despite optimized medical and surgical therapies.[1]
- AHF is associated with frequent hospitalizations, refractory volume overload, severe exertional limitations, and inability to tolerate guideline-directed medical therapy.[1]
- AHF is synonymous with "ACC/AHA stage D," "refractory," or "end-stage" heart failure.
- A broad definition of AHF allows for early referral for AHF therapies.
- AHF therapies range considerably depending on the individual patient. Although heart transplantation may be the gold standard treatment, this is not an option for every patient where medical therapy, durable mechanical circulatory support (MCS), or palliative care may be more appropriate.

Epidemiology

- Patients with AHF comprise an estimated 1% to 10% of the heart failure population[2] and experience high mortality without durable MCS or heart transplantation (medically treated patients had 75% 1-year mortality [REMATCH]).
- As cancer therapies continue to evolve, there exists a growing population of cancer survivors, with **1% to 5% of survivors developing chemotherapy-induced cardiomyopathy** (CCMP). CCMP is defined as symptomatic heart failure without another identifiable etiology in patients with a history of chemotherapy, and in severe cases can require AHF therapies.[3]
- **CCMP patients referred for AHF therapies have favorable survival** compared with patients with AHF of other etiologies.
  - In a retrospective analysis comparing patients receiving MCS, CCMP patients tended to be female (72%), compared to a male predominance in ischemic cardiomyopathy (ICM) or non-ischemic cardiomyopathy (NICM) (87% and 76%) with less comorbidities. CCMP patients more often had biventricular failure.[4]
- Chemotherapy such as anthracyclines at escalating cumulative doses, or in combination with other chemotherapeutics or radiation, is associated with increased risk of incident heart failure.

- Radiation therapy may play pathologic roles in ischemic heart disease, valvular disease, cardiac conduction, pericardial disease, and myocardial fibrosis.[5]
- Monoclonal antibodies and small molecule therapies are innovative techniques that are being used more frequently but are being recognized as a risk for CCMP.[6]

DIAGNOSIS

Clinical Presentation

History
- Classic signs and symptoms of decompensated heart failure include dyspnea at rest or with exertion, orthopnea, lower extremity edema, and weight gain.

Physical Examination
- Vital signs may be notable for tachycardia, tachypnea, and hypotension.
- Patients may have cool and clammy skin with evidence of edema.
- Neck examination may reveal jugular vein distention.
- Pulmonary examination may have coarse rales and dullness to percussion at the base of the lungs, with increased work of breathing.
- Abdominal examination may demonstrate distension with hepatomegaly and/or a positive hepatojugular reflux.
- Cardiac examination may have an audible S_3, functional murmur, and lateral displacement of point of maximal impulse.
- Neurologic assessment may be notable for altered mental status or somnolence.

Diagnostic Testing

Laboratories
- Brain natriuretic peptide (BNP) or N-terminal BNP and high-sensitivity troponin I or T help to assess heart strain and myocardial injury.
- Biochemical assessment of renal function can help identify acute kidney injury and cardiorenal syndrome.
- Hepatic function and coagulation panels are obtained to assess degree of liver congestion, frailty, and synthetic function.[7]

Electrocardiogram
- Electrocardiogram (ECG) may show evidence of left ventricular (LV) or right ventricular (RV) hypertrophy, low voltages, prior myocardial infarction, or arrhythmias such as atrial fibrillation.[7]

Imaging
- Chest imaging may have increased cardiothoracic ratio, interstitial lung edema, or bilateral pleural effusions.
- Transthoracic echocardiography is helpful to characterize the ejection fraction of the left ventricle and classify patients as heart failure with reduced or preserved ejection fraction.
- Echocardiograms and cardiac magnetic resonance imaging (MRI) can also assess for restrictive or constrictive cardiomyopathies and for valvular heart disease. Specific attention to RV function is paramount. These tools play an essential role in defining LV remodeling.[7]

Diagnostic Procedures
- Obtaining invasive hemodynamics can help further stratify patients with acute or chronic heart failure and their candidacy for AHF therapies. This is also useful in patients with worsening organ function despite adequate heart failure therapy.
- Right heart catheterizations assess cardiac filling pressures, pulmonary pressures, and cardiac output. These measurements help assess the adequacy of current medical or mechanical support.
- Left heart catheterizations assess coronary disease and identify if lesions are amenable to treatment with cardiac stents or coronary bypass artery grafting.
- Endomyocardial biopsies may help elucidate the etiology of heart failure. It is a mainstay of posttransplant surveillance for transplant rejection.[7]
- See Table 25-1.

TREATMENT

- A trial of guideline-directed medical therapy should be attempted if the patient is able to tolerate.[7,8]
- Studies have shown benefits of **cardiac resynchronization therapy** (CRT) in CCMP, including improvement in LV ejection fraction.[9]
- Among patients who progress to AHF, temporary or durable MCS may be considered, in addition to cardiac transplantation.
- Indications for durable MCS include frequent heart failure hospitalizations, New York Heart Association (NYHA) Class IIIb-IV symptoms, intolerance of medical therapy, or end-organ dysfunction.

Evaluation for Mechanical Circulatory Support
- MCS support can be distinguished as either temporary or durable.
  - Temporary MCS allows stabilization of CCMP patients as a bridge to recovery or bridge to decision.
  - Temporary MCS includes percutaneous circulatory assist devices (Impella, TandemHeart), intra-aortic balloon pump, or extracorporeal membrane oxygenation (ECMO).
  - Durable MCS includes left ventricular assist devices (LVADs), including the axial-flow HeartMate2 and centrifugal-flow HeartMate3 or HeartWare Ventricular Assist Device (HVAD) as well as total artificial heart.
    - Durable MCS can be stratified as destination therapy or bridge to transplant, depending on patient candidacy for future heart transplantation.
    - As of 2020, all-comer survival with MCS is 80% to 90% at 1 year.[10]
  - Absolute contraindications for durable MCS include irreversible hepatic, renal, neurologic, or psychiatric disease or medical nonadherence.
    - Relative contraindications include obesity, extreme frailty, active substance use, lack of social support, and untreated malignancy.
- Patients with a history of thrombophilia should have a hypercoagulability assessment (Class I, level of evidence [LOE]: C[11]).
- Patients with a history of cancer who are considered free of disease or in long-term remission are candidates for bridge to transplant MCS; care should involve an oncologist (Class I, LOE: C[11]).
- Patients with recently treated or active cancer with life expectancy >2 years may be candidates for destination therapy MCS (Class IIa, LOE: C[11]).

TABLE 25-1 Advanced Heart Failure Clinical Presentation and Diagnostic Workup

Clinical presentation	Physical examination findings	Laboratory findings	Diagnostics
• Functional status decline • Dyspnea at rest • Dyspnea with exertion • Orthopnea • Weight gain • Light-headedness • Dizziness	***Vital Signs*** • Tachycardia • Tachypnea • Hypotension ***Cardiac*** • Jugular venous distention • Audible S3 • Laterally displaced point of maximal impulse ***Pulmonary*** • Coarse rales • Diminished breath sounds • Increased work of breathing ***Abdominal*** • Abdominal distension • Hepatomegaly • Positive hepatojugular reflex ***Extremities*** • Lower extremity edema • Cool extremities	• ↑ BNP or NT-proBNP levels (Congestion) • ↑ Creatinine (Cardiorenal syndrome) • ↑ Liver function tests (Hepatic congestion) • ↑ INR (Impaired hepatic synthesis) • ↑ Lactic acid (Impaired end-organ perfusion)	***Transthoracic Echocardiogram*** • Evaluate systolic function. • Evaluate diastolic function. • Screen for constrictive or restrictive disease. • Assess valvular disease. ***Cardiac MRI*** • Evaluate biventricular function. • Assess for myocardial scarring or evidence of infiltrative disease. ***Right Heart Catheterization*** • Measure cardiac filling pressures. • Measure pulmonary arterial pressures. • Calculate systemic and pulmonary vascular resistance. • Determine cardiac output. ***Left Heart Catheterization*** Evaluate coronary artery disease and potential for revascularization. ***Endomyocardial Biopsy*** • Evaluate cardiomyopathy etiology. • Assess for posttransplant rejection.

BNP, brain natriuretic peptide; INR, international normalized ratio; MRI, magnetic resonance imaging; NT-proBNP, N-terminal pro-brain natriuretic peptide.

- Patients with active malignancy and life expectancy of <2 years should not be candidates for MCS (Class III, LOE: C[11]).
- CCMP patients manifest with **severe biventricular failure** compared to other etiologies.
  - CCMP patients requiring MCS are **more likely to require RV mechanical support** and may have more difficulty weaning from ECMO.[4]
  - CCMP patients had lower pulmonary artery systolic pressures (44.0 mm Hg vs. 51.2 for ICM and 49.4 mm Hg for NICM) but worse indicators of RV function (higher right atrial [RA] pressures, more severe tricuspid regurgitation [TR], higher RA/pulmonary capillary wedge pressure [PCWP]).[4]
- CCMP more often received MCS as destination therapy (33%) compared to patients with ICM (14%) or NICM (23%)[4] and more often required concomitant surgery (most commonly tricuspid repair).
  - Clinical outcomes (mortality, cardiac transplantation, recovery) were no different based on etiology of cardiomyopathy.

Pretransplant Considerations

- Patients being evaluated for heart transplantation range from stable outpatients to the critically ill patient on temporary MCS.
- In CCMP patients being considered for heart transplantation, it is imperative to collaborate with oncologists to assess for risk of malignancy recurrence.[12]
- Heart transplantation may be considered in cancer patients with no evidence of active disease and when the likelihood of recurrence is low. The waiting period after cancer remission for heart transplantation candidacy is individualized based on patient- and malignancy-specific factors (Class I, LOE: C[12]).
- *Disease-Specific Considerations*
  - *Amyloidosis*: The majority of clinical cardiac amyloidosis (>95%) are caused by light chain amyloidosis (AL) and transthyretin amyloidosis (ATTR). Both forms are associated with high mortality because of restrictive biventricular physiology and extracardiac manifestations. Use of LVAD therapy in cardiac amyloid is often limited by small LV cavity size and RV dysfunction. **Heart transplantation is a therapeutic option for end-stage cardiac amyloid**, but remains controversial because of historically poor outcomes in this population. However, more recent studies have revealed similar posttransplant outcomes for amyloid patients compared to other transplant recipients.[13]
    - Among AL amyloid patients, post–heart transplant autologous stem cell transplant (ASCT) has shown success, typically occurring 6 to 12 months later.[14] Patients receiving posttransplant ASCT had similar outcomes to nonamyloid heart transplant recipients.
- Patients undergoing ASCT may need to modify their immunosuppressive regimen to avoid agents that suppress bone marrow (ie, antimetabolites, prophylactic antivirals).
  - *Radiotherapy-induced cardiomyopathy (RT-CMP)*: A relatively rare cardiomyopathy compared to CCMP (0.2% vs. 2% of all AHF).[15]
    - History of chest radiation is thought to be contributory to longer ischemic times during transplantation surgery, often because of more difficult recipient chest dissection.[15]
    - RT-CMP has significantly worse posttransplant outcomes.[15]
    - See Figure 25-1.

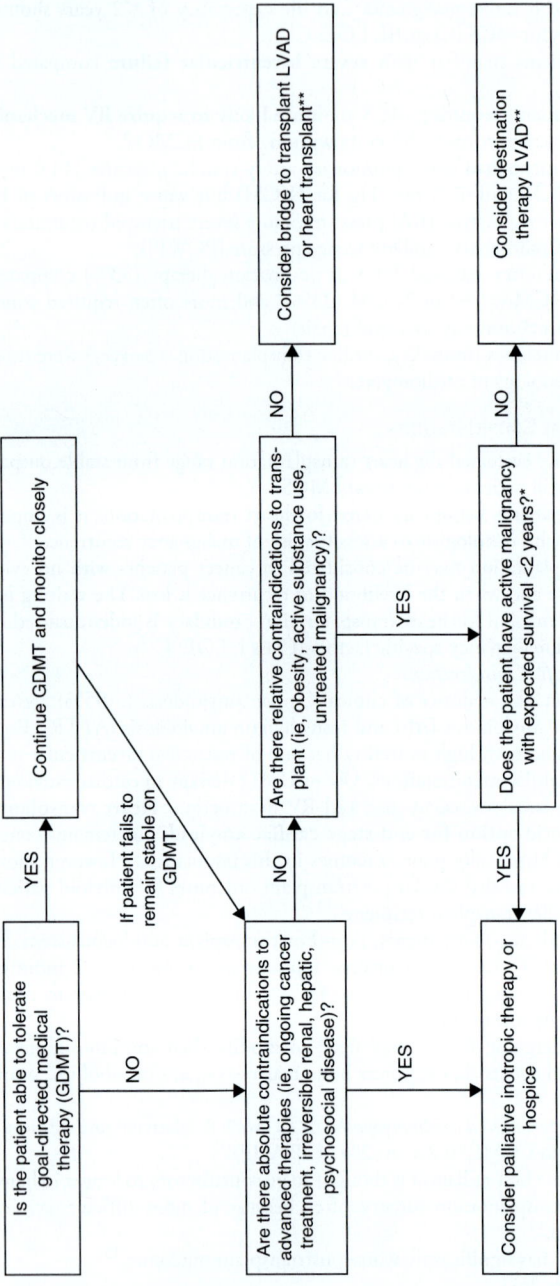

Figure 25-1. Flowchart for decision-making for advanced therapies. ECMO, extracorporeal membrane oxygenation; LVAD, left ventricular assist device.

*All advanced therapy decisions should be made in collaboration with a hematologist/oncologist
**Cancer survivors are more likely to need right ventricular support during ECMO or LVAD implant

Posttransplant Considerations
- *Posttransplant Immunosuppression and Risk for Malignancy*
  - Avoidance of induction immunotherapy should also be considered for transplant recipients with **high malignancy risk**.[16]
  - Calcineurin inhibitors (cyclosporine, tacrolimus) and azathioprine exhibit direct cancer-promoting potential, whereas mycophenolate mofetil and mammalian target of rapamycin (mTOR) inhibitors show antioncogenic properties.[17,18]
    - Calcineurin inhibitors stimulate carcinogenesis by direct inhibition of DNA repair mechanisms and production of interleukin (IL)-2 and transforming growth factor (TGF)-β.[19]
    - Azathioprine increases cancer risk by influencing postreplicative DNA mismatch repair.[20]
    - Azathioprine and cyclosporine directly enhance the carcinogenic effects of ultraviolet radiation.[21]
  - Statin therapy has been associated with a reduction in posttransplant malignancies.[22]
  - Patient-specific immunosuppressive regimens should be considered in recipients with high malignancy risk (older, malignancy history). This includes the use of mTOR inhibitors as a substitute for calcineurin inhibitors.[23,24]
  - Chronic immunosuppression should be minimized in patients at high risk for malignancy, especially as risk of rejection decreases (Class IIa, LOE: C[25]).
  - Reduction of immunosuppression in patients with solid tumors unrelated to the lymphoid system (ie, posttransplant lymphoproliferative disorder [PTLD]) is not supported by current guideline statements (Class I, LOE: C[25]).
- *Posttransplant Malignancies*
  - 50% of transplant patients survive >13 years,[23] with recent trends showing improvements in posttransplant survival.
  - Cancer risk after transplantation is **two to four times higher than the general population**, with the highest risk in thoracic organ transplant recipients.[26]
  - Pathogenesis for posttransplant malignancies includes (a) donor-related transmission, (b) *de novo* development, and (c) recurrence of pretransplant malignancy.[17]
  - See Table 25-2.

Donor-Related Transmission
- There is no consensus for screening transplant donors for malignancy.
- Transplant donor history of malignancy has limited risk to corresponding transplant recipients.
  - Retrospective analysis of United Network for Organ Sharing (UNOS) registry from 1987 to 2016 showed 622/38,781 donors had a history of malignancy. When propensity matched, there was no association between donor malignancy and 10-year mortality (hazard ratio [HR] 1.02 [0.84-1.24]).[27]
  - Donor-related transmission of malignancy is **very rare** in heart transplant recipients (<0.2%) and is thought to be due to the presence of occult malignant cells in the transplanted organ. Potentially transmitted malignancies may include melanoma, renal cell carcinoma, and glioblastoma multiforme.[28]

De Novo Development
- Approximately 10% of heart transplant recipients develop *de novo* malignancy 1 to 5 years posttransplant,[29] which is a significant risk factor for increased mortality.[27]

TABLE 25-2	Post–Heart Transplant Malignancies		
	Donor related	**De novo**	**Recurrence**
Incidence	• Rare (<0.2%)[1]	• Common (~10% at 1-5 years)[2]	• Low
Risk	• No increased risk to recipients from donors with history of malignancy (HR 1.02, 95% CI: 0.84-1.24)[3]	• Variable (5-year survival: lung cancer 21%, lymphoma 32%, prostate cancer 86%)[4]	• Variable (5-year freedom from recurrence ranges from 75% for skin cancer to 100% for colon cancer)[4]
Risk factors	• None	• Recipient age >50 years • Induction therapy • Environmental exposures • Oncogenic viruses • Duration and intensity of immunosuppression[5]	
Types of cancer	• Melanoma • Renal cell carcinoma • Glioblastoma multiforme[1]	• Skin cancer (squamous cell > basal cell) • Lung cancer • Posttransplant lymphoproliferative disorder[4]	• Breast cancer • Lymphoma • Lung cancer • Prostate cancer • Squamous and basal cell cancers[4]
Screening	• No consensus for screening donors for malignancy	• Annual dermatologic examination[6] • Standard population-based screening for breast, colon, and prostate cancer[6]	

CI, confidence interval; HR, hazard ratio.

- ○ Skin cancer is the **most common** posttransplant malignancy, occurring 65 to 250 times more than in the general population, with a predilection for squamous cell carcinoma (SCC) over basal cell carcinoma.
- ○ SCCs tend to be more aggressive with greater metastatic potential in transplant recipients.[30]
- Of those with a *de novo* malignancy after transplant (excluding cutaneous malignancies), lung cancer had the poorest 5-year survival (21%), followed by lymphoma (32%). Prostate cancer had the most favorable prognosis (86%).[31]
- ○ Risk factors for posttransplant malignancy include age of recipient at transplant (>50 years), induction immunosuppression, exposure to carcinogenic agents (sunlight, smoking, diet, alcohol), genetic predisposition, and infection with oncogenic viruses.[17]
- ○ Pathologic mechanisms include impaired immunosurveillance, weakened immune system against oncogenic viruses (human papillomavirus [HPV], Epstein-Barr virus [EBV], human herpesvirus [HHV]-8, hepatitis B virus [HBV], hepatitis C virus [HCV]), and direct carcinogenic effects of immunosuppression.

- PTLD is a spectrum of lymphoproliferative disorders that range from benign lymphoid hyperplasia to lymphoma.[17,32]
  - Incidence varies widely from 1% to 20%, depending on level of immunosuppression and EBV seropositivity.[33]
  - Early-onset PTLD (<1 year posttransplant, 80% of cases)
  - Late-onset PTLD (typically occurring 4 to 5 years posttransplant)
  - Cardiothoracic PTLD is less common overall, but with a higher incidence in heart transplant recipients.[17]
  - Symptoms vary significantly and include "B-symptoms" and intestinal obstruction.
  - Up to 75% of patients present with abdominal findings, often including the distal small bowel. Imaging shows irregular bowel thickening, eccentric mural masses, aneurysmal dilatation, and luminal ulceration.[17,23]
  - Computed tomography (CT), MRI, and positron emission tomography (PET)/CT can all be useful and help delineate PTLD into nodal versus extranodal disease.[17]
  - Treatment includes reduction of immunosuppression (more beneficial in early PTLD), antiviral therapy, and chemotherapy (more beneficial with late PTLD).[17]
  - PTLD should be evaluated and treated at a transplant center by physicians familiar with transplant-associated malignancies (Class I, LOE: C[25]).

Malignancy Recurrence
- Posttransplant recurrence of a pretransplant malignancy among heart transplant patients is **low**. In one study,[31] 5-year freedom from recurrence was: 100% for colon cancer, 96% for prostate cancer, 93% for breast cancer, 89% for lymphoma and lung cancer, and 75% for basal or squamous cell cancers.
- *Posttransplant Cancer Screening*
  - Skin cancer is the most common malignancy affecting transplant recipients.
    - All transplant recipients should partake in preventative behaviors and have annual dermatologic examinations (Class I, LOE: C[25]).
  - Transplant recipients should continue to follow standard screening recommendations regarding breast, colon, and prostate cancer as the general population (Class I, LOE: C[25]).
  - No other screening recommendations are provided by the International Society for Heart and Lung Transplantation (ISHLT) guidelines.
- Special consideration: Checkpoint inhibitors (CPIs) and heart transplantation
  - CPIs have revolutionized cancer treatment, but transplant patients have been excluded from trials of CPIs.
  - In limited studies of heart transplant recipients (62% with melanoma), treatment with CPIs was associated with significant rejection (41%) and mortality (46%),[34] but more data are needed to guide therapy.

OUTCOMES

- In one study of heart transplantations between 1987 and 2011, 453 heart transplants were performed for CCMP compared to 51,312 transplants for other causes.[35]
  - After adjusting for age and gender, CCMP patients had improved survival (HR 1.28, $P = .026$) and did not have a higher risk of death from malignancy.[28]
- In another study of heart transplantations between 2000 and 2008, 232 heart transplants were performed for CCMP compared to 8890 for other causes.[36]

- CCMP patients had higher rates of pretransplant biventricular mechanical support, higher incidence of posttransplant malignancy (5% vs. 2%) (one cancer recurrence, otherwise *de novo*), and higher incidence of infections (22% vs. 14%). CCMP recipients had less rejection (62% vs. 72%). There were no survival differences at 1, 3, or 5 years after transplant.[29]

Summary

- Severe CCMP, when refractory to medical therapy, may necessitate evaluation for AHF therapies, including durable MCS (LVADs) and cardiac transplantation.
- CCMP patients undergoing AHF, when appropriately selected, have been shown to have favorable survival in comparison to other heart failure etiologies.
- Malignancy history plays an integral role in AHF therapies' candidacy given associated prognostic ramifications.
- Cardiac transplantation and chronic immunosuppression are associated with higher risk for posttransplant malignancies, both recurrent and *de novo*. Cardiac transplantation can be considered in patients with malignancy history when the risk of recurrence is low.
- Among cardiac transplant patients with or at risk for malignancy, immunosuppression strategies should consider agents with demonstrated antioncogenic properties (mTOR inhibitors, Mycophenolate MoFetil), while avoiding agents with cancer-promoting properties (calcineurin inhibitors, cyclosporine, induction therapy).

REFERENCES

1. Fang JC, Ewald GA, Allen LA, et al. Advanced (stage D) heart failure: a statement from the Heart Failure Society of America Guidelines Committee. *J Card Fail*. 2015;21(6):519-534.
2. Crespo-Leiro MG, Metra M, Lund LH, et al. Advanced heart failure: a position statement of the Heart Failure Association of the European Society of Cardiology. *Eur J Heart Fail*. 2018;20(11):1505-1535.
3. Oliveira GH, Qattan MY, Al-Kindi S, Park SJ. Advanced heart failure therapies for patients with chemotherapy-induced cardiomyopathy. *Circ Heart Fail*. 2014;7(6):1050-1058.
4. Oliveira GH, Dupont M, Naftel D, et al. Increased need for right ventricular support in patients with chemotherapy-induced cardiomyopathy undergoing mechanical circulatory support: outcomes from the INTERMACS Registry (Interagency Registry for Mechanically Assisted Circulatory Support). *J Am Coll Cardiol*. 2014;63(3):240-248.
5. Lee PJ, Mallik R. Cardiovascular effects of radiation therapy: practical approach to radiation therapy-induced heart disease. *Cardiol Rev*. 2005;13(2):80-86.
6. Foltz IN, Karow M, Wasserman SM. Evolution and emergence of therapeutic monoclonal antibodies: what cardiologists need to know. *Circulation*. 2013;127(22):2222-2230.
7. Higgins AY, O'Halloran TD, Chang JD. Chemotherapy-induced cardiomyopathy. *Heart Fail Rev*. 2015;20(6):721-730.
8. Yancy CW, Jessup M, Bozkurt B, et al. 2017 ACC/AHA/HFSA focused update of the 2013 ACCF/AHA guideline for the management of heart failure: a report of the American College of Cardiology/American Heart Association Task Force on Clinical Practice Guidelines and the Heart Failure Society of America. *J Am Coll Cardiol*. 2017;70(6):776-803.
9. Singh JP, Solomon SD, Fradley MG, et al. Association of cardiac resynchronization therapy with change in left ventricular ejection fraction in patients with chemotherapy-induced cardiomyopathy. *JAMA*. 2019. 322(18):1799-1805.
10. Goldstein DJ, Naka Y, Horstmanshof D, et al. Association of clinical outcomes with left ventricular assist device use by bridge to transplant or destination therapy intent: The Multicenter Study of MagLev Technology in Patients Undergoing Mechanical Circulatory

Support Therapy With HeartMate 3 (MOMENTUM 3) randomized clinical trial. *JAMA Cardiol.* 2020;5(4):411-419.
11. Feldman D, Pamboukian SV, Teuteberg JJ, et al. The 2013 International Society for Heart and Lung Transplantation Guidelines for mechanical circulatory support: executive summary. *J Heart Lung Transplant.* 2013;32(2):157-187.
12. Mehra MR, Canter CE, Hannan MM, et al. The 2016 International Society for Heart Lung Transplantation listing criteria for heart transplantation: a 10-year update. *J Heart Lung Transplant.* 2016;35(1):1-23.
13. Davis MK, Lee PH, Witteles RM. Changing outcomes after heart transplantation in patients with amyloid cardiomyopathy. *J Heart Lung Transplant.* 2015;34(5):658-666.
14. Trachtenberg BH, Kamble RT, Rice L, et al. Delayed autologous stem cell transplantation following cardiac transplantation experience in patients with cardiac amyloidosis. *Am J Transplant.* 2019;19(10):2900-2909.
15. Bianco CM, Al-Kindi SG, Oliveira GH. Advanced heart failure therapies for cancer therapeutics-related cardiac dysfunction. *Heart Fail Clin.* 2017;13(2):327-336.
16. Nair N, Gongora E, Mehra MR. Long-term immunosuppression and malignancy in thoracic transplantation: where is the balance? *J Heart Lung Transplant.* 2014;33(5):461-467.
17. Katabathina VS, Menias CO, Tammisetti VS, et al. Malignancy after solid organ transplantation: comprehensive imaging review. *Radiographics.* 2016;36(5):1390-1407.
18. Sherston SN, Carroll RP, Harden PN, Wood KJ. Predictors of cancer risk in the long-term solid-organ transplant recipient. *Transplantation.* 2014;97(6):605-611.
19. Gutierrez-Dalmau A, Campistol JM. Immunosuppressive therapy and malignancy in organ transplant recipients: a systematic review. *Drugs.* 2007;67(8):1167-1198.
20. Martinez OM, de Gruijl FR. Molecular and immunologic mechanisms of cancer pathogenesis in solid organ transplant recipients. *Am J Transplant.* 2008;8(11):2205-2211.
21. Perrett CM, Walker SL, O'Donovan P, et al. Azathioprine treatment photosensitizes human skin to ultraviolet A radiation. *Br J Dermatol.* 2008;159(1):198-204.
22. Vallakati A, Reddy S, Dunlap ME, Taylor DO. Impact of statin use after heart transplantation: a meta-analysis. *Circ Heart Fail.* 2016;9(10):e003265.
23. Mancini D, Rakita V. Malignancy post heart transplantation: no free lunch. *J Am Coll Cardiol.* 2018;71(1):50-52.
24. Asleh R, Clavell AL, Pereira NL, et al. Incidence of malignancies in patients treated with sirolimus following heart transplantation. *J Am Coll Cardiol.* 2019;73(21):2676-2688.
25. Costanzo MR, Dipchand A, Starling R, et al. The International Society of Heart and Lung Transplantation Guidelines for the care of heart transplant recipients. *J Heart Lung Transplant.* 2010;29(8):914-956.
26. Jaamaa-Holmberg S, Salmela B, Lemström K, Pukkala E, Lommi J. Cancer incidence and mortality after heart transplantation—A population-based national cohort study. *Acta Oncol.* 2019;58(6):859-863.
27. Rudasill SE, Iyengar A, Sanaiha Y, et al. Donor history of malignancy: a limited risk for heart transplant recipients. *Clin Transplant.* 2020;34(2):e13762.
28. Buell JF, Trofe J, Hanaway MJ, et al. Transmission of donor cancer into cardiothoracic transplant recipients. *Surgery.* 2001;130(4):660-666; discussion 666-668.
29. Youn JC, Stehlik J, Wilk AR, et al. Temporal trends of de novo malignancy development after heart transplantation. *J Am Coll Cardiol.* 2018;71(1):40-49.
30. Brewer JD, Colegio OR, Phillips PK, et al. Incidence of and risk factors for skin cancer after heart transplant. *Arch Dermatol.* 2009;145(12):1391-1396.
31. Higgins RS, Brown RN, Chang PP, et al. A multi-institutional study of malignancies after heart transplantation and a comparison with the general United States population. *J Heart Lung Transplant.* 2014;33(5):478-485.
32. Swerdlow SH, Campo E, Pileri SA, et al. The 2016 revision of the World Health Organization classification of lymphoid neoplasms. *Blood.* 2016;127(20):2375-2390.
33. Hayes Jr D, Tumin D, Foraker RE, Tobias JD. Posttransplant lymphoproliferative disease and survival in adult heart transplant recipients. *J Cardiol.* 2017;69(1):144-148.

34. Abdel-Wahab N, Safa H, Abudayyeh A, et al. Checkpoint inhibitor therapy for cancer in solid organ transplantation recipients: an institutional experience and a systematic review of the literature. *J Immunother Cancer*. 2019;7(1):106.
35. Lenneman AJ, Wang L, Wigger M, et al. Heart transplant survival outcomes for adriamycin-dilated cardiomyopathy. *Am J Cardiol*. 2013;111(4):609-612.
36. Oliveira GH, Hardaway BW, Kucheryavaya AY, et al. Characteristics and survival of patients with chemotherapy-induced cardiomyopathy undergoing heart transplantation. *J Heart Lung Transplant*. 2012;31(8):805-810.

INDEX

Note: Page numbers followed by *f* and *t* indicates figure and table respectively.

A

ABCDEs of prevention, 15
Accelerated atherosclerosis, 80–83
    BCR-ABL tyrosine kinase inhibitors, 81–82
    clinical presentation, 83
    general principles, 80–83
    graft-*versus*-host disease, 81
    immune checkpoint inhibitors, 82–83
    management, 83
    nilotinib, 81–82
    radiation therapy, 80–81
Acute coronary syndrome, 83–86
    general principles, 83–84
        cisplatin and platinum compounds, 83–84
        management, 84
        revascularization, thrombocytopenia setting, 84–86, 86*t*
        vascular endothelial growth factor inhibitors, 84
Acute pericarditis, 103–106
    consequences, 106
    definition, 103
    diagnosis, 104–105
    etiology, 103–104, 104*t*
    management, 105–106
Administrative support, role of, 286
Advanced heart failure (AHF) therapies, 315–316, 321–330. *See also* Survivorship, cancer
    definition, 321
    diagnosis, 322
        clinical presentation, 322
        diagnostic procedures, 323
        electrocardiogram, 322
        history, 322
        imaging, 322
        laboratories, 322
        physical examination, 322
    epidemiology, 321–322
    general principles, 321–322
    outcomes, 329–330
    treatment, 323–329
        De Novo development, 327–329
        donor-related transmission, 327
        malignancy recurrence, 329
        mechanical circulatory support, evaluation for, 323–325
        posttransplant considerations, 327–329
        pretransplant considerations, 325
Advanced practice providers, role of, 282–283
AHF therapies. *See* Advanced heart failure (AHF) therapies
Alkylating agents, 8, 11
Amyloid fibril-targeting therapy, 306–307
Amyloidosis, 181, 184, 213–214, 217–218, 287–296
    cardiac magnetic resonance imaging, 294–296, 295*f*
    clinical evaluation, 288–296
    diagnostic testing, 289–292, 293*t*
        cardiac biomarkers, 292
        electrocardiography, 289
        transthoracic echocardiography, 289–292
    epidemiology, 287–288
        light chain amyloidosis, 287–288
        transthyretin amyloidosis, 288
    general principles, 287
    light chain amyloidosis
        epidemiology, 287–288
        history, 288–289
    physical examination, 289
    radiation and surgery, 184
    ^{99m}technetium-labeled bone scintigraphy, 292–294
    transthyretin amyloidosis
        epidemiology, 288
        history, 289
Androgen axis inhibitors, hypertension and, 146
Androgen deprivation therapy, 11
Androgen receptor blockers, 11
Anthracyclines, 11, 210–212
    permissive cardiotoxicity and, 275–276
Anthracycline therapy, 217
Antiandrogens, 11
Anticancer therapies, 9–10*t*
Antineoplastic chemotherapies, 179, 181
Arrhythmias, 150–165
    atrial fibrillation, 150–153
        acute management, 152–153
        anticoagulation, 153
        associated drugs/therapies, 151–152, 151*t*
        definition, 150–151
        diagnosis, 152
    atrioventricular block, 157–160
        associated drugs/therapies, 157–159
        definition, 157
        diagnosis, 159
        management, 159–160
    classification, 150
    definition, 150

Arrhythmias (*continued*)
  general principles, 150
  QT prolongation, 160–163
    associated drugs/therapies, 160–162
    definition, 160
    diagnosis, 162–163
    management, 163
  rhythm disturbances, 150–165
  sinus node dysfunction, 156–157
    associated drugs/therapies, 156–157
    definition, 156
    diagnosis, 157
    management, 157
  supraventricular tachyarrhythmias, 154–156
    associated drugs/therapies, 154
    definition, 154
    diagnosis, 154–156, 155*f*
    management, 156
  ventricular arrhythmias, 163–165
    associated drugs/therapies, 163
    definition, 163
    diagnosis, 164
    diagnostic tests, 165
    management, 164
Aspirin, 19
Atrial fibrillation, 150–153
  acute management, 152–153
  anticoagulation, 153
  associated drugs/therapies, 151–152, 151*t*
  definition, 150–151
  diagnosis, 152
Atrioventricular block, 157–160
  associated drugs/therapies, 157–159
  definition, 157
  diagnosis, 159
  management, 159–160
Autologous stem cell transplantation, 303–305
Autonomic dysfunction, 179–190
  amyloidosis, 181, 184
    radiation and surgery, 184
  anatomy and pathophysiology, 182–184
  antineoplastic chemotherapies, 179, 181
  autonomic nervous system, 182
  background and epidemiology, 179
  classification, 179
  definition, 179
  general principles, 179–182
  neurotoxicity, mechanisms of, 182–184
    antineoplastic agents, 182–184
  paraneoplastic autonomic dysfunction, 182
  paraneoplastic syndromes, 184–190
    cardiovascular diagnostic testing, 186–187
    diagnosis, 184–187
    diagnostic testing, 186–187
    history, 184–186
    lab evaluation, 187
    neurologic diagnostic testing, 187
    orthostasis, differential diagnosis for, 184
    physical examination, 186
    prognosis, 190
    treatment, 187–189
  radiation therapy and surgery, 181–182
Autonomic nervous system, 182

B

B-Blockers, 31
Biomarkers, 208–221
  amyloidosis, 213–214, 217–218
  anthracyclines, 210–212
  anthracycline therapy, 217
  in cancer care, 219–221*t*
  clinical vignettes, 216–221
  C-reactive protein, 209
  definitions, 208
  diagnosis and intervention, 215–216
  general principles, 208–210
  immune checkpoint inhibitors, 213
  integration into cardio-oncology care, 214
  investigational, 209–210
  natriuretic peptides, 208–209
  profiles, 215
  proteasome inhibitors, 213
  trastuzumab, 212
  troponin, 208
  vascular endothelial growth factor inhibitors, 212
  workup, 215
Bisoprolol, 32
Bispecific antibodies, 59
  associated drugs/therapies, 59
  cardiotoxicity, 59, 59*t*
  definition, 59
  epidemiology, 59
  monitoring, 59

C

Cancer-associated thrombosis (CAT), 114–122
  associated drugs/therapies, 115–119, 116*t*
    chemotherapy, 119
    epidermal growth factor receptor inhibitors, 119
    immunomodulatory drugs, 115, 117
    tyrosine kinase inhibitors, 118
    vascular endothelial growth factor inhibitors, 118–119
  definition, 114
  diagnosis, 119–120

epidemiology, 114
general principles, 114, 115*t*
risk factors, 115*t*
treatment, 120–122, 121*t*
  initial, 120
  long-term, 120, 122
Cancer survivorship. *See* Survivorship, cancer
Cancer treatment-related cardiac dysfunction (CTRCD), 203
Carcinoid heart disease, 69–72
  diagnosis, 69–71
  epidemiology/risk factors, 69
  general principles, 69
  laboratory testing, 71–72
  outcome/prognosis, 72
  treatment, 72
Cardiac complications, cancer survivorship, 239–244
  adverse hormonal effects, 243
  conduction disease, 241
  general principles, 239
  heart failure, 241
  lymphedema, 243–244
  myocardial dysfunction, 241
  pain, 244
  pericardial abnormalities, 241
  reproductive considerations, 243
  secondary malignant neoplasms, 243
  structural abnormalities, 241
  valvular abnormalities, 241
  vascular compromise, 240–241
Cardiac dysfunction
  cancer therapy–related, 227–235
  clinical presentation of, 31
    diagnostic testing, 31
    history, 31
    physical examination, 31
  clinical trial for primary prevention, 35–42*t*
  definition of, 26
  drugs and therapies, 26–28
    anthracyclines, 26–27
    cyclophosphamide, 28
    HER-2 inhibitors, 28
    radiation, 28
  epidemiology/risk factors for, 28–31
    anthracyclines, 28–29
    cyclophosphamide, 29–31
    HER-2 inhibitors, 29
    radiation, 31
  general principles, 26
  prevention of, 33–34
  surveillance strategies for, 34, 45
  treatment of, 31–32
    anthracyclines, 31
    cyclophosphamide, 31–32
    HER-2 inhibitors, 31
    radiation therapy, 32
Cardiac dysfunction, cancer therapy–related, 227–235
  gadolinium-based imaging, 230–231, 232–233*t*
  myocardial edema, 230
  myocardial strain, 227, 230
  myocardial T1 mapping, 230
  tissue characterization, 230
Cardiac magnetic resonance (CMR). *See* Magnetic resonance imaging (MRI)
Cardiac masses, 125–138
  classification of, 125, 126*t*
  general principles, 125
  neoplasms, 126–138
    benign primary, 127–134, 128–130*t*, 130*f*
    classification of, 127–138, 128–130*t*, 130*f*
    clinical presentation, 126
    diagnostic testing, 126–127
    lipoma, 133
    lymphoma, 136
    malignant primary, 134–138
    mesothelioma, 136–137
    myxoma, 127, 131–132
    papillary fibroelastoma, 132
    paraganglioma, 133–134
    rhabdomyoma, 133
    sarcomas, 134–136
Cardio-oncology (CO), practical approaches. *See also individual entries*
  ABCDEs of prevention, 15
  alkylating agents, 8, 11
  androgen deprivation therapy, 11
  androgen receptor blockers, 11
  anthracyclines, 11
  antiandrogens, 11
  cardiotoxicity classification, 3*t*–6*t*
  checkpoint inhibitors, 11–12
  chimeric antigen receptor T-Cell therapy, 12
  classification, 2
  coronary vasospasm, 15
  definition, 2
  diagnosis, during cancer therapy, 16–18
  epidemiology, 2
  etiology, 7
  fluoropyrimidine, 12
  general principles, 1
  HER2 targeted therapy, 12
  history, 7–8
  immunomodulatory agents, 13
  ischemic heart disease and. *See* Ischemic heart disease
  left ventricular dysfunction, 15–16
  medications and cardiovascular adverse effects, 14
  nonpharmacologic therapies, 19–20

Cardio-oncology (CO), practical approaches, (*continued*)
  proteasome inhibitors, 13
  radiation, 14–15
  risk factors, 7
  thrombosis, 16
  Torsades de Pointes, 16
  treatment of cardiac diseases, 18–20
  tyrosine kinase inhibitors, 13–14
  vascular diseases in. *See individual entries*
  VEGF receptor inhibitors, 14
Cardioprotective medical therapy, 271–272*t*
Cardiotoxicity classification, 3*t*–6*t*
Cardiovascular toxicities, echocardiography evaluation and, 202–204
  cancer treatment–related cardiac dysfunction, 203
  pericardial disease, 203
  valvular heart disease, 203
  vascular toxicity, 204
CAT. *See* Cancer-associated thrombosis (CAT)
Catheter-directed thrombolysis, 174–175
CCS. *See* Chronic coronary syndrome (CCS)
Checkpoint inhibitors
  permissive cardiotoxicity and, 276–278
Chemotherapy
  for cancer-associated thrombosis, 119
Chimeric antigen receptor T-Cell therapy, 12, 56–58
  associated drugs/therapies, 56
  cardiotoxicity, 58, 58*t*
  definition, 56
  epidemiology, 58
  monitoring, 58
Chronic coronary syndrome (CCS), 92
Chronic graft-*versus*-host disease, 255–256
Colchicine, 105
Constrictive pericarditis, 110–112
  complications, 112
  diagnosis, 111–112
  etiology, 110, 110*t*
  management, 112
Contrast-enhancing agents, 202
Coronary artery calcification, 94–95
Coronary computed tomography angiography, 95–96
Coronary vasospasm, 15
  and 5-fluorouracil, 78–80
    diagnosis, 79
    general principles, 78–79
    management and clinical follow-up, 79–80
C-reactive protein, 209
CTRCD. *See* Cancer treatment-related cardiac dysfunction (CTRCD)

Cyclophosphamide, bortezomib, and dexamethasone (CyBorD), 302
Cytochrome P450 3A4 pathway, 258, 259–264*t*
Cytochrome P450 2C9 pathway, 265–266
Cytochrome P450 2C19 pathway, 265

D

De Novo development, 327–329
Dexrazoxane, 33
Donor-related transmission, 327
Doppler, 199
Droxidopa, 317
Drug-drug interactions, 257–266
  cytochrome P450 3A4 pathway, 258, 259–264*t*
  cytochrome P450 2C9 pathway, 265–266
  cytochrome P450 2C19 pathway, 265
  definitions, 257–258
  general principles, 257–266
  P-glycoprotein, 266
  pharmacodynamic drug interactions, 266

E

Echo techniques, cardiac safety and, 192–205
  cardiovascular toxicities and, 202–204
    cancer treatment–related cardiac dysfunction, 203
    pericardial disease, 203
    valvular heart disease, 203
    vascular toxicity, 204
  contrast-enhancing agents, 202
  Doppler, 199
  echocardiography in surveillance, role of, 192–193
    cardiotoxicity, definition of, 193, 198
    general principles, 192–193
  limitations of, 204, 204–205*t*
  myocardial strain, 202
  three-dimensional imaging, 201
  two-dimensional imaging, 199
Electrocardiography, amyloidosis and, 289
Engraftment, 252
Epidermal growth factor receptor inhibitors, for cancer-associated thrombosis, 119
Eplerenone, 32

F

Fludrocortisone, 317
Fluoropyrimidine, 12

G

Gadolinium-based imaging, 230–231, 232–233*t*

H

Hematopoietic cell transplantation, 249–256
chronic graft-*versus*-host disease, cardiac complications of, 255–256
complications, cardiovascular, 253–255
conditioning regimens and toxicities, 251*t*
immunosuppressant drugs and side effects, 255*t*
indications, 250*t*
overview, 249–252
pretransplant cardiovascular evaluation, 252–253
    cardiovascular optimization, 252–253
    cardiovascular screening, 252
procedures and techniques, 250–252
    collection of hematopoietic cells, 250
    conditioning, 250, 251*t*, 252
    engraftment, 252
    immunosuppression, 252
    infusion of hematopoietic cells, 252
types of, 249
HER2 targeted therapy, 12
Human epidermal growth factor receptor 2 antagonists
permissive cardiotoxicity and, 276
Hypertension, 140–148
cancer therapies associated, 144–147, 148*t*
    androgen axis inhibitors, 146
    immunosuppressants, 146
    non–vascular endothelial growth factor signaling pathway tyrosine kinase inhibitors, 145–146
    platinum-based chemotherapeutic agents, 146
    proteasome inhibitors, 146
    vascular endothelial growth factor signaling pathway inhibitors, 144–145
definition, 140
diagnosis, 140–143
diagnostic testing, 143
epidemiology, 143, 143*t*
general principles, 140
history, 140–141
management of, 147, 148*t*
    antihypertensive drugs, selection of, 147
    on-treatment blood pressure surveillance, 147
    pretreatment evaluation, 147
physical examination, 141–142

I

ICA. *See* Invasive coronary angiogram (ICA)
Immune checkpoint inhibitors, 52, 55, 56*t*, 213
associated drugs/therapies, 55
cardiotoxicity, 55
definition, 52
epidemiology, 55
monitoring, 55
Immunosuppressants, hypertension and, 146
Immunosuppression, 252
Inotersen, 314
Intravascular devices complications, 167–177. *See also* Thrombotic complications
pacemaker and implantable cardioverter defibrillator, 167–172
    general principles, 167
    guidelines/recommendations, 169–171
    radiation considerations, 167–169
    role of leadless pacemaker, 171–172
ports, 172–173
    considerations, 172
    delayed complications, 173
    early complications, 173
    general principles, 172
Invasive coronary angiogram (ICA), 100
Ischemic heart disease, 89–101
chronic coronary syndrome, 92
classification, 90
clinical history, 91–92, 92*t*
definition, 90
diagnosis, 91–99
diagnostic testing, 92–93
epidemiology, 90
etiology, 90–91
general principles, 89–91
invasive imaging and therapeutics, 100–101
    invasive coronary angiogram, 100
    medical therapy for coronary disease, 100
    percutaneous coronary intervention, 100–101
laboratory evaluation, 92
noncardiac surgery, approaches to, 94
noninvasive imaging, 94–99
    coronary artery calcification, 94–95
    coronary computed tomography angiography, 95–96
    myocardial perfusion imaging, 96–98, 98*f*
    stress echocardiogram, 99
risk factors, 91

L

Left ventricular dysfunction, 15–16
  permissive cardiotoxicity and, 270, 273
Light chain amyloidosis, 287–289
  epidemiology, 287–288
  history, 288–289
  treatment strategies, 299–308
    amyloid fibril-targeting therapy, 306–307
    assessment of treatment response, 307–308, 307t
    autologous stem cell transplantation, 303–305
    general principles, 299
    initial therapy, 302–303
    staging, 299–302
    therapy for relapsed/refractory disease, 305–306
Lipoma, 133
Lymphoma, 136

M

Magnetic resonance imaging (MRI), 224–237, 294–296, 295f
  cardiac dysfunction, cancer therapy–related, 227–235
    functional assessment, 227
    gadolinium-based imaging, 230–231, 232–233t
    myocardial edema, 230
    myocardial strain, 227, 230
    myocardial T1 mapping, 230
    tissue characterization, 230
  cardiac tumors, 236–237
  immune checkpoint inhibitor, myocarditis and, 235–236
  infiltrative cardiomyopathy/amyloidosis, 234–235
  overview, 224–225t, 226f
  radiation-induced heart disease, 237
Mechanical circulatory support, evaluation for, 323–325
Mesothelioma, 136–137
Metoprolol, 32
Midodrine, 317
MRI. *See* Magnetic resonance imaging (MRI)
Multidisciplinary team
  administrative support, role of, 286
  advanced practice providers on the C-O team, role of, 282–283
  cardio-oncology research, 285
  collaboration with other disciplines, 280–282
  definition, 280
  nurse coordinators, role of, 283, 284t, 285
Myocardial edema, 230
Myocardial perfusion imaging, 96–98, 98f

Myocardial strain, 201, 227, 230
Myxoma, 127, 131–132

N

Natriuretic peptides, 208–209
NBTE. *See* Nonbacterial thrombotic endocarditis (NBTE)
Neoplasms, cardiac masses, 126–138
  benign primary, 127–134, 128–130t, 130f
  classification of, 127–138, 128–130t, 130f
  clinical presentation, 126
  diagnostic testing, 126–127
  lipoma, 133
  lymphoma, 136
  malignant primary, 134–138
  mesothelioma, 136–137
  myxoma, 127, 131–132
  papillary fibroelastoma, 132
  paraganglioma, 133–134
  rhabdomyoma, 133
  sarcomas, 134–136
Neurotoxicity, mechanisms of, 182–184
  antineoplastic agents, 182–184
Nilotinib, 81
Nonbacterial thrombotic endocarditis (NBTE), 73, 73f
Nonsteroidal anti-inflammatory drugs (NSAIDs), 105
NSAIDs. *See* Nonsteroidal anti-inflammatory drugs (NSAIDs)
Nurse coordinators, role of, 283, 284t, 285

O

Orthostatic hypotension, management of, 316–318, 317t

P

Pacemaker and implantable cardioverter defibrillator (PM/ICD), 167–172
  general principles, 167
  guidelines/recommendations, 169–171
  radiation considerations, 167–169
  role of leadless pacemaker, 171–172
Papillary fibroelastoma, 132
Paraganglioma, 133–134
Paraneoplastic autonomic dysfunction, 182
Paraneoplastic syndromes, 184–190
  diagnosis, 184–187
  diagnostic testing, 186–187
    cardiovascular, 186–187
    neurologic, 187
  history, 184–186
  lab evaluation, 187

orthostasis, differential diagnosis for, 184
physical examination, 186
prognosis, 190
treatment, 187–189
Patisiran, 312
PCI. *See* Percutaneous coronary intervention (PCI)
Percutaneous coronary intervention (PCI), 100–101
Percutaneous suction thrombectomy systems, 175–177
Pericardial disease, 103–112, 203
  acute pericarditis, 103–106
    consequences, 106
    definition, 103
    diagnosis, 104–105
    etiology, 103–104, 104*t*
    management, 105–106
  anatomy of pericardium, 103
  constrictive pericarditis, 110–112
    complications, 112
    diagnosis, 111–112
    etiology, 110, 110*t*
    management, 112
    palliation, 112
  general principles, 103
  pericardial effusions, 106–109
    diagnosis, 107–108
    etiology, 106–107
    management, 108–109
  pericardial tamponade, 109–110
    diagnosis, 110
    pathophysiology, 109
Pericardial effusions, 106–109
  diagnosis, 107–108
  etiology, 106–107
  management, 108–109
Pericardial tamponade, 109–110
  diagnosis, 110
  pathophysiology, 109
Permissive cardiotoxicity, 268–278
  cardioprotective medical therapy, 271–272*t*
  definition, 268–269
  drugs/therapies, 275–278
    anthracyclines, 275–276
    checkpoint inhibitors, 276–278
    human epidermal growth factor receptor 2 antagonists, 276
  early identification, 270, 273
  general principles, 268–269
  left ventricular dysfunction and, 270, 273
  prevention, 269–270
  risk-benefit analysis, 273–274
  stop therapy, indications to, 274–275
P-glycoprotein, 266
Pharmacodynamic drug interactions, 266
PharmD, 257–266
Platinum-based chemotherapeutic agents, hypertension and, 146
PM/ICD. *See* Pacemaker and implantable cardioverter defibrillator (PM/ICD)
Ports, 172–173
  considerations, 172
  delayed complications, 173
  early complications, 173
  general principles, 172
Proteasome inhibitors, 13, 60, 213
  associated drugs/therapies, 60
  cardiotoxicity, 60
  definition, 60
  epidemiology, 60
  hypertension and, 146
  monitoring, 60, 61*f*
Psychological and social complications, cancer survivorship, 244–246
  adult-centered care, transitioning to, 246
  cognitive function, 244–245
  educational achievement, 245
  fatigue, 245
  immunization considerations, 246
  psychiatric issues, 244

Q

QT prolongation, 160–163
  associated drugs/therapies, 160–162
  definition, 160
  diagnosis, 162–163
  management, 163

R

Radiation-induced heart disease, 237
Radiation-induced valvular heart disease, 65–69
  diagnosis, 66–68, 67*f*
  epidemiology/risk factors, 65–66, 65*t*
  general principles, 65–68
  prevention and screening, 68–69
  treatment and prognosis, 68
Relapsed/refractory disease, therapy for, 305–306
Rhabdomyoma, 133
Rhythm disturbances, 150–165
  management of, 318

S

Sarcomas, 134–136
Sinus node dysfunction, 156–157
  associated drugs/therapies, 156–157
  definition, 156
  diagnosis, 157
  management, 157

Small-molecule kinase inhibitors, 48–52, 50–51*t*
  associated drugs/therapies, 48
  cardiotoxicity, 49
  definition, 48
  epidemiology, 48
  monitoring, 49, 52
Social complications. *See* Psychological and social complications, cancer survivorship
Stop therapy, permissive cardiotoxicity and, 274–275
Stress echocardiogram, 99
Sunitinib, 19
Superior vena cava syndrome, 76–78
  diagnosis, 77, 77*t*, 78*f*
  general principles, 76
Supraventricular tachyarrhythmias, 154–156
  associated drugs/therapies, 154
  definition, 154
  diagnosis, 154–156, 155*f*
  management, 156
Survivorship, cancer, 238–246
  advanced heart failure therapies and. *See* Advanced heart failure (AHF) therapies
  cardiac complications, 239–244
    adverse hormonal effects, 243
    conduction disease, 241
    general principles, 239
    heart failure, 241
    lymphedema, 243–244
    myocardial dysfunction, 241
    pain, 244
    pericardial abnormalities, 241
    reproductive considerations, 243
    secondary malignant neoplasms, 243
    structural abnormalities, 241
    valvular abnormalities, 241
    vascular compromise, 240–241
  general principles, 238
  long-term psychological/social issues, 239*t*
  physical issues, long-term, 239*t*
  psychological and social complications, 244–246
    adult-centered care, transitioning to, 246
    cognitive function, 244–245
    educational achievement, 245
    fatigue, 245
    immunization considerations, 246
    psychiatric issues, 244
  standards of, 238
Symptomatic heart failure, management of, 314–315

T

^{99m}Technetium-labeled bone scintigraphy, 292–294
Three-dimensional imaging, 201
Thromboembolism, anticoagulant agents for, 121*t*
Thrombolytics, 174–175
Thrombosis, 16. *See also* Cancer-associated thrombosis (CAT)
Thrombotic complications, 173–177. *See also* Intravascular devices complications
  alternative management, 174–177
    IVC filter, 175
    percutaneous suction thrombectomy systems, 175–177
    stenting, 177
    thrombolytics and catheter-directed thrombolysis, 174–175
  cardiac complications, 174
  general principles, 173
TKI. *See* Tyrosine kinase inhibitors (TKI)
Torsades de Pointes, 16
Transthoracic echocardiography, amyloidosis and, 289–292
Transthyretin amyloidosis, 288–289
  epidemiology, 288
  history, 289
  treatment strategies, 310–318
    advanced heart failure therapies, 315–316
    background, 310
    general principles, 310
    orthostatic hypotension, management of, 316–318
    rhythm disturbances, management of, 318
    stabilizers, 311–312
    staging and prognosis, 311
    symptomatic heart failure, management of, 314–315
    synthesis inhibitors, 312–314
    transthyretin-directed therapy, 311–314
Trastuzumab, 212
Two-dimensional imaging, 199
Tyrosine kinase inhibitors (TKI), 13–14
  for cancer-associated thrombosis, 118

V

Valvular heart disease (VHD), 64–73, 203
  approaches, 64–65
  carcinoid heart disease, 69–72
    diagnosis, 69–71
    epidemiology/risk factors, 69

general principles, 69
laboratory testing, 71–72
outcome/prognosis, 72
treatment, 72
general principles, 64
nonbacterial thrombotic endocarditis, 73, 73f
radiation-induced, 65–69
diagnosis, 66–68, 67f
epidemiology/risk factors, 65–66, 65t
general principles, 65–68
prevention and screening, 68–69
treatment and prognosis, 68
Vascular endothelial growth factor signaling pathway inhibitors, 52, 118–119, 212

associated drugs/therapies, 52
cardiotoxicity, 52, 53t
definition, 52
epidemiology, 52
hypertension and, 144–145
monitoring, 52, 54f
Vascular toxicity, 204
Ventricular arrhythmias, 163–165
associated drugs/therapies, 163
definition, 163
diagnosis, 164
diagnostic tests, 165
management, 164
VHD. *See* Valvular heart disease (VHD)